Healthcare Access

Edited by Amit Agrawal and Srinivas Kosgi

Published in London, United Kingdom

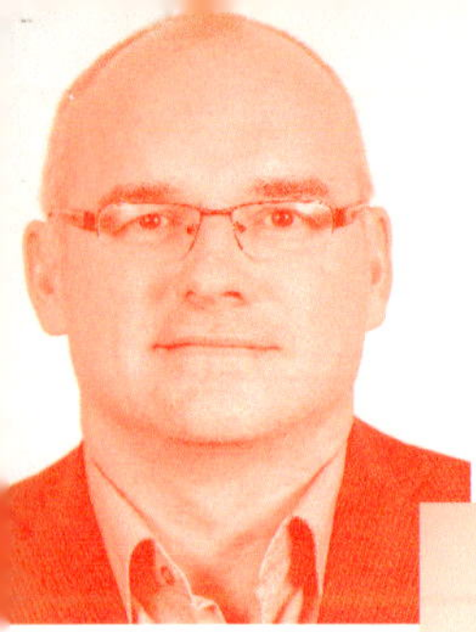
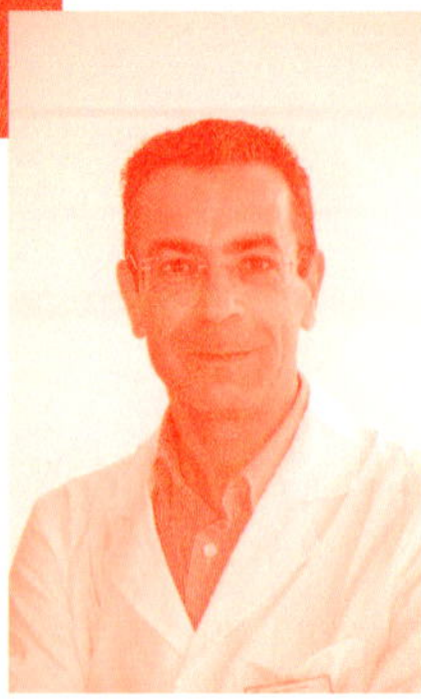
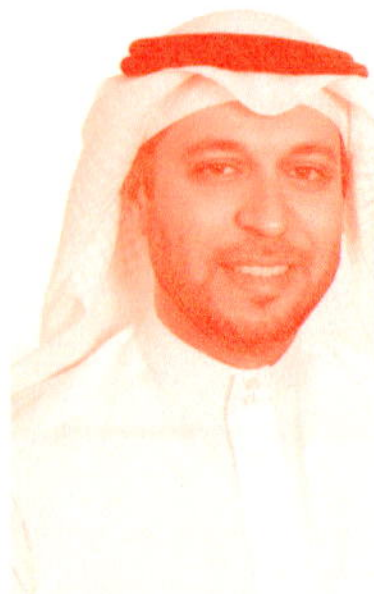
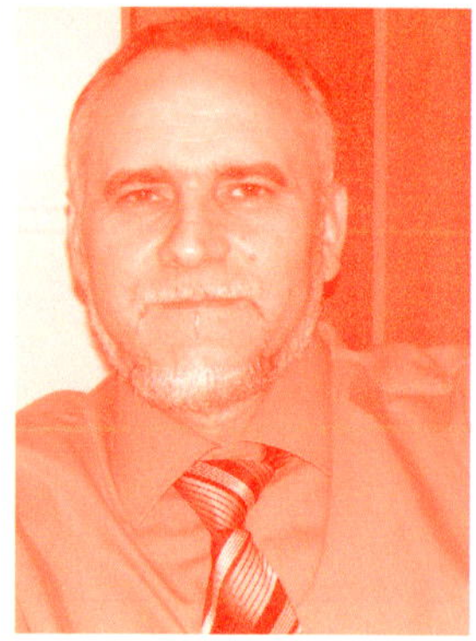
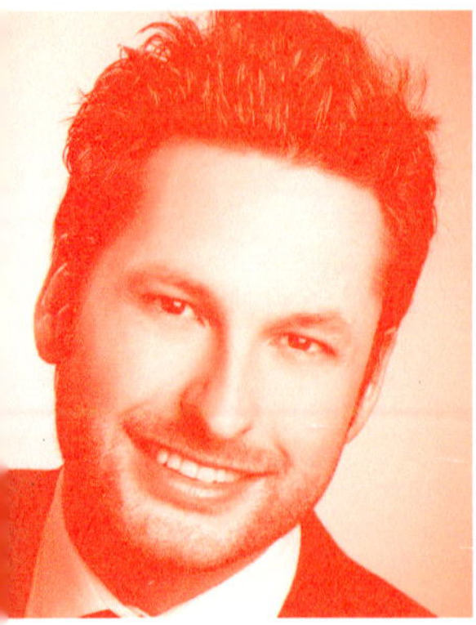
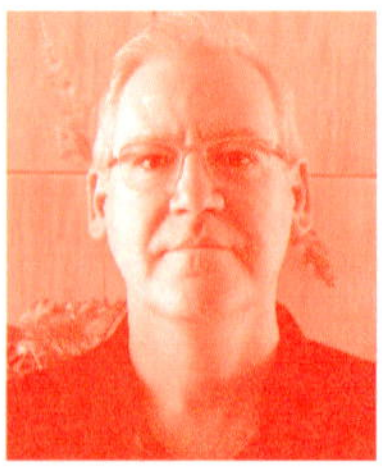
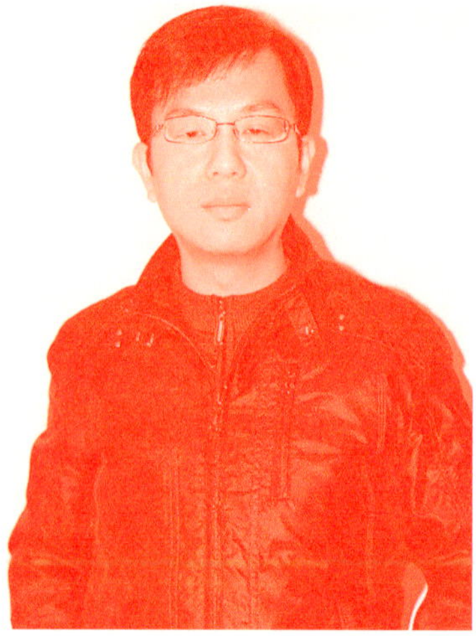

IntechOpen

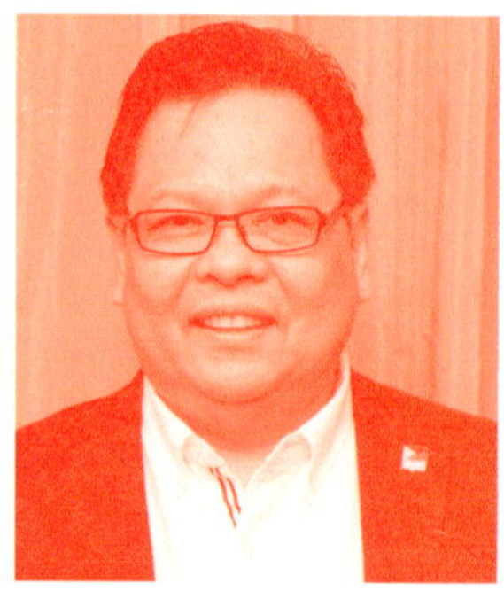
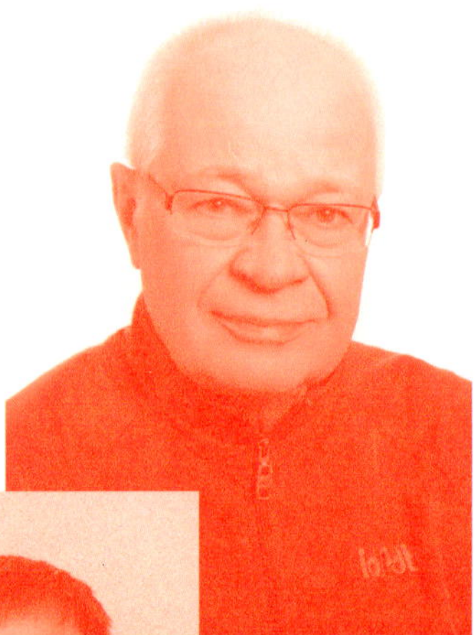
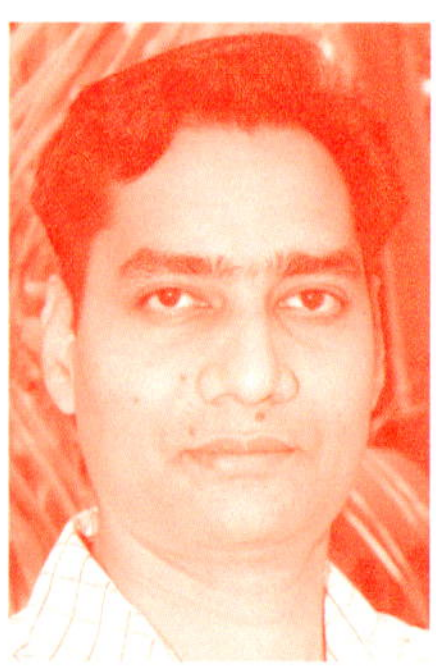
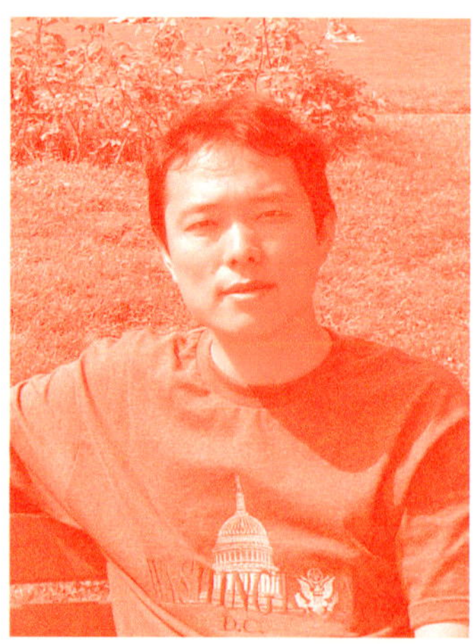
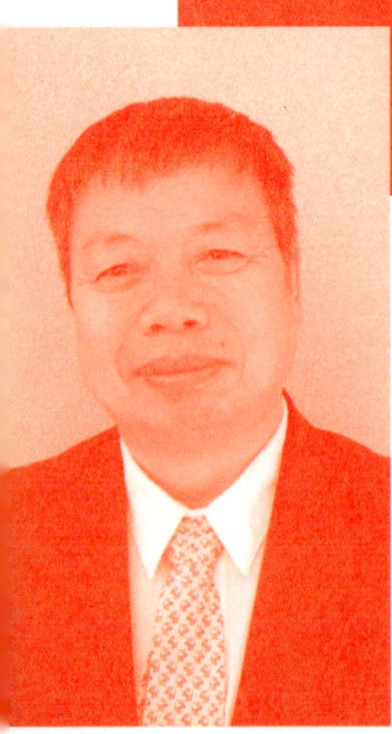
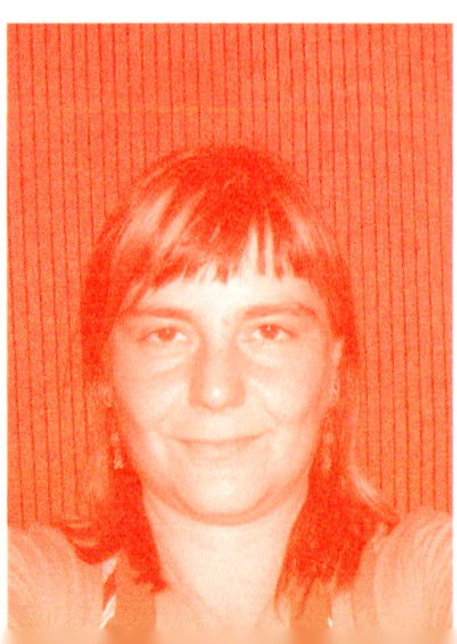

Meet the editors

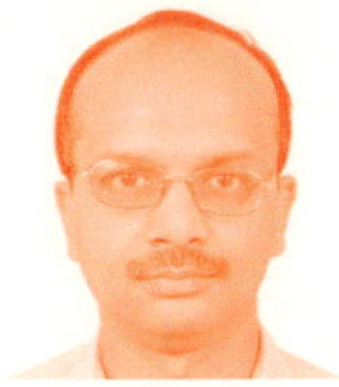

Dr. Agrawal completed his neurosurgery training at the National Institute of Mental Health and Neurosciences, Bangalore, India, in 2003. Dr. Agrawal is a self-motivated, enthusiastic, and results-oriented professional with more than eighteen years of rich experience in research and development, as well as teaching and mentoring in the field of neurosurgery. He is proficient in managing and leading teams for running successful process operations and has experience in developing procedures and service standards of excellence. He has attended and participated in many international and national symposiums and conferences and delivered many lectures. He has published more than 750 scientific articles in various national and international journals. His expertise is in identifying training needs, designing training modules, and executing the same while working with limited resources. He has excellent communication, presentation, and interpersonal skills with proven abilities in teaching and training for various academic and professional courses. Presently he is working at the All India Institute of Medical Sciences, Bhopal, Madhya Pradesh.

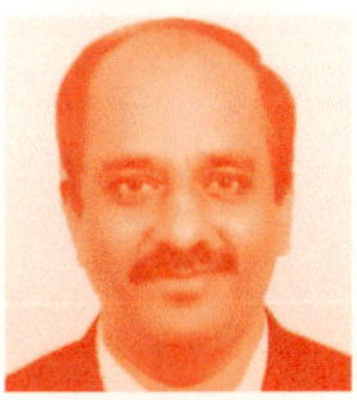

Dr. Srinivas Kosgi is a clinician and academician with sixteen years of experience in the field of psychiatry. He has an excellent track record of working in schizophrenia, forensic psychiatry, child and adolescent psychiatry, de-addiction psychiatry, psychopharmacology, and community psychiatry. His areas of interest are research in thought, language and communication deficits in schizophrenia, and designing treatment strategies for prisoners. Dr. Kosgi has worked in thirty-two multi-center international drug trials. His current functions are developing administrative strategies in improving clinical services in psychiatry hospitals, training postgraduate students in psychiatry, clinical psychology, psychiatric social work, and psychiatric nursing. He currently heads psychiatric hospital services in the capacity of medical superintendent at Dharwad Institute of mental Health and Neuroscience Dharwad, Karnataka. Dr. Kosgi is a pioneer researcher in psychopharmacology and heads the state referral psychiatric hospital as medical superintendent.

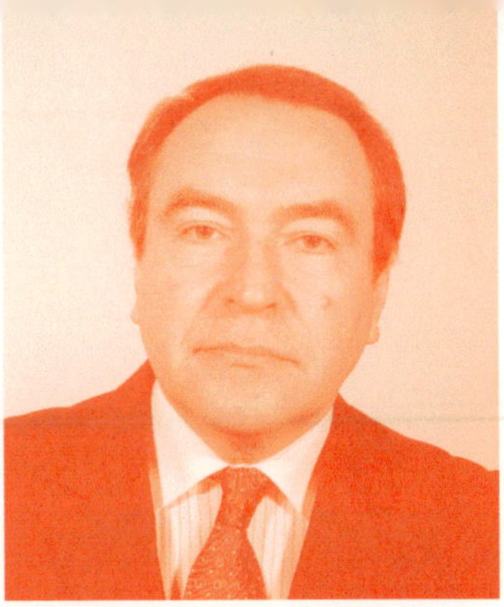
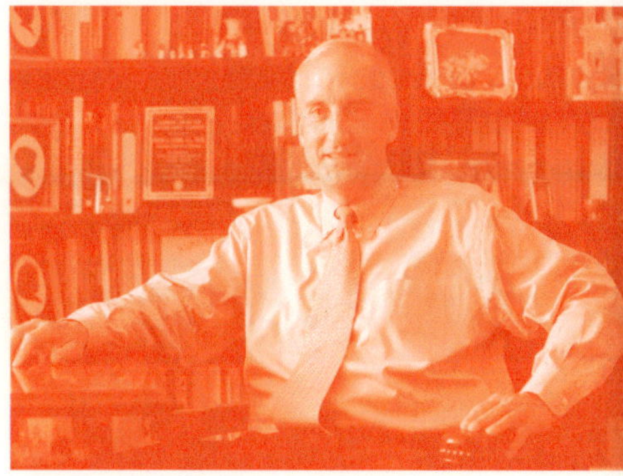
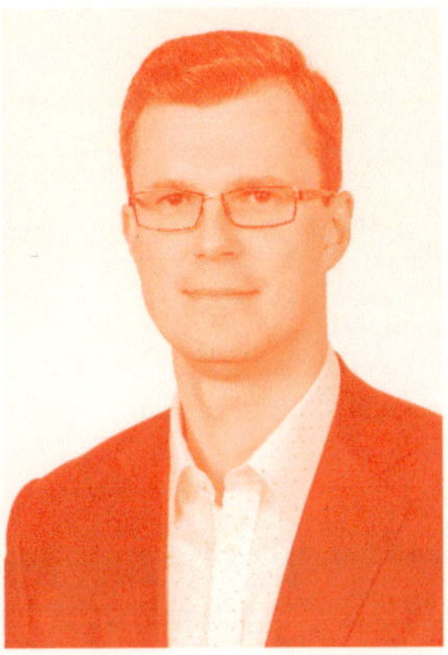
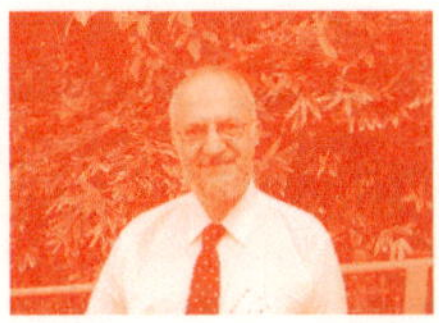
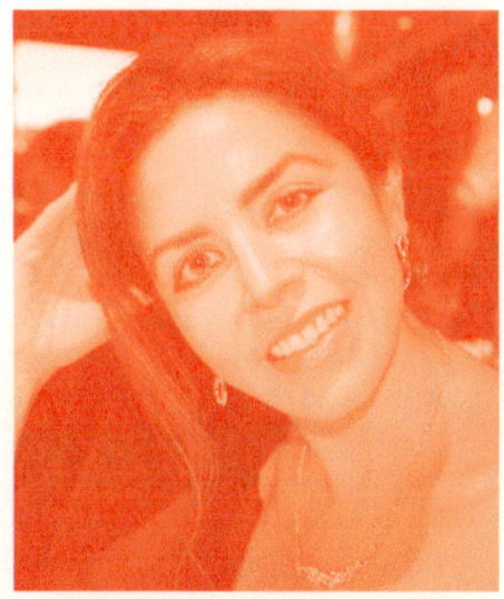

Supporting open minds since 2005

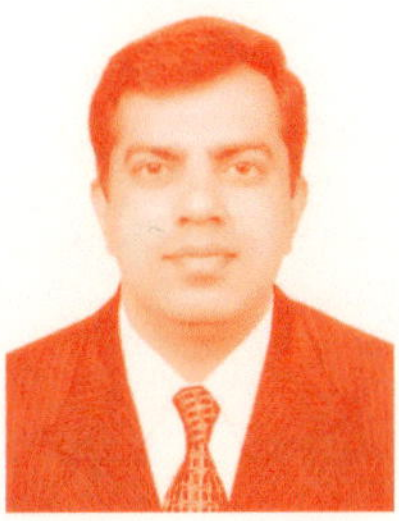
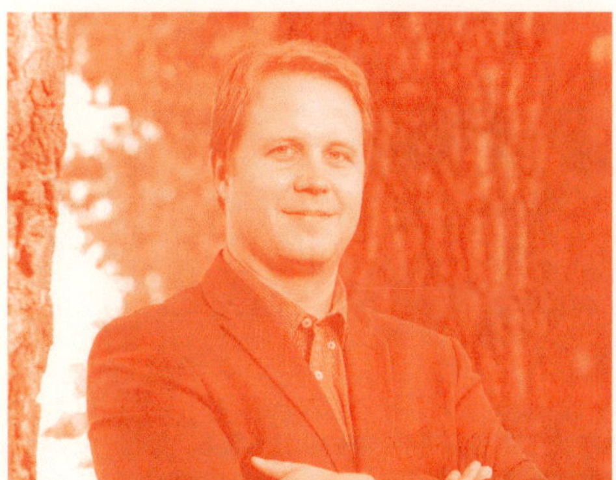
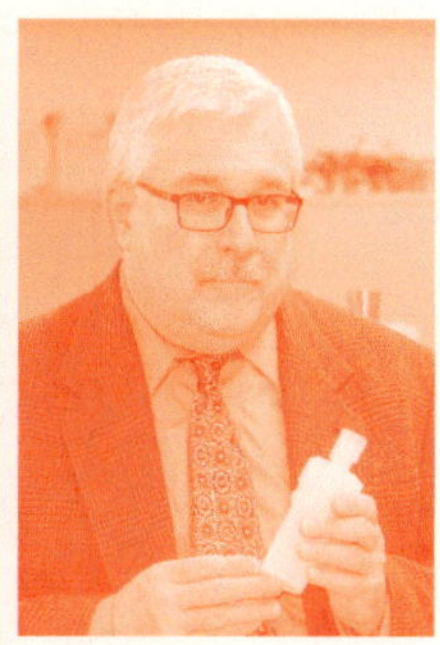
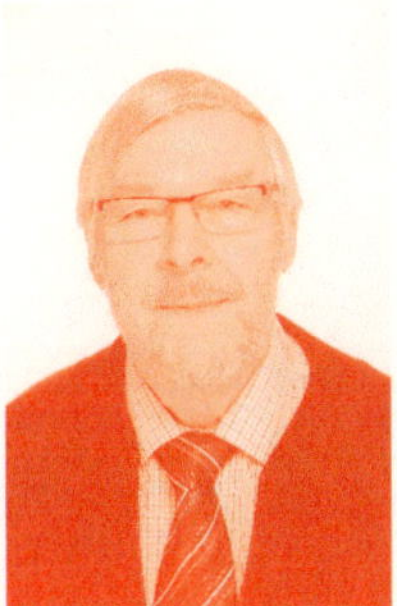
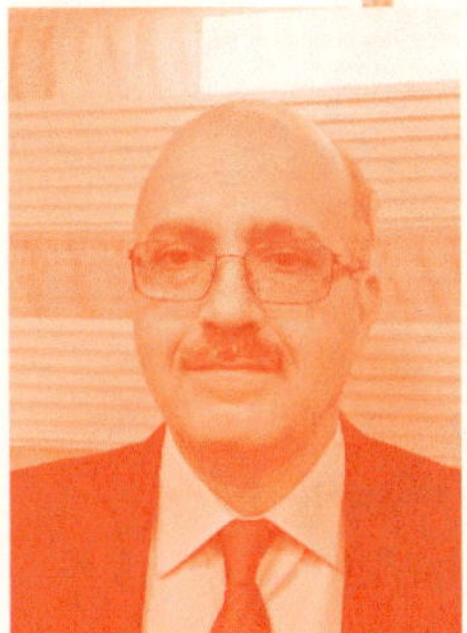
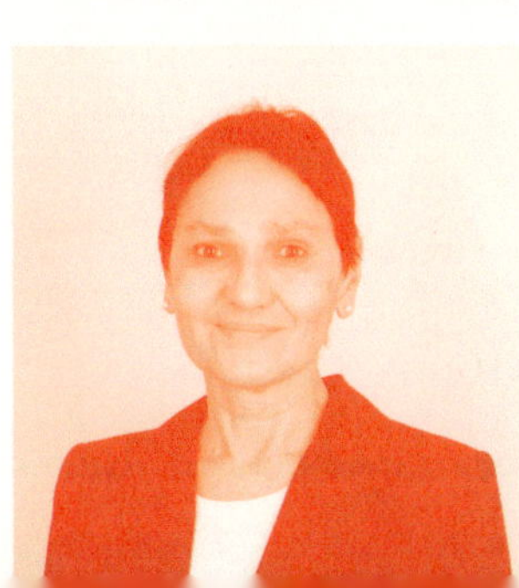
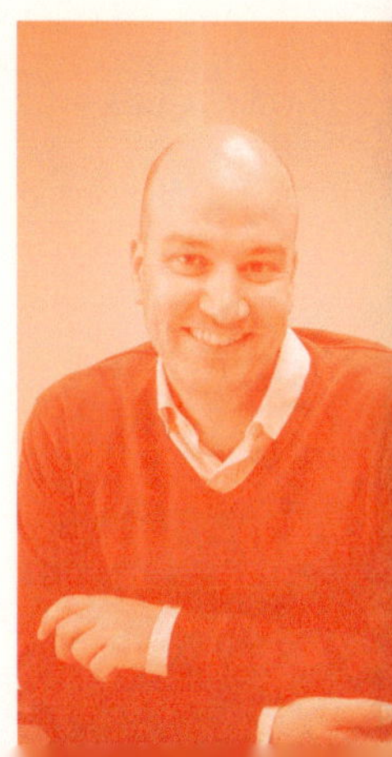

Healthcare Access
http://dx.doi.org/10.5772/intechopen.94675
Edited by Amit Agrawal and Srinivas Kosgi

Contributors
Bryant Bonner, Jesua I. Law, Eric Dacus, Erin Hofmann, Hülya Gül, Isaac Akintoyese Oyekola, Oludele Albert Ajani, Eyitayo Joseph Oyeyipo, Rafael Da Silveira Moreira, Gisele Mariel De Sousa Vasconcelos, Alana Maiara Brito Bibiano, Lucas Fernando Rodrigues dos Santos, Neta Kela-Madar, Esra Zeynep Yıldız, Yüksel Atay, Oktay Pamuk, Bekir Boyacı, Tuncay Göksel, Dilek Yeşim Metin, Servet Gül, Gökberk Devrim, Özlem Topbaş, Habibu Salisu Badamasi, Abdulnasir F.H. Al-Jazairi, Guillaume Alinier, Terry J. Ellapen, Yvonne Paul, Takalani C Muluvhu, Makwena B. Ntjana, Valentina Prevolnik Rupel, Dorjan Marušič, Febronia Kahabuka, Kasusu Klint Nyamuryekung\'E, Priscila Kelly da Silva Neto, Maristela Rodrigues Marinho, Juliana Dias Reis Pessalacia, Sandra Pinto, Marcela Tavares Tavares De Souza, Tatiana Carvalho Reis Martins, Adelakun Edward Odunyemi, Zdeslav Radovčić, Iskra Alexandra Nola, Genesis Chorwe-Sungani, Obeta Mark M. Uchejeso, Nkereuwem Etukudoh, George Athanasiou, Chris Bachtsetzis, Sunny Ibeneme, Nkiruka Ukor, Joseph Okeibunor, Felicitas Zawaira, Makoto Takayama, Alireza Ghorbani, Najeeb Mohammed Al-Shorbaji

First published in London, United Kingdom, 2022 by IntechOpen
IntechOpen is the global imprint of INTECHOPEN LIMITED, registered in England and Wales, registration number: 11086078, 5 Princes Gate Court, London, SW7 2QJ, United Kingdom
Printed in Croatia

British Library Cataloguing-in-Publication Data
A catalogue record for this book is available from the British Library

Additional hard and PDF copies can be obtained from orders@intechopen.com

Healthcare Access
Edited by Amit Agrawal and Srinivas Kosgi
p. cm.
Print ISBN 978-1-83969-566-7
Online ISBN 978-1-83969-567-4
eBook (PDF) ISBN 978-1-83969-568-1

For EU product safety concerns:
IN TECH d.o.o., Prolaz Marije Krucifikse Kozulić 3, 51000 Rijeka, Croatia, info@intechopen.com or visit our website at intechopen.com.

[60] Establishing an evidence base for e-health. Special Theme Issue of the World Health Organization Bulletin, Volume 90(5); 2012 https://www.ncbi.nlm.nih.gov/pmc/issues/209588/ (Accessed 20 June 2021)

[61] Krishna-Harihara S and Akinseinde M. The challenges of implementing digital health in Nigeria 2016; DOI-10.13140/RG.2.2.27417.95849 (Accessed 25 June 2021)

[62] Taylor E, et al. Health IT implementation: challenges and opportunities. In Developing a Strategic Program for Chilean Health Information Technology: Environmental Scan and Key Informant Interviews (pp. 20-28) 2016; RAND Corporation. http://www.jstor.org/stable/10.7249/j.ctt19w739p.11 (Accessed 10 May 2021)

[63] Kazi A M, et al. Current challenges of digital health interventions in Pakistan: mixed methods analysis. J Med Internet Res 2020; 22(9):e21691. doi: 10.2196/21691 (https://www.jmir.org/2020/9/e21691/) (Accessed 15 May 2021)

[64] Mogessie Y G, et al. Digital health and COVID-19: challenges of use and implementation in sub-Saharan Africa. Pan African Medical Journal. 2021; 38:240. doi: 10.11604/pamj.2021.38.240.27948 (https://www.panafrican-med-journal.com/content/article/38/240/full/). (Accessed 30 May 2021)

[65] Whitelaw S, et al. Barriers and facilitators of the uptake of digital health technology in cardiovascular care: a systematic scoping review. European Heart Journal - Digital Health 2021; 2:1, 62-74, https://doi.org/10.1093/ehjdh/ztab005. https://academic.oup.com/ehjdh/article/2/1/62/6128570 (Accessed 10 May 2021)

[66] World Health Organization, Legal frameworks for eHealth: based on the findings of the second global survey on eHealth. (Global Observatory for eHealth Series, v. 5), WHO, 2012. http://whqlibdoc.who.int/publications/2012/9789241503143_eng.pdf. (Accessed 14 May 2021)

[67] James S, et al. (2021), Op Cit.

[68] World Health organization. Ethics and governance of artificial intelligence for health, Op Cit.

[69] United Nations. Universal Declaration of Human Rights. New York: UN, 1948 (https://www.un.org/en/about-us/universal-declaration-of-human-rights (Accessed 2 April 2021)

[70] World Health organization. Directory of eHealth policies survey. https://www.who.int/observatories/global-observatory-for-ehealth/policies (Accessed 10 March 2021)

[71] World Health Organization and the International Telecommunication Union. National eHealth Strategy Toolkit. Geneva: WHO and ITU, 2012. (Accessed 5 April 2021)

Contents

Preface

The concept of healthcare access is continuously evolving. It is globally recognized that healthcare-seeking behavior tends to involve seeking access to multiple healthcare providers. This book covers a range of topics related to healthcare access, including occupational health and safety, occupational hygiene, universal health coverage, economic aspects of healthcare services, issues related to low-resource primary healthcare settings, factors influencing access to reliable healthcare, emergency healthcare access, issues of ethical deliberation in the allocation of resources, patient satisfaction, laboratory services, medical tourism, and healthcare access and usefulness of advanced technologies in healthcare delivery. As an extended responsibility, healthcare providers can create mechanisms to facilitate subjective decision-making in accessing the right kind of healthcare services as well as various options to support financial needs to bear healthcare-related expenses while seeking health and fulfilling the healthcare needs of the population. Adequate healthcare access not only requires the availability of comprehensive healthcare facilities but also affordability and knowledge of the availability of these services. This volume brings together experiences and opinions from global leaders to develop affordable, sustainable, and uniformly available options to access healthcare services.

Dr. Amit Agrawal
Department of Neurosurgery,
All India Institute of Medical Sciences,
Bhopal, India

Dr. Srinivas Kosgi
Department of Psychiatry,
Dharwad Institute of Mental Health and Neurosciences,
Dharwad, India

Section 1

Global Perspective

Chapter 1

The Profession of Biokinetics in South Africa: The Need for Access to the Public Healthcare System

Yvonne Paul, Terry J. Ellapen, Takalani C. Muluvhu and Makwena B. Ntjana

Abstract

This chapter reviews the efficacy of the only South African exercise therapy profession (Biokinetics) in the rehabilitation of non-communicable diseases (NCDs). Biokinetics is a South African exercise therapy profession established in 1983 and which operates in both the pathogenic and fortogenic healthcare paradigms. Unfortunately, the profession of Biokinetics is restricted to the South African private healthcare sector. This chapter describes the scope of the profession of Biokinetics, empirical studies illustrating the efficacy of the profession in addressing society's non-communicable disease epidemic, and the challenges inhibiting the profession from gaining access to the South African public healthcare sector. It is hoped that the presentation and critical appraisal of the empirical evidence which illustrates the contribution of the profession of Biokinetics to the rehabilitation of NCDs justifies the authors' claims for the inclusion of the aforementioned profession in the South African public healthcare sector.

Keywords: Biokinetics, exercise therapy, non-communicable diseases, healthcare

1. Introduction

The profession of Biokinetics is a specialised application of clinical exercise therapy which developed from the South African Universities Physical Education Programme in 1983 [1]. The fundamental roots of the profession of Biokinetics date back to 1934 and form part of the history of the South African Defence Force [2]. In 1934, a resurgence in the study of Physical Education occurred in the South African Defence Force when senior military personnel found that South African recruits were in poor physical conditioning, with poor medical, dental, and psychological health [3–5]. As a result, the South African Defence Force established the *Physical Training Brigade*, a specialised unit aimed at rehabilitating military recruits experiencing medical, educational, dental, physical, social and/or psychological challenges [5, 6]. The multidisciplinary team responsible for the rehabilitation included medical doctors, educators, dentists, physical education instructors, physiotherapists, psychologists, and sociologists [5, 6]. Dr. Danie Craven was the inaugural director of the *Physical Training Brigade* [5]. This historical synopsis places the resurgence of the South African Physical Education programme in the context of military involvement in pioneering South African health and wellness efforts, commemorating the inaugural establishment of the first of the South African multidisciplinary medical rehabilitation team, and the intuitive preliminary South African exercise therapeutic and research based approach to restoring an individual's health and well-being. Biokinetics was born out of the philosophy that *exercise is medicine*. The ground-breaking empirical research of Dr. Danie Craven, Dr. Ernst Jokl and Prof. Gert Lukas Strydom has led to the development of the profession of Biokinetics [1, 7]. Professor Gert Strydom is affectionately known as the *"Father of Biokinetics,"* due to his immense contribution to the establishment and continued advancement of the profession [8].

During the late 1960's a drastic change in the research philosophy of South African exercise rehabilitative medicine occurred, prompted by the inventive research of Gert Lukas Strydom [9]. In his doctoral thesis Mr. Gert Strydom investigated the impact of a habitual structured exercise regime as a therapeutic modality to rehabilitate the functional exercise physiological capacity of coronary heart disease patients [9]. The empirical evidence obtained from the study illustrated that habitual, structured exercise regimes could successful augment cardiac rehabilitation and improve patients' quality of life. The success of these findings encouraged other proponents of the Biokinetics profession, such as FJ Buys and JJ Cilliers, to pursue postgraduate exercise-based rehabilitation credentials in the newly emerging field of Biokinetics [4, 10]. FJ Buys investigated the effects of a structured exercise regime on pre-diabetic and diabetic patients [10], while JJ Cilliers reviewed the effects of structured exercise training on the post-medical rehabilitation of injured soldiers [4]. FJ Buys later became a professor at the Potchefstroom University for Christian Higher Education (now known as North-West University), with JJ Cilliers becoming a prominent professor at Tshwane University of Technology.

2. Scope of profession of Biokinetics

The scope of the profession of biokinetics focuses on enhancing the physical health status and quality of life of a person through a clinical exercise evaluation and subsequent prescription of personalised exercise rehabilitation in the dual context of pathology (pathogenic healthcare paradigm) and physical performance enhancement (fortogenic healthcare paradigm) [11, 12]. The profession of Biokinetics also aggressively campaigns for health and wellness promotion as well as for the prevention of neuro-musculoskeletal injury and NCDs (fortogenic healthcare paradigm), thereby inspiring a positive change in the health and wellness continuum towards optimal well-being [1, 13]. Biokineticists are clinically trained professionals who address *inter-alia* the chronic concerns of NCDs in South Africa and Namibia through structured exercise rehabilitative intervention [14]. In the fortogenic health paradigm a person who is otherwise considered healthy, having no predisposing risk of neuro-musculoskeletal injury and/or NCDs, but who seeks to adopt a physically active lifestyle in order to avoid the onset and/or risk of illness, while simultaneously increasing their quality of life, consults a biokineticist [1, 14].

3. Health dimensions and health paradigms

Strydom *et al.* described the pathogenic healthcare paradigm as being inclusive of both the illness-care dimension and illness prevention dimension (**Figure 1**) [15]. The illness-care dimension involves the presence of disease and/or injury, while the illness prevention dimension involves the predisposing intrinsic risk of prospective disease and/or injury [15]. The illness-care and illness prevention health

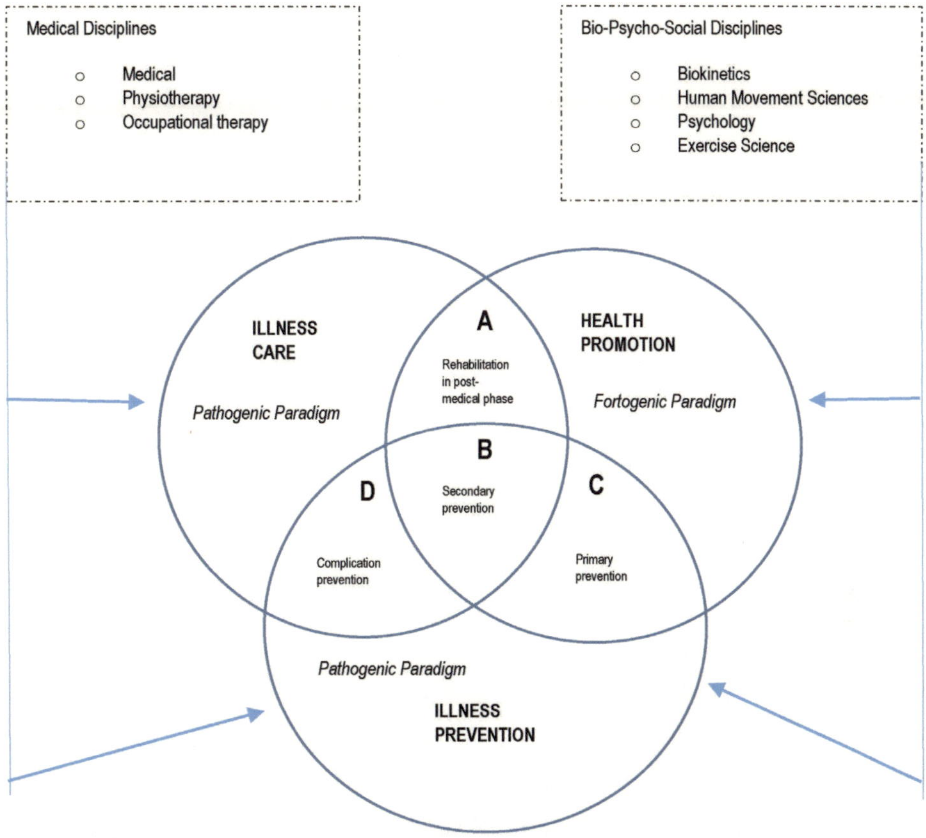

Figure 1.
Articulation of the health dimensions in the health paradigms [15].

dimensions necessitate clinical management by the medical discipline that involves the expertise of the following medical specialists: oncologists, cardiologists, cardiothoracic surgeons, endocrinologists, neurologists, neuro-surgeons and orthopaedic surgeons, general medical practitioners, physiotherapists and nurses [16]. The fortogenic healthcare paradigm is the active attempt to prevent the onset of predisposing risk of neuro-musculoskeletal injury and/or NCDs. The aforementioned three healthcare dimensions actively intersect each other, thereby necessitating the expertise of the aforementioned medical and psycho-social disciplines (biokineticists, dieticians, and psychologists). This dynamic interweaving of the health paradigms encourages interprofessional collaboration [14, 17]. **Figure 1** provides a graphic representation of the dynamic overlap of the different health dimensions and of the interventions of the respective healthcare practitioners [12, 15]. **Table 1** describes the interaction of medical specialists in the rehabilitation of NCDs. The focus of this chapter is to illustrate the value of the profession of Biokinetics to the South African public healthcare sector. As such the chapter will exclusively describe the rehabilitation of NCDs. It must be stressed that Biokinetic rehabilitation also has a strong emphasis on neuro-musculoskeletal rehabilitation.

The aforementioned examples of NCD management provided by a biokineticist illustrate the value of their expertise that can serve both the private and public healthcare sectors. Many patients in the public healthcare sector who experience NCDs receive standardised treatment and do not receive individualised management. The medical and paramedical staff in the public healthcare sector are overworked and therefore prescribe general healthcare management strategies whose

Areas	Non-communicable diseases
Area A displays the overlap between the pathogenic and fortogenic health paradigms, which is known as *final-phase rehabilitation*, or *post medical phase* (Figure 2). During this phase rehabilitation consists exclusively of physical activity and conditioning as the primary therapeutic modality.	An example would be an asthmatic patient who takes prescribed medication, has undergone physiotherapy and, lastly, is referred to a biokineticist [15]. While medication management falls within the purview of a pulmonologist and a pharmacist, the physiotherapist provides acute and sub-acute phases of physical activity rehabilitation and the expertise of the biokineticist improves the asthmatic patient's respiratory (and subsequently cardiorespiratory) function and quality of life, encouraging independent living through structured exercise and physical activity. Ensuring the patient's capacity for, and their improvement in, independent living is also the function of an occupational therapist.
Area B is known as *secondary prevention*, in which a given patient has an injury and/or disease, and has undergone surgical intervention, pharmaceutical management, and is subsequently engaged in final-phase functional rehabilitation in order to prevent deterioration of the predisposing injury (and/or disease) and avoid the development of co-morbidities.	A typical example would be a cardiac artery disease (CAD) patient who has successfully undergone surgery, has been prescribed chronic cardiac medication (to reduce the viscosity of his blood, as well as to control his blood pressure and heart rate). The patient would have completed acute and sub-acute phases of physiotherapy before finally being referred to a biokineticist. The primary goal of the biokineticist is ensure that the patient maintains a controlled and structured physically active lifestyle (within safe clinical exercise physiology guidelines) in order to prevent the recurrence of, and/or development of, co-morbidities. Many cardiac patients have experienced the value of controlled structured clinical exercise regimes but are reluctant to habitually comply with further clinical exercise programmes [15]. As such, many CAD patients continue to be physically active through participation in structured controlled games and sport (*recreational therapy*).[15] Biokineticists should refer these patients to recreational therapists to prescribe games, sport and physical activity regimes [14]. It is, however, imperative that these patients comply with regular biokinetic clinical cardiorespiratory evaluations so as to determine their cardiorespiratory status and the efficacy of exercise therapy. This interaction implies interprofessional collaboration between cardiologists, pharmacists, physiotherapists, biokineticists and recreational therapists.
Area C refers to the scenario in which a healthy, illness free, person is who is not predisposed to any risk of pathology seeks to use physical activity as a proactive protective mechanism against illness and risk of illness (*primary prevention*). Such individuals seek the expertise of biokineticists in order to prescribe a physical activity programme so as to increase their physical conditioning and quality of life. A common example of this would be an apparently healthy person exercising at a health and fitness centre and/or gymnasium (Virgin Active).	
Area D is known as *complication prevention*, which occurs when a patient has no disease and/or injury but is categorised as being at an elevated risk of developing NCDs due to an unhealthy lifestyle (**Figure 1**).	Coronary artery disease, diabetics and obese patients are common examples of individuals who need to adopt lifestyle modifications that include dietary improvements, a reduction in alcohol ingestion, and termination of smoking and regular compliance with structured controlled exercise. Individuals are influenced by both modifiable (nutritional choice, alcohol ingestion abuse, tobacco abuse, physical inactivity, and stress) and non-modifiable (genetic predisposition, age, and gender) risk factors which adversely impact their cardiometabolic profiles. In order to prevent the development of, or advancement of existing NCDs, these patients require the interprofessional collaborative expertise of both the medical and bio-psych-social disciplines [17, 18].

Table 1.
The collaborative interface among the various healthcare professionals while managing non-communicable and neuro-musculoskeletal injuries.

efficacy may not be applicable to all patients suffering from NCDs. The inclusion of skilled practitioners (such as biokineticists) in the public healthcare sector will provide the necessary medical assistance to patients and alleviate the stress placed upon already overworked public healthcare sector staff. The incidence of NCDs and the upsurge in their mortality is of international concern, therefore countries that have skilled professions that are able to assist the present medical workforce in order to better combat NCDs should embrace the aid offered by these healthcare practitioners and include them in the public healthcare management team. The paper encourages the South African Department of Health to include the profession of Biokinetics in the public healthcare registry.

4. Non-communicable diseases

Non-communicable diseases (NCDs) are a group of non-infectious diseases which include chronic diseases of slow progression over a prolonged period of time. These diseases can, however, progress rapidly should they remain untreated and have the potential to lead to premature death. Epidemiological statistics attribute approximately 41 million premature deaths per year globally to NCDs [19], with 85% of the aforementioned mortalities occurring in low to middle income countries such as South Africa [19]. The World Health Organisation has identified four primary non-communicable diseases, which include cardiovascular diseases, respiratory diseases, cancer, and diabetes mellitus as being of particular concern. Collectively, these primary NCDs account for 80% of all deaths attributable to NCDs per year [19]. The individual morality rates of the primary NCDs are: 17.9 million deaths (43.6%) due to cardiovascular diseases, followed by cancer (nine million deaths, 21.9%), respiratory diseases (approximately four million deaths, 9.7%), and diabetes mellitus (approximately one and a half million deaths, 3.6%) [19].

Unhealthy nutritional choices, physical inactivity, alcohol, and tobacco use have been identified as modifiable predisposing risks for mortality related to NCDs. These aforementioned risk factors have been classified as modifiable risk factors, suggesting that if a patient changes their behaviour, this would favourably improve their health status. Regular physical activity of moderate intensity (150 minutes/week) and/or high intensity (75 minutes/week) as recommended by the American College of Sports Medicine has proven successful in improving the risk factors associated with NCDs, thereby improving not only the longevity of patients, but also their quality of life [16, 18, 20].

5. How exercise combats non-communicable diseases

This section will describe the manner in which habitual exercise, through exercise-induced physiological mechanisms, favourably influences the primary mortality agents of NCDs: cardiovascular diseases, chronic respiratory diseases, diabetes mellitus, and cancer.

5.1 Exercise-induced mechanisms for combatting cardiovascular diseases

Empirical exercise physiology literature has shown that habitual physical activity and exercise reduces heart rate and blood pressure, favourable alters high density lipoprotein (HDL) levels, low density lipoprotein (LDL) ratios, total serum cholesterol, excess body mass and body fat [20, 21]. The following exercise-induced physiological mechanisms assist compromised cardiovascular function:

i. Regular exercise improves arterio-venous extraction of oxygen from haemoglobin, which improves cardiorespiratory function. At rest 75–85% of the oxygen bound haemoglobin (oxyhaemoglobin) returns to the heart without having been extracted, while during exercise a larger portion of oxygen (approximately 75%) is extracted from oxyhaemoglobin in order to be used to produce energy. Increased exercise intensity lowers arterial partial pressure extracting more oxygen from oxyhaemoglobin, which becomes a chronic exercise-induced adaptation and prevents an increase in heart rate and blood pressure. This exercise induced mechanism lowers the incidence of cardiac arrest.

ii. Regular exercise and physical activity increase vagal tone, reducing heart rate. This reduction in heart rate affords greater ventricular filling time, thereby increasing end diastolic volume. The increased end diastolic volume in turn contributes to larger stroke volume, where a greater volume of blood being pumped means that a greater volume of oxygen and nutrients is available to the physically active musculature [20].

iii. Regular exercise also decreases arterial blood pressure as measured by the heart rate pressure product (RPP). The rate pressure product (RPP) is the product of the heart rate (HR) multiplied by systolic blood pressure (SBP) [RPP = SBP x HR] [21]. It is the index of myocardial oxygen consumption. As the RPP decreases, greater exercise intensity is required in order to elicit chest pain and/or discomfort (angina pectoris), which allows the patient to perform a greater volume of physical activity, thereby improving their quality of life. Clinically, decreased RPP lowers the myocardial oxygen index, reducing elevated heart rate and blood pressure [21].

iv. Exercise primarily increases venous return through the following hemodynamic mechanisms:

- Habitual physical activity and exercise produces laminar shear stress on the coronary endothelium, which changes the shape of the endothelial cells in the direction of blood flow which in turn stimulates the release of nitric oxide. Nitric oxide diffuses into the endothelium and surrounding smooth muscles producing vasodilation [20].

- Habitual exercise produces better calcium handling in coronary muscles, which decreases coronary vasoconstriction and conversely increases coronary vasodilation. Coronary vasodilation reduces resistance to blood flow thus lowering blood pressure [20].

5.2 Exercise-induced mechanisms for combatting chronic respiratory diseases

Chronic respiratory diseases include both chronic obstructive pulmonary disease, characterised by airway obstruction due to emphysema, and chronic bronchitis (inflammation of the bronchioles). Chronic restrictive pulmonary disease consists of chronic lung disorders that produce fibrosis (scarring) and inflammation, which limits inhalation. The most crucial impediment of patients suffering from chronic obstructive respiratory disease pertains to the hyperinflation exercise response that stems from their constrained exhalation. Hyperinflation could be due to increased airway resistance and reduced lung elasticity recoil. Durstine and

Moore have reported that structured and controlled physical activity can offer the following exercise-induced benefits:

i. Cardiorespiratory reconditioning

ii. Reduced hyperinflation

iii. Enhanced ventilatory efficiency and ventilation-perfusion matching

iv. Increased respiratory muscle strength and endurance

v. Desensitisation to dyspnoea (shortness of breath) and anxiety of physical activity regarding exertion

vi. Improves lung diffusing capacity for carbon monoxide

5.3 Exercise-induced mechanisms for combatting diabetes mellitus

Habitual physical activity and structured exercise reduces the hyperglycaemic state of diabetic patients during and after an exercise session by increasing glucose absorption, which reduces glucose blood concentration.

- Regular exercise increases insulin sensitivity, which necessitates a reduction in exogenous insulin intake [22]. Insulin changes glucose to glycogen, decreasing the diabetic patient's hyperglycaemic state. The enhanced insulin sensitivity allows reduced amounts of insulin to more readily facilitate this function, inhibiting excessive insulin release from the pancreas. This exercise-induced endocrine mechanism limits pancreatic hyperactivity. When a diabetic patient exercises, there is a reduction in insulin secretion, which upregulates the sensitivity of the insulin receptors, enabling them to better recognise the presence of blood glucose, which increases glucose absorption into the exercising muscle [21]. Habitual muscle strength training increases the resting metabolic rate of the patient, increasing blood glucose uptake without augmenting insulin secretion [21].

5.4 Exercise-induced mechanisms for combatting cancer

Habitual exercise rehabilitation of cancer patients is beneficial. For cancer patients who are undergoing treatment, the primary objective of the exercise therapy is to maintain muscle strength, endurance, and functionality. For patients who are in remission, the objective of the exercise therapy is restore prior optimal aerobic fitness, muscle strength, endurance, and functionality. Concurrent aerobic and resistance training have the potential to enhance bone remodelling and inhibit the muscle atrophy that is a side effects of glucocorticoids which are common cancer medications. Durstine and Moore have reported that regular structured exercise therapy has the following exercise-induced benefits for cancer patients:

i. Increases muscle flexibility and joint range of motion

ii. Decreases muscle atrophy

iii. Increases muscle strength and endurance

iv. Increases aerobic fitness

v. Maintains body mass

vi. Facilitates various psychological benefits (alleviates depression, increases self-confidence and body image and improves quality of life) [20].

6. Empirical evidence of Biokinetics research into non-communicable diseases in South Africa

In order to determine whether the profession of Biokinetics has made a scientific rehabilitative contribution to the plight of patients suffering from NCDs in South Africa, the authors reviewed the Biokinetic research related to NCDs. In so

Year	Authors	Title	Journal
2002	Du Plessis, Loots, Brits [23]	Abdominal fat distribution and cardiovascular risk factors in hypertensive females.	South African Journal for Research in Sport, Physical Education and Recreation, 24(1):53-76
2004	Schutte, Huisman, Malan, Van Rooyen, Schutte, Malan, De Ridder [24]	Differences in cardiovascular function of rural and urban African males: the THUSA study.	Cardiovascular Journal of South Africa, 15(4):161-165
2005	Schutte, Kruger, Wissing, Underhav, Vorster [25]	The emergence of the metabolic syndrome in urban obese African women: the POWIRS study.	South African Journal of Science, 101(1):61-67
2006	Shaw & Shaw [26]	Consequence of resistance training on body composition and coronary artery disease risk.	Cardiovascular Journal of South Africa, 17(3):111-116
2006	Schutte, Huisman, Schutte, Malan, Underhav [27]	Cardiovascular function of African women with different BMIs and blood pressures: the POWIRS study.	Cardiovascular Journal of South Africa, 17(1):12-18
2007	Shaw & Shaw [28]	Physical activity and high-density lipoprotein cholesterol in sedentary male smokers: physical activity.	African Journal for Physical Health Education, Recreation and Dance 13(4,): 441-452
2008	Shaw & Shaw [29]	Exercise therapy and its role in glucose maintenance s medicine.	African Journal for Physical Health Education, Recreation and Dance, 14(4): 418-427
2008	Shaw & Shaw [30]	Relationship between resistance training and lipoprotein profiles in sedentary male smokers: cardiovascular topics.	Cardiovascular Journal of Africa, 19(4): 194-197
2008	Shaw, Loots, Lategan, Shaw [31]	Effectiveness of aerobic exercise training in improving pulmonary function in asthmatics.	African Journal for Physical Health Education, Recreation and Dance, 15(1): 150-159
2008	Heilbrunn [32]	Exercise and weight loss in diabetes and coronary artery disease.	South African Journal of Diabetes, 1(1):10-12

Year	Authors	Title	Journal
2009	Moss [33]	Changes in coronary heart disease risk profile of adults with intellectual disabilities following a physical activity intervention.	Journal of Intellect Disability Research, 53(8):735–44.
2009	Shaw, Shaw, Brown [34]	Resistance training and predicted risk of coronary heart disease in sedentary males.	African Journal for Physical Health Education, Recreation and Dance, 15(4) https://doi.org/10.4314/ajpherd.v15i4.47294
2009	Shaw, Shaw, Krasilshchikov [35]	Comparison of aerobic and combined aerobic and resistance training on low-density lipoprotein cholesterol concentrations in men.	Cardiovascular Journal of Africa, 20(5):290-295
2010	Hoebel, De Ridder, Malan [36]	The association between anthropometric parameters, the metabolic syndrome and microalbuminuria in black Africans: the SABPA study.	Cardiovascular Journal of Africa, 21(3):148-152
2010	Shaw, Shaw, Brown, Cilliers [37]	Concurrent resistance and aerobic training as protection against heart disease.	Cardiovascular Journal of Africa, 21(4):196-199
2010	Zeelie, Moss, Kruger [38]	The influence of physical activity on components of metabolic syndrome and vascular function in adolescents: A Narrative Review and Physical Activity.	African Journal for Physical Health Education, Recreation and Dance, 16(2):285-296
2010	Zeelie, Moss, Kruger, Van Rooyen [39]	The impact of a 10-week physical activity intervention programme on selective metabolic syndrome markers in black adolescents.	South African Journal for Research in Sport, Physical Education and Recreation, 32(1): 147-162
2011	Goon, Toriola, Uever, Wuam, Toriola [40]	Prevalence of body weight disorders among adolescent school girls in Tarka, Nigeria.	Minerva Paediatric 63(6):467–71.
2011	Prinsloo, Malan, de Ridder, Potgieter, Steyn [41]	Determining the waist circumference cut off which best predicts the metabolic syndrome components in urban Africans: the SABPA study.	Experimental and Clinical Endocrinology of Diabetes, 119(10):599–603
2012	Botha, Malan, Potgieter, Steyn, De Ridder [42]	Association of waist circumference with perception of own health in urban African males and females: the Sympathetic Activity and Ambulatory Blood Pressure in Africans (SABPA) study: Diabetes Education.	Journal of Endocrinology, Metabolism and Diabetes in South Africa, 17(2):106-112
2012	Du Toit, Kruger, Govender, Henning, Kleynhans, Wood, De Villers, Fletcher, Grant, Van Rooyen [43]	Cardiovascular health screening among South African students.	African Journal for Physical Health Education, Recreation and Dance, 18(1): 159-168

Year	Authors	Title	Journal
2012	Grace, Wilders, Strydom, Ellis [44]	A comparison of the effect of two intervention regimes on coronary prone executives in the South African colliery industry.	Occupational Health Southern Africa, 18(1):15-21
2012	Grace & Semple [45]	The prevalence of cardiovascular disease risk factors in normotensive, pre-hypertensive and hypertensive South African colliery executives.	International Journal of Occupational Medical and Environmental Health. 2012, 25(4):375–82.
2012	Heilbrunn [46]	The CDE biokinetic approach to recreational activities in type 1 diabetes.	South African Journal of Diabetes, 5(4): 25-28
2012	Heilbrunn [47]	Does exercise improve or impair blood glucose control in type 1 diabetes? Report.	South African Journal of Diabetes and Vascular Disease, 9(2):66-69
2012	Reger, Kolwicz, Libonati [48]	Acute exercise exacerbates ischemia-induced diastolic rigour in hypertensive myocardium.	Springer Plus, 2;1:46
2012	Rossouw, Du Plessis, Reynecke [49]	Exercise compliance and health outcome in a chronic disease management programme.	African Journal for Physical Health Education, Recreation and Dance, 18(1):77-89
2012	Semple & Johnson [50]	Allied health professionals and cardiometabolic disease risk screening in the workplace: a study of two companies in Darwin, Australia and physical activity.	African Journal for Physical Health Education, Recreation and Dance, 18(1):65-74
2012	Toriola, Moselakgomo, Shaw, Goon [51]	Overweight, obesity and underweight in rural black South African children: original research.	South African Journal of Clinical Nutrition, 25(2):57–61
2013	Gradidge, Constantinou, Goldberg [52]	Sudden cardiac arrest risk in young athletes.	South African Journal of Sports Medicine. 25(2): 53-54
2013	Goon, Toriola, Shaw, Amusa, Khosa, Shaw [53]	Body fat percent of urban South African children: implications for health and fitness.	West Indian Medical Journal, 62(7): 582–8.
2013	Heilbrunn [54]	The CDE Biokinetic approach to safe exercise prescription in people with complications of diabetes.	South African Journal of Diabetes, 6(1): 19-24
2013	Mathunjwa, Semple, du Preez [55]	A 10-week aerobic exercise program reduces cardiometabolic disease risk in overweight/obese female African university students.	Ethnicity Disability, 23(2):143–8.
2013	Toriola, Moselakgomo, Shaw, Goon, Anyanwu [56]	Are rural South African children abdominally obese?	Pakistani Journal of Medical Science, 29(3): 740–3

Year	Authors	Title	Journal
2014	Ellapen, Essack, Thwala, Van Heerden [57]	Coronary risk profiles among University of Kwa Zulu Natal students.	African Journal of Physiotherapy and Rehabilitative Sciences, 6(1): 21
2014	Mamabolo, Sparks, Moss, Monyeki [58]	The association between dyslipidemia and anthropometric indicators in black and white adolescents residing in Tlokwe Municipality, North-West Province, South Africa: the PAHL study.	African Health Science, 14(4):929–38.
2014	Heilbrunn, Strybos, Mufamadi, Flynn [59]	The Centre for Diabetes 'Why Weight?' weight loss and lifestyle change programme.	South African Journal of Diabetes, 7(2): 19-23
2014	McKersie & Baard [60]	Obesity in 7 - 10-year-old children in urban primary schools in Port Elizabeth.	South African Journal of Sports Medicine, 26(2):55-58
2014	Muluvhu, Mukoma, Amusa, Goon [61]	Screening for components of metabolic syndrome among corporate executives in Gauteng Province, South Africa.	African Journal for Physical Health Education, Recreation and Dance, 20(1):388-399
2016	Heilbrunn & Haddow [62]	Why is activity essential as you get older? : living with diabetes.	Diabetes Lifestyle, 1: 44-47
2017	Van Rooyen & Coopoo [63]	Change in patient nutritional knowledge following coronary artery bypass graft surgery.	Health SA Gesondheid, 22(1): 123-129
2017	Van Rooyen & Coopoo [64]	Physical activity and lifestyle modification in the reduction of cardiovascular disease risk in coronary artery bypass graft patients.	African Journal for Physical Activity and Health Sciences, 23(2): 336-353
2017	Van Rooyen & Coopoo [65]	Comprehensive cardiac rehabilitation and quality of life in coronary artery bypass graft patients.	SA Heart, 14(3): 154-160
2018	Pillay & Rugbeer [66]	Occupational cardiovascular disease risk profile and physical activity categories of university cleaners.	Occupational Health Southern Africa, 24(4):101-104
2018	Van Biljon, McKune, DuBose, Kolanisi, Semple [67]	Do Short-Term Exercise Interventions Improve Cardiometabolic Risk Factors in Children?	Journal of Paediatric, 203:325–329.
2019	Ellapen, Broodryk, Paul, Buys [67]	The effects of exercise on diabetes management.	South African Journal of Diabetes and Vascular Diseases, 16(1): 40–43.
2019	Paul, Ellapen, Barnard, Swanepoel, Hammill, Strydom [68]	Are there sufficient number of exercise therapists in South Africa in order to equitably manage the non-communicable disease epidemic?	International Quarterly in Community Health Education, 39(2): 127–132.

Year	Authors	Title	Journal
2019	Thaane, Motala, McKune [69]	Lifestyle modification in the management of insulin resistance states in overweight/ obesity: the role of exercise training.	Journal of Endocrinology, Metabolism and Diabetes in South Africa, 24(2) 65-69
2020	Ellapen, Barnard, Strydom, Masime, Paul [70]	Comparison between the non-communicable diseases mortality rates between 2010 and 2016 of selected South African countries.	International Quarterly in Community Health Education. http://www. doi:10.1177/0272684X2091658
2021	Hene, Wood, Schwellnus, Jordaan, Laubscher [71]	High Prevalence of Non-Communicable Diseases Risk Factors in 36,074 South African Financial Sector Employees: A Cross-Sectional Study.	Occupational Environmental Medicine, 63(2):159–165

Table 2.
Chronological listing of biokinetics research publications relating to investigations concerning non-communicable diseases.

far as Biokinetics is a uniquely South African profession, the empirical literature published will be focused on the South African population, and in all likelihood be published in South African academic journals, the authors reviewed the Sabinet database. In addition, the PubMed and Medline databases were used to identify international journal publications relating to biokinetics research which was focused on NCDs. This was in order to take both national and international research databases into consideration. The authors identified 599 records from Sabinet and 2241 records from PubMed and Medline using the keyword "biokinetics." All records underwent a three-phase evaluation process, namely: title, abstract, and full text analysis. Inclusion criteria was all biokinetic research concerning NCDs. Records therefore included randomised control trial experiments, observational experiments with and without concurrent controls, review papers, and narrative papers. Exclusion criteria were records unrelated to the profession of Biokinetics (exercise therapy) and to NCDs, biokinetic research related to neuromusculoskeletal injuries and rehabilitation, biokinetic research related to sport performance enhancement, and non-English papers. No time frame was instituted, all appropriates records were interrogated for inclusion. Based on the premise that this was a preliminary literature search in order to determine the involvement of the profession of Biokinetics in NCD research, the quality of the records was not accessed. 51 records complied with the inclusion criteria. Of the 51 records, 3 records were common to both the Sabinet database and to the PubMed and Medline databases. The extraction of the common records left 48 records. These records were classified into 16 experimental observations, two review articles, and 30 NCD profiling studies. Further stratification of the records revealed that there were four common categories: respiratory research (n = 1), cardiovascular research (n = 18), metabolic research (n = 22), and cardiometabolic research (n = 7). These categorises included three of the primary NCD mortality agents: cardiovascular and respiratory diseases, as well as diabetes mellitus (which fell into the category of metabolic diseases). No records concerning research relating to cancer were uncovered. **Table 2** details the Biokinetics research publications relating to NCDs. The efficacy of the empirical findings of the randomised control trials measuring the impact of Biokinetics (exercise therapy) on NCDs were reviewed against Mill's Epidemiological Canons.

7. Experimental research evidence supporting the valuable effects of Biokinetics (exercise therapy) in improving the NCD patient profile

The authors employed Mill's Epidemiological Canons in order to determine the value of experimental research evidence supporting the causal extrapolation of the effect of Biokinetics exercise therapeutic interventions on NCDs [72]. Mill's epidemiological canons have five criteria:

- *Temporal sequence* refers to the sequence of the exposure of the intervention, which must precede the change of the diseased condition within a sufficient time frame in order to make a plausible conclusion. Fourteen (87.5%) of the 16 experimental investigations reported that exercise therapy (Biokinetics interventions) improves the NCD profile of participants. Eight (50%) of these 16 investigations reported that Biokinetic cardiovascular rehabilitation improved the cardiac profile of participants [26, 32, 33, 35, 37, 44, 64, 65]. Five (43.7%) investigations illustrated that Biokinetic exercise therapy interventions improve metabolic risk profiles of NCDs patient [29, 39, 47, 55, 67]. One (6.25%) study showed that exercise improved pulmonary function of NCD patients [31].

- *Strength of association* refers to the clinical meaningful difference between the disease and the intervention. Fourteen (87.5%) of the 16 investigations indicated a strong association between Biokinetic exercise therapy and improved NCD profiles (**Table 2**).

- *Consistency of results* refers to the consistent observation of the association between the outcome of the intervention and the disease. Fourteen (87.5%) of the 16 experimental studies indicated that Biokinetic exercise therapy had a positive outcome on the NCD profiles of participants (**Table 2**).

- *Biological plausibility* refers to the clinical explanation of the observed outcome of the intervention in regard to the disease. The 14 studies that reported favourable outcomes proposed credible reasons for these improvements (**Table 2**).

- *Dose response* refers to the volume of intervention required to produce a specific outcome on the disease. There is, however, no consensus pertaining to the amount or volume of Biokinetic exercise therapy needed to produce beneficial outcomes. It is recommended that prospective experimental research be conducted in order to determine the dose response regarding intensity, duration, and frequency of exercise therapy for NCD patients. This new research will help medical practitioners and exercise therapists determine the adequate dose response to exercise.

8. The need to include Biokinetics in the public health sector and challenges facing inclusion

Non-communicable diseases are increasingly prevalent within South Africa [73]. Physical inactivity is recognised internationally as a significant modifiable risk factor contributing to the increased prevalence of NCDs [74]. The integration of physical activity programmes into the primary health care system through multidisciplinary platforms is thus advocated for and envisioned to be more cost-effective than current practices. However, within the current primary health care setting of

South Africa, there is an absence of Biokinetics professionals. These professionals, whose scope of practice is to improve physical functioning and health through exercise, are ideally suited to developing and implementing physical activity programmes in the public sector. Despite the evident need for such interventions, the role of the Biokineticist has not yet been incorporated into the national public healthcare system.

8.1 Role of Biokinetics in the public sector

In South Africa, while research in this field is ongoing, preliminary results are however promising and provide an alternative strategy beyond pharmaceutical medication regarding the management of NCDs. Effectively, the profession of Biokinetics advocates structured exercise interventions as a cheaper alternative to current pharmacological and medical strategies employed in the treatment of NCDs [69, 73]. The inclusion of Biokinetics in the public sector will assist in accomplishing the following strategies, as defined by the Department of Health: [75].

- Prevent NCDs and promote health and wellness at population, community, and individual levels.
- Improve control of NCDs through the strengthening and reform of healthcare systems.
- Monitor NCDs and their main risk factors, as well as conducting innovative experimental research validating the efficacy of exercise therapy.

Other benefits that Biokinetics offers to the public sector include:

- Counselling/educating patients while they are waiting for chronic medication.
- Support in the assessment of risk factors for NCDs.
- Provision of services aimed at preventing (fortogenic healthcare paradigm) and managing (pathogenic healthcare paradigm) NCDs through lifestyle education and exercise–based activities.
- Prescription of home-based physical activity programmes that are cost-effective.
- Visiting communities using mobile health clinics in order to educate people and evaluate risk factors for NCDs.
- Organising community activities after having assessed physical working capacity and risk factors.
- Offering rehabilitation programmes for chronic diseases and injuries in a hospital environment in concert with the treatment offered by physiotherapists and doctors.
- Supporting non-clinical phase rehabilitation and physical strengthening of patients.

8.2 Challenges for the inclusion of the profession of Biokinetics into the South African public healthcare sector

These challenges include a lack of recognition for the invaluable role that the profession of Biokinetics can play in the South African public healthcare sector, coupled with the inaccessibility of national funding for Biokinetics positions by the South African Department of Health and a lack of policy regarding strategic planning relating to the inclusion of the profession of Biokinetics in regards to the prevention (fortogenic healthcare paradigm) and management of NCDs (pathogenic healthcare paradigm). The mobilisation of these solutions so as to overcome these challenges is fundamental for the inclusion of the profession of Biokinetics into the public healthcare sector and for the funding of multidisciplinary community health programmes supporting education regarding physical activity interventions and its role in improving health at all levels of society.

9. Conclusion

The profession of Biokinetics is an exercise therapy vocation that advocates habitual physical activity and exercises as an adjunct to other management strategies adopted within a multi-disciplinary healthcare support team. At present, the profession of Biokinetics is only operational in the private healthcare sector in South Africa. Biokinetics has shown to be a valuable adjunct therapeutic modality both in the pathogenic and fortogenic healthcare paradigms. Numerous experimental research studies have been undertaken illustrating the efficacy of Biokinetic exercise therapy programmes in managing NCDs and improving the quality of life of patients. The inclusion of Biokinetics holds significant promise in helping to better manage the NCD epidemic in the South African public healthcare sector. Exercise therapy is a substantially more cost-effective alternative to other healthcare management strategies as concerns the ongoing management of NCDs within the South African population. The profession of Biokinetics is comparable to the South African professions of Physiotherapy and Occupational Therapy who also prescribe exercise and human movement activity as a rehabilitative modality, however these professions are allowed to function within the South African healthcare public sector. Internationally, clinical exercise physiologists, clinical kinesiologists and exercise specialist (scientists) who have an analogous scope of profession to that of Biokinetics function within both the private and public healthcare sector. As such the authors strongly recommend the inclusion of the profession of Biokinetics into the South African public healthcare sector.

Author details

Yvonne Paul, Terry J. Ellapen*, Takalani C. Muluvhu and Makwena B. Ntjana
Tshwane University of Technology, Pretoria, South Africa

*Address all correspondence to: ellapentj@tut.ac.za

References

[1] Ellapen TJ & Swanepoel M. (2017). The Evolution of the Profession of Biokinetics. South African Journal of Research in Sport Physical Education Recreation, 39(1): 41-50.

[2] Jooste M. (1954). 'n Bepnopte oorsig van die ontwikkeling van Liggaamlike Opvoeding in Suid-Afrika (1652-1936). Deel 1. *VIGOR*, 7(3), 32-34.

[3] Geyer GJ. (1969). Liggaamlike opleiding in die Unie-Verdedigingsmag (1912-1946). University of Pretoria. Verhandeling MA.

[4] Cilliers JJ. (1985). Die bydae van geprogrammerde inoefening in na-mediese fisieke rehabilitasie van beseerdes uit die miltere operasionele gebied. 'n Proefskrif ingelewer ter verkryging van die graad Doctor Philosophiae in Liggaamlike Opvoedkunde aan die Potchefstroomse Universiteit vir Christelike Hoer Onderwys.

[5] Malan DDJ & Strydom GL. (2007). The evolution of physical education at the North-West University- a multifaceted historical development. *African Journal for Physical, Health Education, Recreation and Dance*, September (Supplement), 1-22.

[6] Ellapen TJ, Paul Y, Qumbu BT, Swanepoel M, De Ridder JH, Opperman M, Strydom GL. (2019). Do we need a common name for the study of Physical Activity in South Africa? A narrative review. *African Journal for Physical Activity and Health Science*, 25(1): 27-41.

[7] Strydom GL. (2005). Biokinetics – The development of a health profession from physical education: A historical perspective. *South African Journal for Research in Sport, Physical Education and Recreation*, 27(2): 113-128.

[8] Ellapen TJ, Paul Y, Swanepoel M, Hammill HV. (2020). Professor Gert Lukas Strydom: The Father of the Biokinetics profession in South Africa. *African Journal for Physical Activity and Health Science*, 26(1): 71-80.

[9] Strydom GL. (1968). Die invloed van oefening op die kardiovaskulere fiksheid van koronere-trombose pasiente. 'n Proefskrif ingelewer ter verkryging van die graad Doctor Philosophiae in Liggaamlike Opvoedkunde aan die Potchefstroomse Universiteit vir Christelike Hoer Onderwys.

[10] Buys FJ. (1970). Die invloed van progressief verswaarde oefening of pre-diabetiesie en diabetiesie pasiente. 'n Proefskrif ingelewer ter verkryging van die graad Doctor Philosophiae in Liggaamlike Opvoedkunde aan die Potchefstroomse Universiteit vir Christelike Hoer Onderwys.

[11] HPCSA (Health Professions Council of South Africa). *No 1746: Regulations defining the scope of practise for the profession of Biokinetics*, 2013. Available from http://www.hpcsa.ac.za Accessed: 2016/03/15.

[12] Ellapen TJ, Swanepoel M, Hammill HV, Paul Y, Strydom GL. (2018). Biokinetics a South African Health Profession Evolving From Physical Education And Sport. InTech Publishers.

[13] Robbins G, Powers D & Burgess S. (1991). *A wellness way of life*. Dubuque, IA: WM.C Brown Publishers.

[14] BASA. (2017). *Biokinetics Association of South Africa: Guidelines for Biokineticists*, 2017. Available from http://www.biokinetics.org.za. Accessed on 2017/10/31.

[15] Strydom GL, Wilders CJ, Moss SJ, Bruwer E. (2009). A conceptual

framework of Biokinetic procedures and referral system: An integrated protocol for the various health paradigms. *African Journal for Physical, Health Education, Recreation and Dance,* 15(4), 641-649.

[16] ACSM. American College of Sports Medicine, ACSM's guidelines for exercise testing and prescription, (6th Ed.). Philadelphia, Lippincott & Wilkins, 2001.

[17] Hall J. (2013). Scope of Professions of Physiotherapy, Podiatry and Biokinetics: Overlap identification. *Physiotherapy, Podiatry and Biokinetics News*, 8.

[18] Ehrman JK, Gordon PM, Visich PS, Keteyian SJ. (2013). *Clinical Exercise Physiology* (3rd Ed.) New York: Human Kinetics, 10-13.

[19] WHO. World Health Organization (2021). Non-communicable diseases. (www.who.com)

[20] Durstine JL & Moore GE. (2003). ACSM's Exercise Management for Persons with Chronic Diseases and Disabilities (2nd Edition). Human Kinetics Champion. South Africa. Department of Health. Strategic Plan for the Prevention and Control of Non-Communicable Diseases 2013-17.

[21] McArdle WD, Katch FI, Katch VL. (2003). Exercise Physiology: Nutrition, Energy and Human Performance (7th Ed.) Lippincott Williams & Wilkins.

[22] Melzer K. (2011). Carbohydrates and fat utilization during rest and physical activity. *European e-Journal of Clinical Nutrition and Metabolism*, 6: e45-e52.

[23] Du Plessis, Loots JM, Brits JS. (2002). Abdominal fat distribution and cardiovascular risk factors in hypertensive females. *South African Journal for Research in Sport, Physical Education and Recreation*, 24(1):53-76.

[24] Schutte R, Huisman HW, Malan L, Van Rooyen JM, Schutte AE, Malan NT, De Ridder HJ. (2004). Differences in cardiovascular function of rural and urban African males: the THUSA study: cardiovascular topics. *Cardiovascular Journal of South Africa*, 15(4):161-165.

[25] Schutte AE, Kruger HS, Wissing MP, Underhav MP, Vorster HH. (2005). The emergence of the metabolic syndrome in urban obese African women: the POWIRS study: research article. *South African Journal of Science*, 101(1):61-67.

[26] Shaw I & Shaw BS. (2006). Consequence of resistance training on body composition and coronary artery disease risk: cardiovascular topic. *Cardiovascular Journal of South Africa*, (173):111-116.

[27] Schutte R, Huisman HW, Schutte AE, Malan NT, Underhav C. (2006). Cardiovascular function of African women with different BMIs and blood pressures: the POWIRS study: cardiovascular topics. *Cardiovascular Journal of South Africa*, 17(1):12-18.

[28] Shaw BS & Shaw I. (2007). Physical activity and high-density lipoprotein cholesterol in sedentary male smokers: physical activity. *African Journal for Physical Health Education, Recreation and Dance,* 13(4): 441-452.

[29] Shaw BS & Shaw I. (2008). Exercise therapy and its role in glucose maintenance s medicine. *African Journal for Physical Health Education, Recreation and Dance*, 14(4): 418-427.

[30] Shaw I, Shaw BS. (2008). Relationship between resistance training and lipoprotein profiles in sedentary male smokers: cardiovascular topics. *Cardiovascular Journal of Africa*, 19(4): 194-197.

[31] Shaw I, Loots JM, Lategan L, Shaw BS. (2009). Effectiveness of aerobic exercise training in improving pulmonary function in asthmatics: exercise physiology. *African Journal for Physical Health Education, Recreation and Dance*, 15(1): 150-159.

[32] Heilbrunn A. (2008). Exercise and weight loss in diabetes and coronary artery disease. *South African Journal of Diabetes*, 1(1):10-12.

[33] Moss SJ. (2009). Changes in coronary heart disease risk profile of adults with intellectual disabilities following a physical activity intervention. *Journal of Intellect Disability Research*, 53(8):735-44.

[34] Shaw BS, Shaw I, Brown GA. (2009). Resistance training and predicted risk of coronary heart disease in sedentary males: biokinetics 3(1): *African Journal for Physical Health Education, recreation and Dance,* 15(4). https://doi.org/10.4314/ajpherd.v15i4.47294.

[35] Shaw I, Shaw BS, Krasilshchikov O. (2009). Comparison of aerobic and combined aerobic and resistance training on low-density lipoprotein cholesterol concentrations in men: cardiovascular topic. *Cardiovascular Journal of Africa*, 20(5):290-295.

[36] Hoebel S, De Ridder JH, Malan L. (2010). The association between anthropometric parameters, the metabolic syndrome and microalbuminuria in black Africans: the SABPA study: cardiovascular topics. *Cardiovascular Journal of Africa*, 21(3):148-152.

[37] Shaw I, Shaw BS, Brown GA, Cilliers JF. (2010). Concurrent resistance and aerobic training as protection against heart disease: cardiovascular topics. *Cardiovascular Journal of Africa*, 21(4):196-199.

[38] Zeelie A, Moss SJ, Kruger HS. (2010). The influence of physical activity on components of metabolic syndrome and vascular function in adolescents: A Narrative Review and Physical Activity. *African Journal for Physical Health Education, Recreation and Dance*, 16(2):285-296.

[39] Zeelie A, Moss SJ, Kruger HS, Van Rooyen JM. (2010). The impact of a 10-week physical activity intervention programme on selective metabolic syndrome markers in black adolescents. *South African Journal for Research in Sport, Physical Education and Recreation*, 32(1): 147-162.

[40] Goon DT, Toriola AL, Uever JN, Wuam S, Toriola OM. (2011). Prevalence of body weight disorders among adolescent school girls in Tarka, Nigeria. *Minerva Paediatric*, 63(6):467-71.

[41] Prinsloo J, Malan L, de Ridder JH, Potgieter JC, Steyn HS. (2011). Determining the waist circumference cut off which best predicts the metabolic syndrome components in urban Africans: the SABPA study. *Experimental and Clinical Endocrinology of Diabetes*, 119(10):599-603.

[42] Botha J, Malan, L Potgieter CJ, Steyn HS, De Ridder JH. (2012). Association of waist circumference with perception of own health in urban African males and females: the Sympathetic Activity and Ambulatory Blood Pressure in Africans (SABPA) study: Diabetes Education. *Journal of Endocrinology, Metabolism and Diabetes in South Africa*, 17(2):106-112.

[43] Du Toit PJ, Kruger PE, Govender C, Henning E, Kleynhans M, Wood P, De Villers N, Fletcher L, Grant CC, Van Rooyen JM. (2012). Cardiovascular health screening among South African

students. *African Journal for Physical Health Education, Recreation and Dance*, 18(1): 159-168.

[44] Grace, JM, Wilders CJ, Strydom, GL, Ellis SM. (2012). A comparison of the effect of two intervention regimes on coronary prone executives in the South African colliery industry: original research. *Occupational Health Southern Africa*, 18(1):15-21.

[45] Grace J & Semple S. (2012). The prevalence of cardiovascular disease risk factors in normotensive, pre-hypertensive and hypertensive South African colliery executives. *International Journal of Occupational Medical and Environmental Health*, 25(4):375-82.

[46] Heilbrunn A. (2012). The CDE biokinetic approach to recreational activities in type 1 diabetes. *South African Journal of Diabetes*, 5(4): 25-28.

[47] Heilbrunn A. (2012). Does exercise improve or impair blood glucose control in type 1 diabetes? Report. *South African Journal of Diabetes and Vascular Disease*, 9(2):66-69.

[48] Reger PO, Kolwicz SC, Libonati JR. (2012). Acute exercise exacerbates ischemia-induced diastolic rigor in hypertensive myocardium. *Springer Plus*, (1):46.

[49] Rossouw F, Du Plessis R, Reynecke, F. (2012). Exercise compliance and health outcome in a chronic disease management programme. *African Journal for Physical Health Education, Recreation and Dance*, 18(1):77-89.

[50] Semple SJ & Johnson L. (2012). Allied health professionals and cardiometabolic disease risk screening in the workplace: a study of two companies in Darwin, Australia and physical activity. *African Journal for Physical Health Education, Recreation and Dance*, 18(1):65-74.

[51] Toriola AL, Moselakgomo VK, Shaw BS, Goon DT. (2012). Overweight, obesity and underweight in rural black South African children: original research. *South African Journal of Clinical Nutrition*, 25(2):57-61.

[52] Gradidge PJL, Constantinou D, Goldberg L. (2013). Sudden cardiac arrest risk in young athletes. *South African Journal of Sports Medicine*, 25(2):53-54.

[53] Goon DT, Toriola AL, Shaw BS, Amusa LO, Khosa B, Shaw I. (2013). Body fat percent of urban South African children: implications for health and fitness. *West Indian Medical Journal*, 62(7): 582-8.

[54] Heilbrunn, A. (2013). The CDE Biokinetic approach to safe exercise prescription in people with complications of diabetes. *South African Journal of Diabetes*, 6(1): 19-24.

[55] Mathunjwa ML, Semple SJ, du Preez C. (2013). A 10-week aerobic exercise program reduces cardiometabolic disease risk in overweight/obese female African university students. *Ethnic Disability*, 23(2):143-8.

[56] Toriola A, Moselakgomo V, Shaw B, Goon D, Anyanwu F. (2013). Are rural South African children abdominally obese? *Pakistani Journal of Medical Science*, 29(3): 740-3.

[57] Ellapen TJ, Essack FM, Thwala S, Van Heerden HJ. (2014). Coronary risk profiles among University of Kwa Zulu Natal students. *African Journal of Physiotherapy and Rehabilitative Sciences*, 6(1): 21.

[58] Mamabolo RL, Sparks M, Moss SJ, Monyeki MA. (2014). The association between dyslipidemia and anthropometric indicators in black and white adolescents residing in Tlokwe

Municipality, North-West Province, South Africa: the PAHL study. *African Health Science*, 14(4):929-38.

[59] Heilbrunn A, Strybos S, Mufamadi V, Flynn R. (2014). The Centre for Diabetes 'Why Weight?' weight loss and lifestyle change programme. *South African Journal of Diabetes*, 7(2): 19-23.

[60] McKersie J & Baard ML. (2014). Obesity in 7 - 10-year-old children in urban primary schools in Port Elizabeth. *South African Journal of Sports Medicine*, 26(2):55-58.

[61] Muluvhu TC, Mukoma G, Amusa LO, Goon DT. (2014). Screening for components of metabolic syndrome among corporate executives in Gauteng Province, South Africa. *African Journal for Physical Health Education, Recreation and Dance*, 20(1):388-399.

[62] Heilbrunn A & Haddow G. (2016). Why is activity essential as you get older? : living with diabetes. *Diabetes Lifestyle*, 1: 44-47.

[63] Van Rooyen L & Coopoo Y. (2017). Change in patient nutritional knowledge following coronary artery bypass graft surgery. *Health SA Gesondheid*, 22(1): 123-129.

[64] Van Rooyen L & Coopoo Y. (2017). Physical activity and lifestyle modification in the reduction of cardiovascular disease risk in coronary artery bypass graft patients. *African Journal for Physical Activity and Health Sciences*, 23(2): 336-353.

[65] Van Rooyen & Coopoo Y. (2017). Comprehensive cardiac rehabilitation and quality of life in coronary artery bypass graft patients. *SA Heart*, 14(3): 154-160.

[66] Pillay TE & Rugbeer N. (2018). Occupational cardiovascular disease risk profile and physical activity categories of university cleaners. *Occupational Health Southern Africa*, 24(4):101-104.

[67] Van Biljon A, McKune AJ, DuBose KD, Kolanisi U, Semple SJ. (2018). Do Short-Term Exercise Interventions Improve Cardiometabolic Risk Factors in Children? *Journal of Paediatric*, 203:325-329.

[68] Ellapen TJ, Broodryk A, Paul Y, Buys P. (2019). The effects of exercise on diabetes management. *South African Journal of Diabetes and Vascular Diseases*, 16(1): 40-43.

[69] Paul Y, Ellapen TJ, Barnard M, Swanepoel M, Hammill HV, Strydom GL. (2019). Are there sufficient number of exercise therapists in South Africa in order to equitably manage the non-communicable disease epidemic? *International Quarterly in Community Health Education*, 39(2): 127-132.

[70] Thaane T, Motala AA, McKune AJ. (2019). Lifestyle modification in the management of insulin resistance states in overweight/obesity: the role of exercise training. *Journal of Endocrinology, Metabolism and Diabetes in South Africa*, 24(2) 65-69.

[71] Ellapen TJ, Barnard M, Strydom GL, Masime KM, Paul Y. (2020). Comparison between the non-communicable diseases mortality rates between 2010 and 2016 of selected South African countries. *International Quarterly in Community Health Education*. http://www. doi:10.1177/0272684X2091658

[72] Hene N, Wood P, Schwellnus M, Jordaan E, Laubscher RJ. (2021). High Prevalence of Non-Communicable Diseases Risk Factors in 36,074 South African Financial Sector Employees: A Cross-Sectional Study. *Occupational Environmental Medicine*, 63(2):159-165.

[73] Evans, R W, Smith, T, Kay, P, McWade, D, Angouras, N, van Aarde, R F, Arkell, R, Lambert, E V, & van der Schyff, N. (2016). The need for biokineticists in the South African public health care system. *South African Journal of Sports Medicine*, *28*(3), 85-86. https://dx.doi.org/10.17159/2078-516x/2016/v28i3a1310

[74] Steyn K, Fourie J, Temple N. (eds). Chronic diseases of lifestyle in South Africa: 1995-2005. Technical Report. Cape Town: *South African Medical Research Council*, May 2006:33-47. Available from: http://www.mrc.ac.za/noncomm/cdl1995-2005.pdf

[75] Department of Health. 2013. Available from: http://www.hsrc.ac.za/uploads/pageContent/3893/NCDs%20STRAT%20P LAN%20%20CONTENT%208%20april%20proof.pdf

Chapter 2

Structure, Processes and Results in Healthcare System in Slovenia

Valentina Prevolnik Rupel and Dorjan Marušič

Abstract

Achieving high quality in the provision of healthcare services represents a basic factor in meeting the healthcare needs of the individuals. Accessibility to health services in Slovenia over the last two decades has been presented according to some of the core values of quality and safety: performance, quality and patient-centeredness. The focus of the chapter is on three pillars of health system quality: structure, processes, and outcomes. In each part, we presented the standard practice and state of the art, but also the main achievements in the last decade. In the structural part, we highlight the investment in equipment and human resources and in the process part, the role of the primary level as a gatekeeper with the secondary and tertiary level. The results section concentrates on the measurement of the results in healthcare; the use of quality indicators and PROMs is discussed, the role of quality strategy and health technology assessment in the Slovenian healthcare system is presented.

Keywords: health-related quality of life, patient-centeredness, integrated care, strategy, structure, processes results, indicators

1. Introduction

Basic motivation for healthcare system upgrading should be citizen's centeredness. By positioning citizen in the center, the whole chain of healthcare from promotion, prevention, and protection to diagnostics, treatment and rehabilitation is challenged to meet real healthcare needs of individuals. Immediate access to healthcare services with highest possible quality is crucial to achieve high health-related quality of life.

We decided to review provision of healthcare services in Slovenia in this millennium from the quality perspective. Considering performance, safety, timeliness, efficiency, equality and patient-centeredness as main values of quality and safety of healthcare system we projected them in the three pillars: structure, processes, and outcomes.

In the selection and description of the structural indicators, we aimed to highlight financing, equipment and human resources as the basis for physical accessibility – the availability of services enables the citizens to reach them within reasonable distance from home and within relatively short time. The analysis of the financing system presents the economic dimension acting as a support to physical accessibility and describes people's ability to pay for services without financial hardship.

With procedural indicators our focus was on the major processes in Slovenia which can act as good practices in the implementation of integrated healthcare through a specific role of the primary level as gatekeeper and forming integrated care pathways with the secondary and tertiary level. Cases are presented which offered the solutions and supported the move of the healthcare towards more result-oriented system, such as accreditation process and introduction of RheumaHelper application.

The final part of the chapter concentrates on the measurement of the results in healthcare. Quality indicators and PROMs are presented; existing registries containing data on patients' health status, medical and case-mix variables that can serve as source to obtain useful information and ensure the baseline comparability of treatment populations and intervention factors. Quality strategy and status of health technology assessment is presented as well as a pilot project to implement outcome indicators through national tender.

Throughout the chapter we tried to objectively present the main structural, procedural and result-oriented developments and on the other hand, present the main achievement and implemented solutions in the last decade that are exceptional when evaluating them in the current moment with a critical time distance.

2. Structure

2.1 Financing

The financial and economic crisis starting in 2008 significantly affected Slovenia. The crisis resulted in a severe economic contraction of 7.8% of real gross domestic product (GDP) in 2009 in comparison to 4.4% across the EU28. After 2013, GDP grew continuously. According to Eurostat database, Slovenia's GDP increased for 47.1% in a period 2005–2017; in 2017 reached 43 billion EUR. In comparison, in the same period GDP of EU countries increased for 32.6%.

Total health expenditures (THE) as a percentage of GDP have been increasing steadily since 2000. In 2000 they amounted to 7.8%, and then increased to 8.8% in 2013 and start decreasing thereafter, reaching 8.21% of GDP in 2019. The main explanation for the decrease was the strong growth of GDP after 2013, which was not followed with the comparable growth of THE.

Three main sources of financing the healthcare system are compulsory health insurance, transfers from the central and local budgets, voluntary complementary health insurance and out-of-pocket expenditures paid directly by the citizens. Compulsory health insurance is carried out by a single payer Health Insurance Institute of Slovenia (HIIS) and represents the main public sources of financing; it accounted for 66% of THE in 2019. Complementary health insurance premiums (13.5% of THE) and out-of-pocket payments (13.6%) represent the main private sources of funding.

Public health expenditures as a share of THE have decreased slowly; they ranged between 70 and 74%, reaching 71.8% in 2019. The most important part of public health expenditures is compulsory health insurance, representing between 91 and 96%.

Consequently, there has been an increase in private health expenditure. The slow increase started in 2000 where they amounted to 27.1% of THE, and then reached as high as 28.9% in 2014 and 29% in 2018. In 2019, they amounted to 28.2% [1].

OOP payments as % of THE do not have a clear trend and have been relatively stable amounting to around 12% between 2000 and 2019. In 2018, they amounted to 11.9% [2].

The role of complementary health insurance has been unclear and source of numerous debates as it acts as co-insurance, covering share of each healthcare service in the basic benefit package. Although this makes the basic benefit package largely undefined (as almost each healthcare service from the package is partially covered also from complementary insurance) and causes inefficiencies in the healthcare system, complementary health insurance acted as a protection in economic downturns. In recession, the share of coverage from complementary insurance increased for many healthcare services, enabling complementary insurance to act without loss; the consequences are of course higher premiums for complementary insurance causing higher inequities as the premiums are in absolute terms and equal for all [3]. These inequities, however, have largely been counteracted with a measure introduced in 2012, when the automatic coverage of claims by socially vulnerable are directly covered by central budget [4].

2.2 Payment mechanisms

The total budget for health services is divided among the providers through the negotiation process with main stakeholders, being Health Insurance Institute of Slovenia on behalf of the patients, Ministry of Health on behalf of the Government and the providers of healthcare services. When the allocation of the funds is agreed, the defined models are applied for fund allocation. This procedure clearly defines provider budgets as well as the healthcare services they have to provide and which will be paid for by compulsory health insurance. In contrast, there are no predefined limits for private health expenditure. The general agreement with special agreements for different groups of healthcare providers are the key products of the first phase of contracting processes, which create the fundament for direct contracting negotiations between the Health Insurance Institute of Slovenia and each provider.

The second stage of purchasing of health services involves Health Insurance Institute of Slovenia and the specific provider within the public healthcare network. Definition of the general agreement includes special agreements for various groups of healthcare providers, on basis of which the contracts between the Health Insurance Institute of Slovenia and each provider are concluded. The contracts specify the type and volume of services, but also the prices, methods of payments and other important elements, such as supervision and quality monitoring. With the exception of some of the programs (outpatient care, surgeries, dialysis services and the transplantation program), the reimbursement of provided services is prospectively defined and capped in way that healthcare services exceeding the negotiated amount are not paid by the Health Insurance Institute of Slovenia. If a provider produces fewer services than determined by the contract, he is reimbursed according to the actually provided services. Voluntary health insurance companies do not participate in the negotiation process to define the general agreement and special agreements for different groups of healthcare providers, but are mandated to reimburse the total value of the provided health services covered by complementary health insurance according to the annual plan negotiated in the general agreement. The relative value of voluntary health insurance coverage for different health services is defined by law.

Payment mechanisms used in Slovenia differ according to the health service category. In primary health care, a combination of capitation and fee-for-service is used. The planned income of the family medicine in the amount of 132,000 EUR at the annual level is divided into the capitation income (approximately 50%) and fee-for-service income (approximately 50%).

The capitation income is defined according to the number and age structure of the registered persons. Doctors with an above-average number of registered persons (more than 29,231 capitation coefficients per year) receive more funds than family physicians with a below average number of persons registered. Capitation is paid in a flat rate.

The other half of the income - the service part - depends on the services provided. Although the program of services is planned (27,488 coefficients per family physician per year), however, in order to obtain the whole service part of the revenue, it is sufficient to perform half of the planned services (13,000 coefficients). The acute care services (coefficients – relative prices) are listed in a catalog. One coefficient is worth around 2.5 EUR, depending on the value of the total annual budget for family physicians [5].

Outpatient care is paid on a fee-for-service basis. The payment is based on the planned (and realized) number of "points", which historically reflect the estimated costs of the provided services. Each specialty has a defined set of services (short visit, expanded visit, ultrasound etc.) and each service is assigned a cost weight expressed in the number of points. These points reflect the labor costs (medical doctor specialist, nurse, administrative and laboratory staff), material costs, depreciation, and a separate informatization costs.

Acute inpatient care is paid on DRG basis and non-acute inpatient care on bed day of stay.

2.3 Network of providers

The Slovene healthcare system remains relatively centralized, as the responsibilities of municipalities have not been fully implemented. The Ministry of Health has the task of planning healthcare ensuring equal access to healthcare services and equal patient rights for all citizens. All administrative and regulatory functions of the system are managed at the national level, whereas municipalities have a task to execute the policies and strategies in the area. Compulsory health insurance is centrally managed and administered by Health Insurance Institute of Slovenia. The professional chambers and organizations also operate at the state level or through their regional branches. Municipalities seem to be making limited use of autonomy they gained to plan health services. Consequently, the de facto devolution in planning primary health care from the central government to local communities has not yet occurred.

Primary care falls under the jurisdiction of municipalities, which are responsible for health policy development at the local level. Municipalities are the owners of the community-level primary health care centers that occur all over the country. Primary health care centers are established and owned by municipalities, which are responsible for their functioning and for ensuring sufficient funds for the maintenances of the centers. All employees receive their salary in line with the general contract, which is valid for all employees in the public sector. Primary health care centers provide emergency medical aid, GP/family medicine, and healthcare for women, children and teenagers, community nursing, laboratory and other diagnostic facilities, preventive and curative dental care for children and adults, physiotherapy and ambulance services. Primary care practitioners in Slovenia include family physicians, pediatricians, gynecologists, community nurses, midwives, dentists, pharmacists, therapists, psychologists or psychiatrists and other profiles necessary to deliver care. Family physicians and nurses are the initial contact with patients, who are in need of care. Community nurses support the patients through health promotion and prevention activities, curative, long-term and palliative care. Patients are entitled to select their own physician from among the physicians operating at the primary health care level (i.e. in primary health care centers). Slovenia operates a typical gatekeeping system, and patients need a referral from their family physician to be treated by a specialist. International organizations (such as the WHO and the World Bank) have played a key role in establishing a family medicine model based on the English and Dutch models. The International Survey on the Benefits of Primary Health Care "Monitoring Primary Health Care" assessed 77 indicators for 2009 and 2010 and included, among others, the areas of governance, staff development, accessibility, continuity, coordination and scope. Indicators for Slovenia show that primary health care is very good and better than in neighboring countries [6].

A total of 30 public and private hospitals provide care in Slovenia. There are 10 general hospitals, 2 university hospitals, 5 mental health hospitals and 13 specialized hospitals (3 of them are private). Upon the referral by family physician, the patients can freely choose their secondary care provider. Most of outpatient care and inpatient care is offered in the hospitals. Most of the hospitals are public owned by the state. They are non-profit organizations. Private hospitals, on the other hand, are profit organizations, privately owned. They can receive concession from the Ministry of Health and can make a contracts with the Health Insurance Institute of Slovenia, who would pay them for the care provided. Tertiary care is provided by University Medical Centers located in Ljubljana and Maribor, the Institute of Oncology, the University Clinic of Respiratory and Allergic Diseases Golnik, the Psychiatric Clinic Ljubljana and the University Rehabilitation Institute [7].

According to the number of beds for acute treatment per 1,000 inhabitants, Slovenia has been close to EU-15 average since the early 1990s, in contrast to the countries of Central and Eastern Europe, which have drastically reduced the number of beds. The number of acute hospital beds and the average length of stay have decreased since the early 2000s. Such a development is due to many factors: the introduction of new payment systems, (e.g. bed-days payment was replaced by Diagnosis-Related Groups (DRG) payment in inpatient care); during the economic crisis the prices of healthcare services were reduced; and there was a significant increase in the provision of day care (from 11.1% of all hospital cases in 2005 to 30% in 2013). The number of beds is currently similar to the EU average and the average length of stay is low at 6.8 days. Still, bed occupancy rates are below the EU average, indicating an overextended network at the secondary level. The data would require urgent strategic measures to streamline the network, subspecialize and connect operators [7].

With regard to the number of days in acute treatment, the number of dismissals and the number of outpatient visits, Slovenia does not deviate from the EU-15 average. Slovenia has the lowest number of private beds for acute treatment per 1,000 inhabitants in the EU28.

Outpatient specialist services are paid on a fee-for-service basis, whereas inpatient care is covered (in theory) by fixed allocations and DRG. In practice, however, hospitals are still financed according to historical volumes, meaning that they are not really limited by the DRG-based budget limit. Although the primary care system is strong, particularly since 2011 when the government upgraded family medicine practices and increased the emphasis on prevention and care coordination, service organization and delivery overall are highly fragmented. Waiting lists represent the biggest challenge, and they have translated into an elevated unmet need due to waiting. Share of people reporting unmet needs was higher than EU average according to Eurostat data: 3.5% of people in 2017 and 2.9% of people in 2019 reported unmet needs [8]. The large increase of unmet needs in 2017 is not due to sudden change, but rather to a change in question supporting the calculation of the unmet needs indicator. Presumably, the unmet needs were higher than reported already before 2017.

2.4 Human resources

Despite a steady increase in the number of physicians, partly driven by migration from neighboring countries, Slovenia has one of the lowest physician densities in the EU. In 2018, Slovenia ranked a modest 17th among the twenty-one Member States with 326 physicians per 100,000. In terms of the numbers of nurses (383 per 100,000) medical technician (645 per 100,000) and graduate midwife, Slovenia ranked in the first third among the EU countries and in terms of the number of dentists (72.5 per 100,000 inhabitants) just below the EU average. There are high geographical variations among the number of medical staff: while the number of physicians is highest in Central Slovenia statistical region (463 per 100,000), it is lowest in the Coastal-Karst region (136 per 100,000) [9].

In 2020, the number of general practitioners and pediatricians still lagged behind most EU countries, leading to problems of access and over-referrals to specialist care in some parts of the country. Nurse density was slightly above the EU average. Slovenia tried to solve the lack of medical doctors by opening second medical faculty Maribor in 2003. Also, provision has been made for foreign doctors to practice in Slovenia. Still, the issue of lack of physician has not been solved, especially in some defined specializations, such as primary care and anesthesiology. Due to these difficulties, the question of task-shifting has been analyzed and the scope of practice for community nurses has been widened to optimize patient-centered care. The model practices were introduced, described in the processes, unfortunately the evaluation of their introduction has never been conducted.

2.5 Health information structure

According to the Digital Economy and Society Index (DESI), Slovenia performs very well. More specifically, it ranks very high in the use of provision of access to open data and e-health services (it ranks 6 among EU members) and in the area of electronic prescriptions (number 3 among EU member states). Electronic prescriptions are used by 98% by all family physicians [10]. The e-prescription system has improved interoperability and transparency. The e-registry of patient data and patient summaries the registry of healthcare providers, e-referral system and the e-booking system are implemented. zVem patient portal, which enables patients to see their own medical data is active and used. The current epidemics further increased the use of the implemented solutions, especially zVem portal, which is used for vaccination applications, alongside other lists.

3. Processes

3.1 Referral system

Slovenia operates a gatekeeping system whereby patients require a referral from their family physician in order to access specialist care. Family physicians may refer their patients to a particular outpatient specialist or to hospital diagnostics and treatment units. Physicians may also advise patients on which specialist or institution they would recommend, but, ultimately, patients make the final decision themselves. Patients can choose their secondary or tertiary provider anywhere in the country every time they are given a referral. Specialist services without referral by family physician are paid out of pocket. The same goes for family physicians and other private providers without contract with HIIS or for those services not included in the basic benefits package covered by the compulsory insurance scheme.

If patients select a private provider who does not have a contract with the HIIS, they are required to cover the cost of these services in full themselves [11].

3.2 Integrated care and model practices

The National Health Plan [12] "seeks to strengthen primary care and provide greater access to comprehensive and quality treatment through better care integration and a more adequate professional skill-mix across care levels". The upgrading of family medicine practices in 2011 was an innovative government initiative to improve care coordination and the management of chronic diseases. Upgraded primary health care teams or 'model practices' include a designated nurse who has a part time responsibility to screen for chronic disease risk factors, preventive counseling and care coordination. Additional nurse received specific training including screening for chronic disease risk factors and preventive counseling for patients aged 30 and over, as well as the care coordination of all registered patients with a stable chronic disease. Following the asthma and chronic obstructive pulmonary disease (COPD) modules [13], training was expanded to include the arterial hypertension, coronary disease, diabetes [14], and osteoporosis and prevention modules [15]. The purpose of family medicine "Model practices" operation is to improve the quality of work with an active approach in the promotion of health, screening for the most current health problems of the adult population and systematic management and monitoring of patients with stable chronic diseases. The new way of increased the accessibility of the whole population to high-quality and safe healthcare.

By 2014, about half of all primary care provision was in such 'model practices' and by 2018 most practices included an additional nurse. Annual costs for model practices are estimated to 13 million EUR, the effects of their functioning have not been evaluated yet.

3.3 Transitions from inpatient to outpatient care

Many of the diagnostic and treatment procedures that years ago required hospitalization may be performed today on an outpatient basis: day hospital, outpatient surgery, home hospitalization, tele-health, etc. This is a trend that can increase efficiency and lower costs without losing quality.

Secondary care services are provided by specialists' office in hospitals, private specialists with concessions and in health centers on primary level. On average, a patient has 6.7 outpatient contacts per year. Between 2006 and 2015, this number increased by 0.1 contacts or by 1.5%. Slovenia reaches 88.8% of EU23 [16].

The number of acute hospital beds and the average length of stay have consequently been decreasing since the early 2000s. In 2017, Slovenia had 450 acute hospital beds per 100,000 inhabitants (504.3 in EU 28) with the average length of stay 7.0 days (7.5 days in EU15) [16]. There are more reasons for this besides shift from inpatient to outpatient care, among them also the shift from bed-day payments to case-based (DRG) payments, tariff reductions and rationalization during the crisis; however, shifting from inpatient to outpatient care is one of the reasons. To replace inpatient care with outpatient care forms, various financial incentives have been introduced since 2010. The percentage of day-care cases has risen from 11.1% in 2005 to 30% of all hospital cases in 2013. A particular success re transition from inpatient to outpatient care has been a cataract surgery - with 97.9% cases in outpatient care Slovenia is among the highest in the EU [14]. The quality indicator of the share of one-day surgery determines the number of procedures performed as one-day surgeries (excluding overnight hospitalizations) according to the total number of procedures performed in hospital. One-day surgery helps to redirect resources to less intensive care environments and to reducing the occupancy of hospital beds. At the same time, it brings faster recovery and return to work as well as lower proportion of hospital infections. The indicator shows the shares of one-day surgeries in some selected procedures: the proportion of one-day surgery in knee arthroscopy has increased from 41.3% in 2009 to 54.4% in 2019; in operations of inguinal hernia from 11.6% in 2009 to 15.0% in 2019; tonsillectomy and/or adenoidectomy from 0.25% in 2009 to 0.82% in 2019; cholecystectomy from 0.12% in 2009 to only 0.21% in 2019 and varicose vein surgery from 3,6% in 2009 to 49,2% in 2019 [17].

3.4 RheumaHelper, mobile assistant for rheumatology

In 2013, the mobile application RheumaHelper was implemented as a tool to easily and quickly check the disease activity and with a classification criterion for main rheumatological diseases. In Slovenia it is used by virtually every rheumatologist.

Each year the application is upgraded with new criteria and disease activity calculators, thus expanding the range of usability. Continuous updates of the application with new criteria and disease activity calculators give the doctor access to the latest treatment guidelines and new methods in practice, leading to faster training of doctors and better-quality care. The doctor's app monitors everywhere, allowing you to make quick but quality decisions regardless of the situation, as the source with verified information is available in your pocket. Care decisions are thus always well supported, ensuring a higher quality of work. In the future, the aim is to add integration with hospital systems, where calculated values could be stored in an electronic medical card.

In Slovenia, the app has been used more than 700,000 times by 2016. The app is translated into 6 languages and active in more than 120 countries. In just 3 years, the app has become a global leader, with more than 4,500 rheumatologists using it in more than 40,000 times a month. Nowadays, it is used by more than 7.000 rheumatologists worldwide.

In 2015, the app also received the portal award Healthline.com in the category of best applications for rheumatoid arthritis [18].

3.5 Patient engagement and empowerment

There are numerous patient organizations in Slovenia, and they often actively participate in the drafting of policies and regulations in their specific area. All proposed laws and regulations in Slovenia, also in healthcare area, undergo a public debate phase, in which individuals can participate directly. Patient organizations play a crucial role in public debates and often bring issue in the debates, based on own experiences which result in improved legislation.

Decisions about purchasing of healthcare services are made through negotiations between the key partners in healthcare: providers of healthcare services, the HIIS and the Ministry of Health. HIIS acts on behalf of the patients; however, as a main buyer and payer of healthcare services, it often has to follow the goals that may not be completely in line with the patients' interests. Patients hence participate in the process only indirectly, bringing their suggestions and concerns in the debate through any of the partners.

Every person covered by compulsory health insurance has the right to choose a personal physician without administrative and/or territorial constraints within the country. Moreover, insured people also have the right to choose a personal gynecologist and dentist. There is only one insurer offering compulsory health insurance, the HIIS. Complementary insurance is offered by three insurance companies, which patients can freely choose from. These companies also offer supplementary insurance packages, as do other insurance companies; however, the supplementary insurance market in Slovenia is rather small.

The Patient Rights Act [19] is mainly concerned with individual rights which must be respected by all healthcare providers, public or private. Patient Rights Act importantly limits these rights by stating that their execution must take into account the right to healthcare services as determined in other laws and by taking into account modern medical doctrine and standards. There are 13 patient rights representatives in Slovenia as well as the Commission for the Protection of Patient Rights. They report regularly to Ministry of Health which monitors the protection of patients' rights.

Health literacy is an important determinant of health. It encompasses the knowledge, motivation, and competencies of individuals to access, understand, judge, and apply health information to day-to-day decisions related to health promotion, disease prevention, and healthcare. Health literacy is a key to empowering and actively participating individuals in caring for their own health.

Since October 2019, the project Raising Health Literacy in Slovenia (ZaPiS) has been running. It is implemented by the Ministry of Health of the Republic of Slovenia and the National Institute of Public Health. The purpose of the project is to raise the health literacy of the population of Slovenia, with an emphasis on connecting all key structures that can contribute to better health of the population. With the planned activities, we will be able to adequately address the changed health needs of people and make better use of new communication opportunities. Project activities will include both the health literacy aspect at the individual level and organizational health literacy. The latter involves the implementation of strategies in healthcare institutions that make it easier for patients to understand health information, navigate their healthcare system, integrate into the healthcare process and take care of their own health [20].

3.6 Accreditation process

The accreditation procedure of healthcare providers in Slovenia is voluntary. Providers are accredited by internationally recognized organizations independent of the Ministry of Health or the HIIS (e.g. Det Norske Veritas International Accreditation Standards, Accreditation Canada International). The accreditation processes are financially supported by HIIS. The accreditation is valid for three years and then needs to be renewed. All hospitals in Slovenia obtained internationally acquired accreditation; the last hospital obtained it in 2018. Additionally to hospitals, accreditation is becoming more popular also among providers of outpatient care and in healthcare centers at primary level. The data on accreditation is published on the Ministry of Health website [21].

4. Results

4.1 Quality indicators and PROM

Slovenia introduced healthcare quality indicators in 2010. The chosen indicators were selected form a number of sources, such as OECD Healthcare Quality Indicators project and WHO Performance Assessment Tool for Quality Improvement in Hospitals. Additionally, some indicators were proposed and developed by the Ministry of Health and the Medical Chamber. The results are published every year in a special report on quality indicators and are publicly accessible on the Ministry of Health webpage; the last report covers year 2019 [15]. Altogether, there are 30 indicators; one in patient-centered care, four in promotion, prevention and primary care (hospital admissions), seven in communicable diseases, 12 in healthcare efficiency, five in patient safety and an indicator for hand hygiene. Patient-reported outcome measures have been launched in 2009 and 2010 in National Tender, but later on not systematically introduced [22].

4.1.1 Patient-centered indicators

The share of exclusively breastfed newborns has decreased significantly, by almost 17 percentage points, in the last decade. In 2019, the share of exclusively breastfed healthy newborns in Slovenian maternity hospitals was thus only 69.9%. The differences between hospitals are large; they range from 16% of exclusively breastfed newborns in Postojna to 96% in Ptuj, while the shares in most of the hospitals range between 60 and 80%.

4.1.2 Promotion, prevention and primary care indicators

Hospital admission rate due to chronic diseases is used in pulmonary disease (COPD), heart failure, asthma and arterial hypertension. These indicators reflect the quality of primary care. In 2019, the hospital admission rate for asthma was 32.7 and has been declining since 2016. The hospital admission rate for COPD was 113.1, heart failure 285.9 and arterial hypertension 47.9. In all chronic disease a general downward trend can be noticed in the last decade.

4.1.3 Communicable diseases

The indicators on communicable diseases report proportions of vaccinated children against measles, diphtheria, tetanus, whooping cough and hepatitis B. Vaccination against these diseases has been relatively high at the national level for several years in a row, higher than 90% (except for hepatitis B), there are no major deviations. This provides good protection against the spread of the aforementioned infectious diseases in Slovenia. The vaccination of elderly aged 65 years and more reached 12.9%, which is among the lowest levels in EU.

Further indicators in this category report incidence rates of measles, whooping cough and chronic hepatitis B. While the incidence rate in measles and chronic hepatitis B are low, the incidence rate for whooping cough was relatively high in 2017 and 2018, above 10%. Among the possible causes relatively rapid decline in immunity after vaccination, change in the causative agent, and lower performance of a newer (acellular) whooping cough vaccine are mentioned. Therefore, many countries have introduced boosting doses in adolescence, booster doses at least once in adulthood and vaccination of pregnant women.

4.1.4 Healthcare efficiency

The pressure ulcer quality indicator shows the rate of hospital ulcers. The differences in the percentage of ulcers acquired differ widely among hospital and ranges from 0 to 23%. Further indicator in this category refer to waiting times for computer tomography – the legal framework for monitoring waiting times was established in 2008 by the Patient Rights Act [19] and the Regulation on maximum waiting times for individual health rights [23]. On 1 May 2011, National Institute for Public Health published data on the waiting lists for selected healthcare services for the first time. There were 24,819 patients waiting for 60 defined services. The list of 60 services was slightly changed on 1 September 2012, and then there were no further changes until 1 May 2016, when one more service was added to the list. In August 2018, the whole operational system of reporting was replaced, and at the same time, the list of services, their coding and the reporting methodology have been completely changed. For example, data on physiotherapy treatment are no longer monitored and 58 services from previous system now correspond to 400 new services. The service code translator has not yet been officially published; however, the data could potentially be compared if it existed.

Between 1 January 2015 and 1 January 2020, the number of patients waiting for first visit increased by 54.1%. There were total of 403,811 patients on waiting lists on 1 January 2020, among them 165,201 or 40.9% waited longer than allowed. 71.3% of all patients were waiting for outpatient specialist services and the rest were waiting for diagnostic procedures or day care. The estimated financial value for provision of services for all patients on waiting list was 120.4 mio EUR, and the estimated value of service provision for patients waiting longer than allowed was 44.7 mio EUR [24].

A series of indicators on efficiency of the surgical processes include utilization of operating theaters for hospital and outpatient procedures, share of canceled procedures, average length of stay for selected procedures (cholecystectomy, pneumonia, hip replacement etc.), indicators connected to diabetes (hospital admissions because of diabetes, amputations due to diabetes), indicators connected to newborns. The first one is injuries in vaginal delivery: in 2019 a total of 17 cases of third- or fourth-degree of such injuries were reported during childbirth. The share of cesarean sections has increased significantly in the last decade, but remains below EU average. Both the proportion of elective and emergency cesarean sections increased. In 2019, the proportion of Cesarean sections at the gestational age of 37 was 17.2 percent, lowest in general hospital Jesenice (9.1%) and highest at 30.5%, in Trbovlje.

Very important indicators are post-surgical deep vein thrombosis and lung embolism. The rate of cases of pulmonary embolism per 100,000 admissions due to hip or knee endoprosthesis has been decreasing constantly in the last decade while the data on the lung embolism are less clear, stills showing a slight general decreasing trend. The use of antimicrobials is monitored as well.

4.1.5 Patient and personnel safety

Patient and personnel safety report data on the injuries with sharp objects, falls, foreign bodies in the body after the surgery, methicillin resistant *Staphylococcus aureus* (MRSA) and post-surgical sepsis. Hand hygiene has been improving, but can improve further: overall consistency of hand hygiene has reached 77.5% in 2019.

4.2 Quality strategy

The first National Strategy for Health Quality and Safety was launched in 2010. Its aim was to assure systematic and continuous development of improvements in healthcare system. The strategy defined numerous strategic objectives, such as the development of quality management systems, the development of a clinical culture of safety and quality within and the development and implementation of education programmes in quality and safety. During the period of the strategy, most hospitals and many other providers accredited their quality management systems through one of the international standards. According to the evaluation [25], National Strategy did not play a sufficient role in the practical implementation of other measures. A new strategy has not yet been formed, also due to a lack of political will. On a positive note, the National Healthcare Plan includes several objectives in the area of quality, such as strengthening of training in quality and safety and patient communication and an update of the quality indicators. Furthermore, several projects, such as ZaPIS [20] or a standardized patient experience measurement in outpatient consultations was set up and survey of patient experiences in hospital care was updated [26].

4.3 Registries

Cancer registries are a service for the systematic collection, storage, analysis, interpretation and presentation of data on cancer patients, their disease and treatment in Slovenia. Cancer reporting is mandatory and legal. More detailed information can be ordered by doctors, researchers and the general public using a special form.

The Cancer Registry is one of the oldest population registries in Europe. It was established in 1950 at the Ljubljana Oncology Institute as a special service for collecting and processing data on all new cases of cancer (incidence) and on the survival of cancer patients. The Cancer Registry of the Republic of Slovenia has been a regular member of the International Association of Cancer Registries since its establishment in 1968, and from the very beginning also of the European Cancer Registry Association [27].

The Healthcare Databases Act entered into force in August 2000. The list of databases and registers is defined as an annex, which facilitates the possible amendment of the lists. The annex includes 40 records and 35 registers. Each collection has a defined purpose, reports, data reporter, controller, and data delivery method and data retention time [28].

The endoprosthesis registry contains extended information about the patient, the provider, the prosthesis, the operation, or the reoperation. The collection is managed for: monitoring the survival (time from insertion to removal) of inserted hip and knee endoprostheses, ensuring quality control of endoprosthetic operations, enabling rapid detection of lower quality endoprostheses, indirect reduction of costs of primary and revision hip and knee endoprostheses and as a basis for clinical and epidemiological studies and expert analyzes. The registry manager is hospital Valdoltra, which prepares an annual report on the basis of data sent on an ongoing basis by all providers and other legal and natural persons, regardless of the concession, who perform the arthroplasty medical activity [29].

4.4 National tender and health-related quality of life

The national tender for hip, hernia, varicose vein and carpal tunnel operations was introduced as a mechanism for lowering prices, measuring outcomes and increasing the efficiency of performed health services. The national tender conducted in 2009 increased the availability of tendered health programs, as 13% more services were provided for the same funds due to lower prices offered by the providers. The effects of the national tender 2009 were the basis for further activities of the HIIS in the implementation of purchasing function. Namely, even in the years of the relative lack of additional financial resources, the HIIS tried to increase the accessibility of insured persons to health services in various ways. Based on the tender HIIS managed to increase the number of the surgeries by 6.6% (increase in the number of surgeries from 12,695 to 13,536) and achieve 4.5% savings. At the same time, national tender enabled control over the safety and quality of health services as for the first time a generic measure for health-related quality of life (EQ-5D) was used to measure changes in the health status of the patients [30]. Further quality indicators were introduced as well, but were unfortunately never analyzed. The results of the EQ-5D analyses represented a very good concept for national implementation, but could not offer deep enough insight to provide recommendations on the reorganization of the health network or the limitation of the scope of services at an individual provider. Unfortunately, HIIS abandoned the national tender after two years of pressure from public providers, and today it does not monitor the results of treatment and the quality of treatment when distributing funds.

4.5 Health technology assessment (HTA)

HTA framework in Slovenia has not been established at the national level. The need to formalize HTA for all health technologies has been known and various initiatives have been present in the system to introduce it. The most developed level of HTA is present in the area of pharmaceuticals, while with other health technologies, HTA process is much more unclear, irregular and unsystematic [31]. HTA in pharmaceuticals is conducted by HIIS. HIIS passed the Rules on inclusion of medicines in the list [32], which define the types of the analysis that can be used, timelines, and decision criteria that are to be followed in the assessment process. The criteria, according to which the pharmaceuticals are evaluated, are clinical effectiveness, safety and cost-effectiveness. Adaptation of the study results to Slovenian setting is demanded and the analysis should use Slovenian data as much as possible.

Consulting body to HIIS, called Pharmaceutical Reimbursement Commission, makes recommendations on the placement of the pharmaceuticals on the positive or intermediate list [31]. These are based on the presented relative therapeutic value and incremental cost-effectiveness ratio of the drug. The latter must be expressed in marginal costs per quality-adjusted life-year (QALY). The threshold for the acceptance of the pharmaceuticals into the public financing is set to 25,000 EUR [33]. The Pharmaceutical Reimbursement Commission members are physicians and clinical pharmacists as well as other experts with systemic knowledge in the field of drugs. Their recommendations are independent.

Other healthcare technologies, especially healthcare services programmes, are introduced through Health Council. Health Council is the highest advisory body to the Minister of Health. It gives recommendations on introducing new technologies to the Minister, who makes the final decision on their introduction. Upon his decision, the suggestion is made to the HIIS for its public financing and HIIS can make a decision to reimburse the use of new technology or not. The recommendations to the Minister of Health are based on the criteria defined in Procedures on handling the applications for new healthcare programs [34]. The protocol is quite complex and long and consists of several questions on the technology, its safety, target population, clinical effectiveness, costs, and organizational issues. Cost-effectiveness is not included in the protocol.

5. Conclusion

Slovenia is committed to universality, accessibility, solidarity and equality, which are all fundamental values of EU health systems. In the last two decades, measures to maintain the achieved level of development and attempts to accelerate the introduction of innovative solutions to move upwards from the position of the golden mean of the development of EU health systems have continued. Given the high level of development of the healthcare system in Slovenia, the chapter focuses on the presentation of success in introducing pilot solutions, lack of perseverance in evaluating pilots before their national implementation and persistent maintenance of implemented system practices. While promoting the quality and safety of the health system and ensuring greater prosperity and faster development, it will be necessary to ensure more appropriate investment in health. Taking into account all the successful steps of upgrading the healthcare system, investments in staff, knowledge and innovation will be needed in finding a balance between the wishes and real health needs of citizens. Healthcare is a complex system, so comprehensive and systemic solutions are needed; most of them already exist at home.

Author details

Valentina Prevolnik Rupel[1*] and Dorjan Marušič[2]

1 Institute for Economic Research, Ljubljana, Slovenia

2 Health Centre Celjenje, Koper, Slovenia

*Address all correspondence to: rupelv@ier.si

References

[1] Health Insurance Institute of Slovenia. Poslovno poročilo za leto 2005-2020 [Internet]. Zavod za zdravstveno zavarovanje Slovenije, 2021. Available from: https://www.zzzs.si/zzzs-api/e-gradiva/vsa-gradiva/?vrsta=BR39YG226&cHash=5f4a5a05a80acdc92f131e53fe711160 [Accessed: 2021-04-15]

[2] Eurostat data, https://appsso.eurostat.ec.europa.eu/nui/submitViewTableAction.do

[3] Ministry of Health of Republic of Slovenia. Nadgradnja zdravstvenega sistema do leta 2020 [Upgrading Health Care System by 2020] [Internet]. Ministrstvo za zdravje Republike Slovenije, 2011. Available from: http://www.ds-rs.si/sites/default/files/file/dokumenti/Dsvet/DS_s35_t3_G1.pdf [Accessed: 2021-04-15]

[4] Health Care and Health Insurance Act [Zakon o zdravstvenem varstvu in zdravstvenem zavarovanju]. Official Gazette of the Republic of Slovenia, No. 72/06 and updates. Available from: http://pisrs.si/Pis.web/pregledPredpisa?id=ZAKO213 [Accessed: 2021-04-15]

[5] Švab I, Homar V, editors. Support for the development of the primary care system in Hungary. Ljubljana: Institute for development of Family medicine; 2021. 454 p.

[6] Kringos D, Boerma W, Bourgueil Y, et al. The strength of primary care in Europe: an international comparative study. Br J Gen Pract. 2013;63(616):e742-e750. DOI:10.3399/bjgp13X674422

[7] Albreht T, Pribaković Brinovec R, Jošar D, Poldrugovac M, Kostnapfel T, Zaletel M, Panteli D, Maresso A. Slovenia: Health system review. Health Systems in Transition, 2016; 18(3):1-207. Available from: https://www.euro.who.int/__data/assets/pdf_file/0018/312147/HiT-Slovenia_rev3.pdf [Accessed: 2021-04-16]

[8] Eurostat data, https://ec.europa.eu/eurostat/data/database [Accessed: 2021-05-10]

[9] NIPH. Zdravstveni statistični letopis za leto 2019 [Yearbook in Health Care for 2019] [Internet]. National Institute for Public Health. Available from: https://www.nijz.si/sl/publikacije/zdravstveni-statisticni-letopis-2019 [Accessed: 2021-04-20]

[10] Better. Client stories: Ministry of Health of Republic of Slovenia [Internet]. Available from: https://www.google.com/search?q=98+per+cent+of+Slovenian+general+practitioners+use+e-prescription&rlz=1C1CAFB_enSI691SI698&oq=98+per+cent+of+Slovenian+general+practitioners+use+e-prescription&aqs=chrome..69i57.6901j0j15&sourceid=chrome&ie=UTF-8 [Accessed: 2021-04-19]

[11] Health Insurance Institute of Slovenia. Right to specialist and hospital healthcare [Internet]. Zavod za zdravstveno zavarovanje Slovenije, 2021. Available from: https://zavarovanec.zzzs.si/wps/portal/portali/azos/pravice_zdravstvenih_storitev/pravice_specialisticne/ [Accessed: 2021-04-28]

[12] Resolution on the National Health Care Plan 2016-2025 »Together for Health« [Resolucija o nacionalnem planu zdravstvenega varstva 2016-2025 »Skupaj za družbo zdravja«]. Official Gazette of the Republic of Slovenia, No. 25/16. Available from: http://pisrs.si/Pis.web/pregledPredpisa?id=RESO102 [Accessed: 2021-04-29]

[13] Poplas-Susič T, Švab I, Klančar D, Petek D, Vodopivec-Jamšek V, Bulc M,

et al. Screening and registering patients with asthma and COPD in Slovenian primary care: first results. Slovenian Journal of Public Health. 2015;54:161-167. DOI: 10.1515/sjph-2015-0023

[14] Petek D, Mlakar M. Quality of care for patients with diabetes mellitus type 2 in 'model practices' in Slovenia–first results. Slovenian Journal of Public Health. 2016;55:179-184. DOI: 10.1515/sjph-2016-0023

[15] Petek Šter M, Šter B. Pomen izobraževanja diplomiranih medicinskih sester v referenčnih ambulantah: primer arterijske hipertenzije. Obzornik zdravstvene nege. 2015;49:52-59. DOI: 10.14528/snr.2015.49.1.46

[16] OECD. Health at a Glance 2019: OECD Indicators, 2019. Paris: OECD Publishing; 2021. Available from: https://doi.org/10.1787/4dd50c09-en. [Accessed: 2021-05-03]

[17] Perko D, Borovničar A, editors. Kazalniki kakovosi v zdravstvu – letno poročilo za leto 2019 [Quality indicators in healthcare – annual report for year 2019]. Ljubljana: National Institute for Public Health Ministry of Health of Republic of Slovenia; 2020. Available from: https://www.gov.si/assets/ministrstva/MZ/DOKUMENTI/Dostopnost-in-varnost-zdravstvenega-varstva/Kakovost-zdravstvenega-varstva/Porocila/Kazalniki-kakovosti-v-zdravstvu-2019.pdf [Accessed: 2021-05-07]

[18] Zajc T. Zmagovalna dobra praksa: Rheumahelper - spodbuda k oblikovanju podobnih orodij tudi za druge specialnosti [Winning good practice: Rheumahelper – incentive to form similar tools also for other specialties]. Ljubljana: Medicina danes; 28.02.2016. Available from: https://www.medicina-danes.si/8841936/ZMAGOVALNA-DOBRA-PRAKSA-Rheumahelper-spodbuda-k-oblikovanju-podobnih-orodij-tudi-za-druge-specialnosti [Accessed: 2021-05-09]

[19] Patients' Rights Act [Zakon o pacientovih pravicah]. Official Gazette of the Republic of Slovenia, No. 15/08, 55/17 and 177/20. Available from: http://pisrs.si/Pis.web/preglesPredpisa?id=ZAKO4281 [Accessed: 2021-05-07]

[20] NIPH. Project Increasing health literacy in Slovenia (ZaPiS) [Projekt Dvig zdravstvene pismenosti v Sloveniji (ZaPiS)]. [Internet]. National Institute of Public Health, 2021. Available from: https://www.nijz.si/sl/projekt-zapis-dvig-zdravstvene-pismenosti-v-sloveniji [Accessed: 2021-04-15]

[21] Ministry of Health. Kakovost zdravstvenega varstva [Quality of Health Care] [Internet]. Ministrstvo za zdravje Republike Slovenije, 2021. Available from: https://www.gov.si/teme/kakovost-zdravstvenega-varstva/ [Accessed: 2021-05-09]

[22] Prevolnik Rupel V, Erker R, Divjak M. Comparing Quality of Life of General Population and Orthopedic Patients in Slovenia. Value in Health Regional Issues, 2020; 22: 93-98. DOI: 10.1016/j.vhri.2020.07.575

[23] Rules on the referral of patients, the management of waiting lists, and the maximum permissible waiting times [Pravilnik o naročanju in upravljanju čakalnih seznamov ter najdaljših dopustnih čakalnih dobah], Official Gazette of the Republic of Slovenia, No 3/2018 and 201/2020. Available from: http://www.pisrs.si/Pis.web/pregledPredpisa?id=PRAV13238 [Accessed: 2021-04-21]

[24] Simčič B, Kuhar M, Marušič D. Nedopustno čakajoči - dosežen je novi rekord! Razsežnosti problema pravočasne zdravstvene obravnave [Number of waiting above permissible waiting time – a new record is set! Viewpoints on the problem of timely health services]. Dnevnik. 2018; 68:14-15. Available from: https://www.

dnevnik.si/1042842229 [Accessed: 2021-05-03]

[25] Pantelli D, et al. Analysis of the Health System in Slovenia: Purchasing and Payment Review. Final Report. Ljubljana: European Observatory on Health Systems and Policies; 2016. Available from: https://www.euro.who.int/en/countries/slovenia/publications/slovenia-health-system-review-reports/analysis-of-the-health-systems-in-slovenia-purchasing-and-payment-2016 [Accessed: 2021-05-17]

[26] NIPH. Project PREMs. [Internet]. National Institute of Public Health, 2021. Available from: https://www.nijz.si/sl/prems [Accessed: 2021-04-15]

[27] Institute of Oncology Ljubljana. Register raka Republike Slovenije in drugi registry [Cancer Registry of the Republic of Slovenia and other registries] [Internet]. Onkološki Inštitut, 2021. Available from: https://www.onko-i.si/rrs [Accessed: 2021-05-12]

[28] Healthcare Databases Act [Zakon o zbirkah podatkov s področja zdravstvenega varstva]. Official Gazette of the Republic of Slovenia, No 61/2010. Available from: http://pisrs.si/Pis.web/pregledPredpisa?id=ZAKO1419 [Accessed: 2021-04-24]

[29] Orthopedic Hospital Valdoltra. Register Endoprotetike Slovenije [Registry of Endoprosthetic of the Republic of Slovenia] [Internet]. Ortopedska bolnišnica Valdoltra, 2021. Available from: https://www.ob-valdoltra.si/sl/raziskovalna-dejavnost/register-endoprotetike-slovenije [Accessed: 2021-04-26]

[30] Prevolnik Rupel V, Ogorevc M. Use of the EQ-5D Instrument and Value Scale in Comparing Health States of Patients in Four Health Care Programs among Health Care Providers. Value in Health Regional Issues. 2014;4:95-99. DOI: 10.1016/j.vhri.2014.07.001

[31] Prevolnik Rupel V. Current Implementation of Health Technology Assessment in Healthcare System in Slovenia. Int J Technol Assess Health Care. 2017;33:360-364. DOI: 10.1017/S0266462317000083.

[32] Rules on inclusion of medicines on the list [Pravilnik o razvrščanju zdravil na listo]. Official Gazette of the Republic of Slovenia, No 35/2013, 3 April 2013. Available from: http://www. pisrs.si/Pis.web/pregledPredpisa?id=PRAV11493. [Accessed: 2021-04-22]

[33] Health Insurance Institute of Slovenia. Decision on incremental cost effectiveness ratio. Ljubljana: Zavod za zdravstveno zavarovanje Slovenije; 2013. Available from: http://www. zzzs.si/zzzs/info/egradiva.nsf/0/de161d25a238859cc1257c1d0026d7f9/ $FILE/Podpisan%20sklep%20ICER.pdf [Accessed: 2021-05-14]

[34] Ministry of Health of Republic of Slovenia. Postopek obravnave vlog za nove zdravstvene programe [Procedures on handling the applications for new health care programmes]. Ljubljana: Ministry of Health; 2015. Available from: https://www.gov.si/assets/ministrstva/MZ/DOKUMENTI/O-ministrstvu/Zdravstveni-svet/Postopek-obravnave-vlog-za-nove-zdravstvene-programe.pdf [Accessed: 2021-05-14]

Chapter 3

Demand for Health and Healthcare

Alireza Ghorbani

Abstract

Healthy human beings are the center of sustainable development, and human beings have long sought to maintain and improve their health by increasing their health reserves. In general, the use of services or the demand for medical services has a vital role in improving the level of health of each person. The demand for healthcare is a demand derived from the demand for health and is influenced by several factors, including price, income, population, etc.

Keywords: Healthcare Services, Demand, Demand Curve, Price, Health Economics

1. Introduction

When people are asked why health is important, many are unable to answer it. The reason for this may be due to their lack of awareness of the importance of health and the consequent lack of proper self-care. Health can generally be considered an essential basis of life, but many people still do things that show that health is not a priority in their lives. They spend a lot of time on the opportunities they find but do not spend time learning what is good for them to exercise or stay healthy; they spend their budget on Nonsignificant things. But for a more nutritious diet, they pay less.

According to the World Health Organization's definition, health is a state of complete physical, mental and social well-being and not only the absence of disease or infirmity. This definition of health has been given more attention since 1978 at the UN Summit in Almaty. Due to the considerable differences in the level of health in different countries of the world, the members of this organization were required to provide Primary Health Care by providing an essential package aimed at reducing the health gap between different countries and with the goal of Health for All by the year 2000. Undoubtedly, one of the most critical concerns and challenges that different countries have faced in providing primary health care to their population has been the lack of resources in the face of the growing need to receive this care during all these years.

So from the perspective of health economists, health is a durable good, or type of capital, that provides services. The flow of services produced from the stock of health capital is consumed continuously over an individual's lifetime. Each person is assumed to be endowed with a given stock of health at the birth time, such as a year. Over the period, the stock of health depreciates with age and maybe promoted by investments in Health services. Death occurs when an individual's stock of health falls below a critical minimum level.

2. Demand

To request a product or service, you must ask for it, afford it, and have a specific plan for purchasing it. Desires are, in fact, the unlimited desires and inclinations that people have for goods and services. Imagine being able to afford something if you could afford it or it was not so expensive. When we make choices, scarcity guarantees that many of our desires will never be met. Demand reflects our plan and vision for the demands that will be met. The amount of goods and services that the consumer plans to buy depends on many factors: commodity prices, related commodity prices, personal income, expected future prices, population, advertising, and preferences.

We must first discuss the relationship between the demand for a good or service and the price. All other factors influencing demand must be kept constant to study this relationship called the Citrus Paribus principle. The demand for a good or service is inversely related to its price; as the price increases, the demand for it decreases, and vice versa. Of course, the rate of demand response to price changes is not the same for all goods, which will be discussed in the topic of elasticity [1].

2.1 Demand curve

The demand curve is a geometric location of points where the dependent variable is the rate of use of a good, and the independent variable is the price of that good; in general, the demand curve shows the maximum demand for a good at different prices and also represent the ultimate price for a certain amount of a good. Usually, the price variable is shown on the y axis and the amount of goods or services on the x-axis (**Figure 1**).

This shows the maximum amount someone is willing to pay for a small increment in consumption rate. Care should be taken in using the "demand" to mean the amount of consumption of a particular good or service at a specific price and to use it to mean a range of corresponding values in the price range (for example, one point on the demand curve versus the whole Points on the curve). The demand for a good or service is a function of its relative price and buyers' income. The demand curve is a two-dimensional representation of this process. Responding to price changes is moving along the demand curve and responding to changes in revenue as the entire demand curve changes and shifts (**Figure 2**). Some of the characteristics of the demand side that should always be kept in mind when using the demand curve in healthcare, especially when making normative statements about well-being, are: Uncertainty

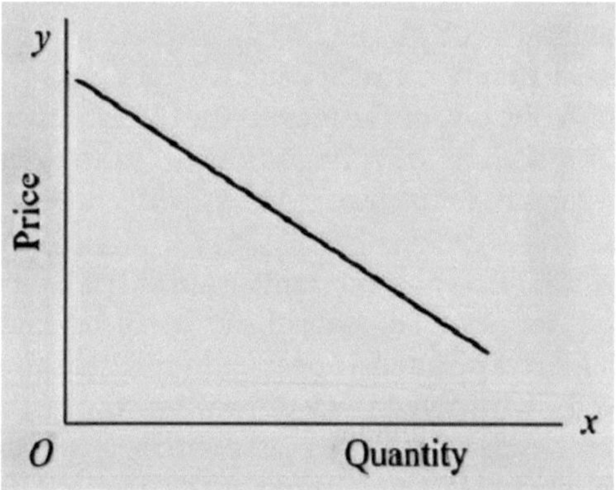

Figure 1.
Demand curve.

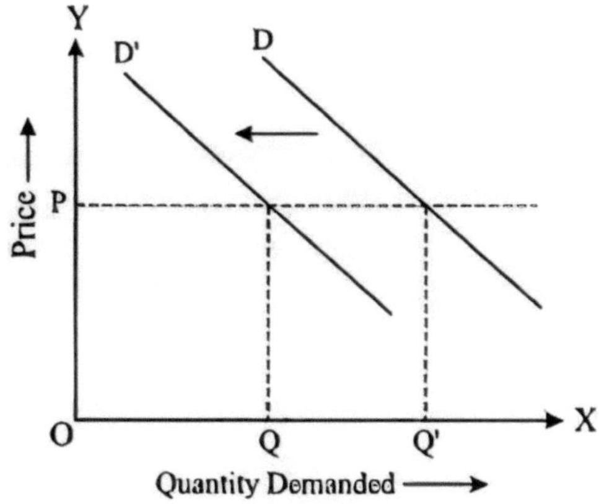

Figure 2.
Change in demand curve.

on the part of the consumer about the likelihood of future illness; Side effects, the effectiveness of treatment methods and their possible cost. When sick, people experience anxiety, disability, suffering, and pain that may not be considered in the theory of desirability; It is also important to note that there may be an external demand for care and treatment of a person in addition to their need; And the fact that the price at which the applicant responds to the service or goods may in no way be an accurate reflection of the final cost of providing that product or service to the service provider.

We can also consider the demand curve as a payment ability curve that measures the ultimate benefit. This curve shows the highest price a person is willing and able to pay for the last unit purchased. If there are fewer goods available, the highest price that a person is willing and able to pay for a larger unit will be high. But as the quantity of available goods increases, the ultimate benefit of each additional unit decreases, and the highest price offered on the demand curve decreases.

In addition to the price of the product in question, which is inversely related to the demand for that product, we can examine the relationship between the demand for a product and other factors in the space of the demand curve.

Prices of other goods: The amount of goods or services that consumers plan to buy depends in part on the prices of other goods and services. In this case, there are two types of goods: substitute goods and complementary goods. Two substitute goods can be used instead of each other, and if the price of one of them increases, the demand for that product will decrease, and people will be more likely to demand a substitute product. For example, if beef and chicken are two substitutes, as the price of beef increases, so makes the demand for chicken.

A complementary good is a good that is used with another commodity, and if the price of one of these commodities increases, in addition to the demand for that commodity, the demand for the other commodity also decreases.

Income: Assuming other factors are constant when people's incomes increase, they buy more goods and services, and vice versa. Demand increases as income increases are normal goods, and goods for which demand decreases as income increases are called inferior goods. But in general, it can be said that the demand for health goods and services has little to do with income. Because medical goods and services provide their health reserves, and as a result, people's income cannot have a significant impact on demand for these goods. However, rising incomes will increase the demand for luxury medical services.

Population: Demand also depends on the size and age structure of the population. If the population increases, the demand for all goods and services increases, and the population decrease. The demand for goods and services decreases. At the same time, as other factors remain constant, as the population in a particular age group increases, so makes the demand for goods and services used by that age group.

Consumer's Preferences: Demand also depends on consumer preferences. Preferences are people's tastes and attitudes towards different goods and services. Preferences are formed based on previous experiences, genetic factors, propaganda, religious beliefs, and other cultural and social factors [2, 3].

2.2 Medical goods

Medical care consists of countless goods and services that maintain, improve, or restore a person's health. For example, a young man may have wrist surgery to repair a torn tendon so he can return to work, an older woman may have cataract surgery to improve her vision, or a parent may have to Bring their child to a healthcare center for an annual dental checkup to prevent future problems. Prescription drugs, prescription glasses, and dentures are examples of medical supplies, while surgeries, periodic physical examinations, and visits to medical professionals are examples of medical services. Preventive and medical care are heterogeneous, making it difficult to measure and quantify medical care units accurately. Medical care services have four characteristics that distinguish these from other goods and services: intangibility, inseparability, inventory, and inconsistency.

Intangibility means that the five senses are incapable of evaluating medical services. Unlike new shoes, a vegetable salad dinner, or a new cell phone, the consumer cannot see, taste, or touch medical services. Indivisibility also means that the production and consumption of a medical service take place simultaneously. For example, when you see an ophthalmologist for an examination, you use ophthalmic services right at the time of production. In addition, a patient is often seen as both a producer and a consumer. Inventory is directly related to inseparability. Because the production and consumption of a medical service occur simultaneously, healthcare providers cannot store or maintain medical services. For example, a physiotherapist cannot provide a list of different physiotherapy services to meet demand during busy times. Finally, inconsistency means that the variety, composition, and quality of medical services are very different. Although different people may see a doctor simultaneously, there are various reasons for visiting a doctor. One person may see a doctor because of a typical physical problem, while another may see a doctor because of a heart attack. The combination of prescribed medical care or the frequency of its use can vary significantly from person to person and at different times [4, 5].

Demand for healthcare: Demand requires people to seek a service they can afford and are willing to pay for it. The need for healthcare is the care that doctors believe is essential for a person to stay healthy or healthy. Sometimes, patients think they need healthcare, but doctors believe they cannot benefit from such care. Sometimes the doctor believes that there is a medical need, but the patient does not consult his doctor because he prefers not to receive treatment or that he has not recognized the need. Even if patients have as much knowledge as doctors, their demands may be different from their needs.

The following factors affect the demand for healthcare:

I. Needs (based on patient perception)

II. Patient preferences

III. Price or cost of use

IV. Income

V. transportation cost

VI. waiting time

VII. Quality of care (based on patient perception)

The use of healthcare depends on demand and availability. If planners allocate resources based on need rather than demand, they may find themselves in a situation where some services are underused, and some services are overused.

Just as the healthcare market is different from other commodities, so is the demand for healthcare different from the simple demand model. One of the differences is that healthcare is not demanded because it is self-satisfying. After all, healthcare itself does not lead to satisfaction. Instead, healthcare is in demand because people are satisfied with their activities when they are healthy. So the demand for healthcare is a derived demand.

Patients' perceptions of their need and capacity to benefit from healthcare are strongly influenced by physicians and healthcare providers. Although in economics, it is assumed that consumers can make informed decisions about their consumption patterns, healthcare consumers delegate this decision-making power to healthcare workers who are more aware of them. This phenomenon is due to information asymmetry between healthcare providers and patients, which carries the risk of induced demand by providers to increase revenue. Another complication stems from the fact that healthcare is highly heterogeneous. Each patient has a relatively different combination of pain and symptoms. Therefore each patient needs to purchase a fairly different package of care that both the patient and the physician have uncertainty about its effectiveness in meeting the need.

Another critical difference is that many health services are paid for by third parties. Payments by third parties or insurance companies Although they significantly increase people's purchasing power for healthcare, it is also important to note that they can lead to ethical risks and increase demand for services that patients may not need.

Demand for healthcare depends on the level of consumption of an individual in case of illness; the amount of consumption can differ according to the factors affecting the demand, such as income, service price, education, norms, social traditions, and quality. A person's decision to use or use services is related to his or her illness/injury status rather than healthcare. Developing countries are focused on promoting healthcare as an essential policy to improve health outcomes and fulfill international obligations and universal coverage of health services. However, many policies have focused more on improving physical access than on the demand-side healthcare needs pattern. In low-income countries, allocating scarce financial resources is based on clear criteria for the impact of investment in the health sector on service demand.

In these countries, due to the lack or weakness of social security systems, the occurrence of the disease leads to increased health costs and reduced labor productivity and leads to a loss of household welfare. In developed countries, due to insurance, many health services are used with minimal consumer participation in the payment; however, in developing countries, concerns about less use of health services, to the extent of supply. Or poor access is associated. However, even in health services, due to various barriers on the demand side, related to the cost of treatment, travel costs, and quality of services, the rate of exploitation is low. Also, the importance of a person's health status in a clinical context is related to the analysis and social evaluation of a person's health and social environment. Studies have shown that the risk of death is related to people's perception of the health importance of maintaining it. Since one of the priorities of health policymakers is to improve people's health, various factors that directly and indirectly affect the demand for health services should be examined more carefully. Identifying the factors influencing individuals' decision to request healthcare services and choosing from different providers. Therefore, evaluating the determinants of demand for health services will introduce and implement appropriate incentive schemes to encourage better health services. Because health is one of the essential components of human capital and healthy human beings are the center of sustainable development, health can significantly increase the ability of individuals to perform various activities, including productive activities. As a result, people are looking for health. At the individual level, health is mainly influenced by multiple factors such as biological factors, lifestyle, purchased non-medical services, purchased medical services and goods, and different socio-economic characteristics. People's understanding and expectation of healthcare quality are essential because the perceived quality of health services often affects health services' behavior and consumption patterns [6].

2.3 Derived demand for healthcare

Grossman used human capital theory to explain the demand for healthcare. According to human capital theory, people invest in themselves through education and health to increase their income. Grossman proposed an approach in which many important aspects of the demand for health services differ from the traditional demand approach:

1. That consumers are looking for health and demand health services to achieve it.

2. To achieve health, consumers buy health services from the market and combine them with their efforts to improve health, such as diet and exercise.

3. The health gained lasts more than a period and is not immediately depreciated to be analyzed as a capital good.

4. Most notably, health can be considered as both a consumer good and a capital good. From the people's point of view, health is a consumer product because it makes them feel better. As a capital good, it is also suitable for people's health because it increases the number of healthy days of life to work and earn money. **Figure 3** provides a simple diagram that explains the concept of health capital. Just as one thinks that cars or laptops are capital goods that use the flow of their services over time, one can also understand the savings of one's health capital, the outcome of which is "healthy days". Outflow may be considered as one dimension of healthy days or measured in several dimensions of physical, mental health, and limited activity. People consume a range of health inputs, including healthcare inputs, diet, exercise, and time, so they invest in health savings. These investments help maintain or improve consumers' health reserves, providing them with healthy days. Over time, health reserves may either grow, remain constant, or decrease with age due to illness or injury. As mentioned in Box 3, many technologies may generate

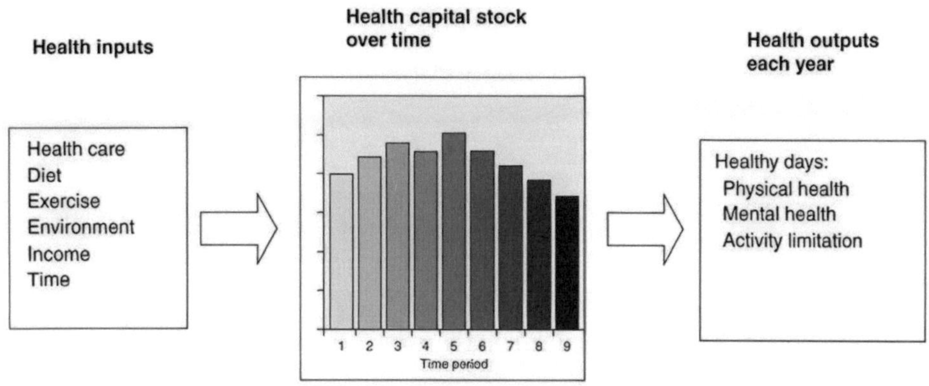

Figure 3.
Investing in health.

health capital, using different amounts of time or health goods and services. **Figure 3** shows how the ultimate goal of "healthy days" guides consumer decisions about the amount, time, and cost of investing in health storage. We will see that the prices of healthcare, the rate of wages of individuals, and their productivity in the production of health determine how resources are allocated between health capital and other goods and services that people buy. Consider a consumer who buys market inputs (e.g., medical care, food, clothing) and combines them with his or her own time to generate a health capital reserve that increases his or her utility [2].

2.4 Price elasticity of demand

As an economic principle, the price of a good and the demand for that good are inversely related. That is, the higher the price of a commodity, the less demand there is for that commodity, and the lower the price of a good, the greater the demand for it. Price elasticity of demand shows that a one percent change in a good price causes a few percent changes in the demand. For example, if the price of a car rises by one percent, the demand for it will fall by a few percent, and vice versa, if the price of a vehicle falls by one percent, the demand will increase by a few percent.

Three things can happen when we calculate the price elasticity for a commodity:

a. When a one percent change in the price of a commodity occurs, the demand for that commodity changes by more than one percent. These types of goods are very price sensitive.

b. When a one percent change in a good price causes the demand for that good to change by less than one percent, this type of product is called inelastic. Demand for this type of goods shows a mild reaction to price changes.

c. The third case is when a one percent change in the price of a good causes a one percent change in the demand for that good.

If there is an inverse relationship between price and demand, demand elasticity will always be negative because the percentage change in one face or denominator is a negative fraction. Therefore, after calculating the price elasticity of demand, if the result, regardless of the negative sign of the number, becomes more than one, the

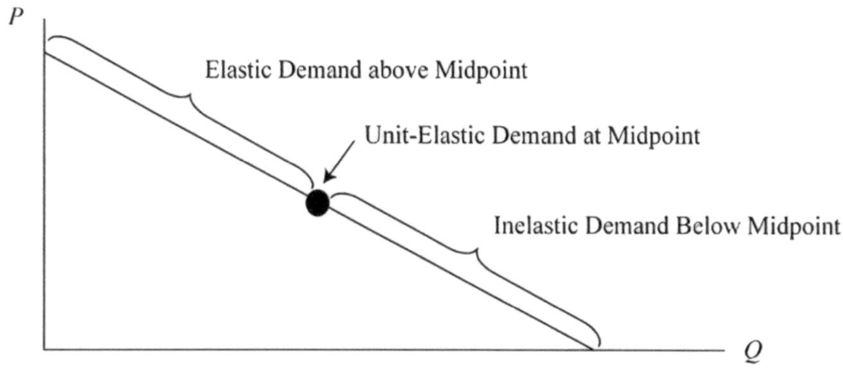

Figure 4.
Types of elasticity.

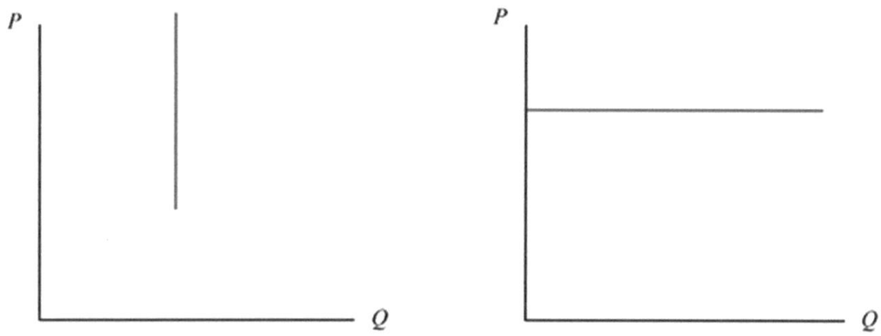

Figure 5.
Marginal modes in demand elasticity.

commodity with elasticity is less than one, the good without elasticity, and if it is equal to one, the good has a single elasticity.

Although the price elasticity of a commodity can be determined only by collecting price information and calculating, some factors affect this ratio.

2.5 Factors affecting the price elasticity of demand

Alternative goods: The more alternative goods there are, the higher the price elasticity of that product. That is, when the price changes, the demand for that product changes more drastically. Also, price changes in a product cause a shift in the demand for alternative goods. In the healthcare sector, there are usually few alternatives to a health or medical intervention.

Complementary goods: When a product has a supplement, a change in the price of a complementary product causes a change in the demand for another product. Maternal and child care can be mentioned as complementary goods in the field of health (**Figure 4**).

Commodity prices: In general, if the price of a commodity is very low, the amount of demand does not react to price changes. But high-priced products are attractive. On the other hand, different results are obtained depending on the price at which the demand elasticity is calculated. As mentioned initially, the price of a product has an inverse relationship with the amount of demand. When the price is precisely in the middle of the demand curve of a commodity, the commodity has a single elasticity. Also, if the price is less than the midpoint, the product in that range is unattractive. If the price is above the midpoint, the product will be pulled. You can see this in the chart below.

Marginal modes in demand elasticity: There are also two cases in which the product is completely elastic or completely non-elastic. If the good is fully elastic, the demand for that good will be zero if there is a slight change in the price of the good. Perhaps this is the case for a salesperson in a highly competitive market. If the good is completely inelastic, demand is a fixed figure, regardless of the price range. You can see these modes in **Figure 5**.

Author details

Alireza Ghorbani
Health Economics, Sabzevar University of Medical Sciences, Sabzevar, Iran

*Address all correspondence to: ghorbania1474@yahoo.com

References

[1] Culyer, A. J. (2008). *The Dictionary of Health Economics*: Edward Elgar.

[2] Folland, S., Goodman, A. C., Charles, A., & Stano, M. (2017). *The Economics of Health and Health Care*: Taylor & Francis Group.

[3] Gu, T., Li, D., & Li, L. (2020). The Elderly's demand for community-based care services and its determinants: A comparison of the elderly in the affordable housing community and commercial housing Community of China. Journal of Healthcare Engineering, 2020, 1840543. doi:10.1155/2020/1840543

[4] Santerre, R. E., & Neun, S. P. (2013). *Health Economics: Theory, Insights, and Industry Studies*: South-Western, Cengage Learning.

[5] Wellay, T., Gebreslassie, M., Mesele, M., Gebretinsae, H., Ayele, B., Tewelde, A., & Zewedie, Y. (2018). Demand for health care service and associated factors among patients in the community of Tsegedie District, northern Ethiopia. BMC Health Services Research, *18*(1), 697. doi:10.1186/s12913-018-3490-2

[6] Wonderling, D. (2005). *Introduction to Health Economics*: McGraw-Hill Education.

Chapter 4

Shared Decision-Making towards a Higher Quality of Care: Is This the Norm?

George Athanasiou and Chris Bachtsetzis

Abstract

Patient-doctor relationship has traditionally been paternalistic, in which the doctor decided on behalf of the patient. It focused mainly between the patient who called for help and the doctor whose decisions had to be silently observed and followed by the patient. In this paternalistic model, the physician used his skills to choose the necessary interventions and treatments that were likely to restore the health of the patient. All the information given to the patient was selected to encourage them to consent to the doctor's decisions. This definition of the asymmetric or unbalanced interaction between physicians and patients has begun to be questioned over the last 20 years. There has been a shift from this direction to one where the patient is more informed, empowered, and independent - a move from a "paternalistic" to a more "complementary" relationship. Critics suggested a more active, autonomous patient-centered role which supports greater patient control, reduced doctors' dominance, and a more mutual participation. This approach has been described as one where the doctor attempts to enter the patient's world to see the disease with the eyes of the patient and is becoming the predominant model in clinical practice today.

Keywords: Shared Decision-Making, Doctor-Patient Relationship, Informed Decision, Patient involvement, Measuring shared decision-making

1. Introduction

The relationship between the patients and the doctors has been dependent through the centuries on the medical situation and the social scene. This relationship was predominantly between a patient seeking help for an illness or symptom and a doctor whose decisions were silently complied with by the patient. The patient-doctor relationship has traditionally been paternalistic, in which the doctor took all decisions on behalf of the patient. Nevertheless, there has been a shift from this direction to one where the patient is more informed, empowered and independent - a move from a "paternalistic" to a more "complementary" relationship. In this 'mutualistic' relationship, the patient is more empowered, informed, and autonomous [1].

This paternalistic doctor-patient relationship focused mainly on the patient, who called for help, and the doctor, whose decisions had to be silently observed and followed by the patient. In this paternalistic model, the physician used his skills to choose the necessary interventions and treatments that were likely to restore the health of the patient. All the information given to the patient was selected to encourage them to consent to the doctor's decisions. This definition of an asymmetric or unbalanced interaction between physician and patient has begun to be questioned over the last 20 years. The critics suggested a more active, autonomous and, therefore, a more patient-centered role which supports greater patient control, reduced doctors' dominance, and a more mutual participation. This patient-centered approach has been described as one where the doctor attempts to enter the patient's world to see the disease with the eyes of the patient and has become the predominant model in clinical practice today [2].

2. Historic pathway

In Ancient Egypt, the doctor-patient relationship was that of a priest-supplicant relationship, retaining the ideology of a parent-figure to manipulate events on behalf of the patient [3]. Such healers used rationality, theology, magic, and mysticism in their care of external and visible disorders. This type of relationship may be defined as activity-passivity type of relationship. This relationship was not changed for years, as there were no technical advances or the appropriate social circumstances to require such a change. During the Greek enlightenment in the 5th century BC, medicine shifted to a naturalistic observation with the elements of trial and error. Based on the Hippocratic Oath, the doctor provided regimen which had to be to the benefit of the patient, irrespective of gender and age. The needs, the well-being and the best interest of the patient were above the doctor's self-interest, respecting confidentiality. This doctor-patient relationship under the Hippocratic approach was based on a guidance-cooperation and mutual participation. During the Medieval times, the doctor, was in a glorious, high ranking position in society, filled with magical powers. The patient was regarded as helpless infants. The relationship between doctor and patient weakened and deteriorated and resembled the activity-passivity model of the ancient times, with the era of witch hunting and incarcerating the mentally ill [2].

The social and cultural changes brought in the transition period of the Renaissance movement and the period towards the French Revolution encompassed innovative flowering of an increased demand for equality, liberalism, and dignity. This, inevitably, led to changes in the doctor-patient relationship from the activity-passivity model to a more guidance-co-operation model [2, 4].

In the 18th century, Medicine was based on symptoms and thus the model of illness was developed. Hospitals emerged to treat ill patients following the foundation of professional nursing by Florence Nightingale. With the development of microbiology and surgery, Medicine focused, not on the symptom but the biomedical model of diagnosis. The expert clinical and anatomical knowledge, the knowledge of the patient's body and the necessity of physically examining the patient, evolved the doctor as an active participant, with the patient becoming more dependent as a result. The relationship resulted in a dominant doctor and a passive patient, i.e. an activity-passivity (paternalistic) model [2].

3. Doctor-patient relationship: the models

There are three models of the doctor-patient relationship as proposed by [4]:

The model of activity-passivity: A paternalistic model with limited interaction, as the patient is unable to actively contribute, as they are regarded as helpless requiring the doctor's expert knowledge. Treatment is commenced "irrespective of the patient's contribution and regardless of the outcome". This doctor-patient relationship focused mainly between the patient who called for help and the doctor whose decisions had to be silently observed and followed by the patient. In this paternalistic model of doctor-patient relationship, the physician uses his skills to choose the necessary interventions and treatments that are likely to restore the health of the patient. All the information given to the patient is selected to encourage them to consent to the doctor's decisions.

The model of guidance-co-operation: This takes into account that, despite the fact that the patient is ill, they are conscious and thus have feelings and aspirations of their own. The patient is, therefore, ready, and willing to "cooperate" and obey to their guidance without question.

The model of mutual participation: This model, also advocated by [5], considers that the doctor does not know exactly what is best for the patient. It is argued that there is an equal interaction between the doctor and the patient, having equal power, mutual independence, and equal satisfaction with mutual participation between this relationship. This model has elements of mutual and equal partnership, without power or control of any member of this relationship upon the other. This gives a greater emphasis on patient-centered medicine.

4. Patient-centeredness

As suggested by [6] the patient-centered medicine is a "two-person medicine" with both the doctor and the patient having their integral part in this relationship, and cannot be considered separately, as they are influencing each other all the time. Mead and Bower [7] underline that a large number of variables can potentially influence the patient-centeredness. The so-called "shapers", these variables may impact this relationship. Such variables include cultural norms, socioeconomic background, and societal expectations, such as norms relating to gender, the medical training of doctors, etc. For example, it is more socially acceptable for females to discuss feelings and emotions than males. On the other hand, ethnic differences, presence of third parties, workload pressures or time-limitations may create barriers to effective communication and limit possibilities for full negotiation in this doctor-patient relationship.

5. Shared decision-making process

In recent days, there is a shift of interest and additional research on this new doctor-patient relationship. This new alliance is based on co-operation rather than confrontation, in which the doctor must "understand the patient as a unique human being" [8]. Thus, patient-centered care has replaced the one-sided, doctor-dominated relationship in which the exercise of power distorts the decision-making process for both parties. This decision-making is based on a two-way process in which both the patient and the doctor share the information and the responsibility for decision-making. It applies to most visits, as the majority of treatment decisions include several options, even if one of the options is a no-action or non-treatment. The shared decision-making (SDM) process has begun to be at the center of healthcare. Coulter and Collins [9] define SMD as *a process in which clinicians and patients work together [...] sharing information about options [...] with the aim of reaching mutual agreement on the best course of action.*

SDM includes at least one patient and one healthcare provider. Both parties take steps to actively participate in the decision-making process, share information and personal values, and together they come to a shared responsibility decision [10, 11]. This process is indicated when there are multiple possible treatments and the alternatives have different and uncertain results, as is the case of most chronic diseases or if the outcome of the treatment is considered to be subjectively significant [12]. Furthermore, it might help the patient and the healthcare professional to conclude to a mutual agreement on treatment or other long-term decisions [13]. Chewning et al. [14] argue that greater patient involvement in management decisions is associated with fewer conflicting decisions, which can be considered moderate to patient satisfaction. SDM is associated with feelings of autonomy, control, and individual capacity from the patient. Actions for the implementation of SDM are becoming increasingly important and their results should be evaluated and measured.

5.1 The stages of SDM

Elwyn et al. [15] define SDM with the following steps:

1. Definition/explanation of the problem in simple terms

2. Presentation and explanation of the different possible management options - this should include all possible choices, including no decision-making or watchful waiting. The patient should know an equipoise or equilibrium position where there is no right or wrong decision, only a preferred option.

3. Discussion of the benefits/disadvantages (benefits/risks/costs) - these should be explained along with all possibilities (if known), so as the patient can weigh their options.

4. Clarification of patient preferences - the attitudes, concerns and expectations of each individual should be explored.

5. Discussion of the patient's capacity - the patient should be aware that he/she does not need to make the decision on his/her own, but that family members or friends are invited to participate, as appropriate. The doctor should support the decision-making process so that the patient does not feel destitute.

6. Presentation of the data (what is known) and recommendations - the physician should present the available data through his/her clinical experience and advise the patient in the joint decision-making process.

7. Clarification and checking the understanding of the patients - the patient should have the opportunity to ask questions or ask for more information if necessary.

8. Discussion about possible postponement of the decision - Some patients will make the decision at this time. For others, it may be better to make a decision at a later stage until all possible options are considered without time pressure. It should be possible to re-examine the problem at a later stage (e.g. at the next appointment).

5.2 The pros and cons

The perceived potential benefits when applying SDM are multiple and include the improvement of patient's knowledge and self-esteem, even though not all of them are conclusively proven. It also improves patient's risk perception and reduces their anxiety. It is worth noting that the main drawbacks cited are usually based on clinicians' perceptions rather than an evidence base. Not all patients request it and not all consultations are suited to such approach as it takes more time and requires special training from the doctor's side [16].

A recent systematic review by [17] looked into the barriers and facilitators of SDM in clinical practice. It was found that the most commonly identified facilitators were positive impact on the clinical process, provider motivation, and positive impact on patient important outcomes. On the other side, common barriers were time constraints, lack of applicability due to the characteristics of the population, and the clinical situation.

6. Is shared decision-making the norm nowadays?

If the benefits of SDM are not conclusively proven, with not all patients wanting it and being potentially time consuming, why are doctors encouraged through the health systems to engage in such a practice? Whether research findings are conclusive or not, there are some other convincing reasons. In the UK, practicing SDM is supported and encouraged by the General Medical Council, General Dental Council, and government policy. It is considered as an ethical and legal imperative and underpins government legislation [18]. The National Health System (NHS) of the UK, has recognized the importance of patient involvement in treatment decision and adopted SDM into the redesigned health-system through a recent Health and Social Care Act. The government has provided the legislation for SDM to become the norm. With the mantra 'no decision about me without me', SDM is now a statutory requirement for the commissioning board of the NHS and local clinical commissioning groups [19, 20].

In order to support developments in this area, a Shared Decision-Making Collaborative has been established in 2015. It comprises members from the statutory sector, patient and voluntary sector organizations and academia committed to thinking collectively about the role of SDM in UK health systems [21]. Throughout Europe there is an increasing awareness that patients should be allowed to play a crucial role in decision-making and care management. WHO is encouraging SDM practices as innovative strategies to support patient-centered health services and promote patient rights [22]. WHO indicates that most research on SDM in Europe has occurred in Northern European countries, however, the SDM approach may fit also the Mediterranean region with different socioeconomic and cultural factors and lower degree of patient empowerment and communication.

SDM is of international importance and is currently promoted in many health systems. The reasons for these changes include the expansion of patients' knowledge on different conditions and treatments through the internet and mass media and the increasing number of therapeutic options available. The increased preference for more active patient involvement, by both, the patient and the physician is also a key factor [23]. According to [24] SDM requires collaboration between patients and healthcare professionals who work together to select the appropriate management, treatment and support, based on patient preferences and needs, physician experience and evidence-based data. It can improve patient involvement in healthcare and help provide effective services.

One recent study by [25] on SDM in mental health services, reveals that this application is a continuous, dynamic, and difficult process that requires every mental health professional to internalize his characteristics, facilitate patient involvement, and create a culture of trust in the management process of treatment.

It is reported that SDM balances the power and responsibility for creating safe care. This balance requires continuous thinking and evaluation of patient resources, constraints and need for assistance to give them the power (patient empowerment) and responsibility to be able to manage the different needs during various phases of illness and management. The patient's functionality may change over time, so, in order to ensure safe care, mental health professionals must always compensate for the strength and responsibility that the patient cannot maintain.

The main provisions for the implementation of SDM are that health professionals recognize that different medical situations require different approaches, as well as accepting SDMs as a key element of good practice [26]. It is understandable that healthcare professionals know that facilitating patient participation is important, as many patients either do not want to, or, are unable to participate in the recovery process. Grol et al. [27] report that patients need flexible services to accommodate their changing needs. It was argued that when patients have severe symptoms, they need care and less responsibility. When they have fewer symptoms, there is a growing need for empowerment, active participation, and more responsibility for decision-making. Most patients want to be more informed about their health status, investigation, and management options than they are routinely given by health professionals, and many would like a greater share in the process of making decisions about how they will be treated. Bastiaens et al. [28] have shown that, patients are dissatisfied when they are not being properly informed about their condition and the options for treating it. However, not all patients want to share in making the decisions. For example, older people or those with life-threatening conditions tend to be more likely to prefer to delegate decision-making to the doctor as described by [29].

As suggested, different cultures or settings may influence the degree of patient involvement in decision making. A survey [29] showed that a more paternalistic view of the doctor–patient relationship prevailed in Poland and Spain than Germany, Italy, Slovenia, Spain, Sweden, Switzerland and the United Kingdom. 91% of Swiss and 87% of Germans felt that the patient should have a key role in their management decision, either by sharing responsibility with the doctor or by being the primary decision-maker. This percentage was much lower in Polish and Spanish patients - 59% and 44% respectively.

Clinicians should always try to find patient preferences through effective communication. Stevenson et al. [30] highlighted that they need to encourage patients if they are to play an active role in decisions about their care. As a result of this encouragement, patients become more involved, their knowledge improves, their anxiety lessens, and they feel more satisfied. Encouraging patients to play an active role in decisions regarding their healthcare can ensure better compliance to their treatment and management appropriately tailored to the individual.

6.1 How to evaluate the process of shared decision-making

SDM can be categorized and evaluated at its various stages, namely, before the decision (e.g. role preferences), during the decision-making process (e.g. observed or perceived physician behavior) or the outcome of decisions (e.g. conflict of decisions, satisfaction). The process may also be evaluated by an external observer, the patient, or the physician. Measuring SDM using observational tools is laborious, costly and not conductive to rapid data feedback.

The OPTION instrument ("Observing Patient Involvement in Decision Making") is an important tool for assessing the extent to which clinicians actively involve patients in decision-making [31]. Barr et al. [32] emphasize that this is the most frequently used instrument for measuring patient involvement from an observer's viewpoint. It has been developed to evaluate shared decision making specifically in the context of general practice, but it is intended to be generic enough for use in all types of consultations in clinical practice. The OPTION scale is designed to assess the overall shared decision-making process. In summary, it examines whether problems are well defined, whether options are formulated, information provided, patient understanding, and role preference evaluated, and decisions examined from both the professional and patient perspectives [33]. Recently it has, been revised in a shorter form, which evaluates the SDM process from its observer's viewpoint to just five OPTION-5 elements. Another way to measure and evaluate SMD is the CollaboRATE scale [34]. This is a fast and frugal a three-item patient-reported measure of SDM. It is applicable to a wide range of clinical settings, especially in the primary care setting where varied and unanticipated decisions are made [35, 36].

However, there are only two ways to evaluate the perceptions of both the patient and the doctor using the same process and these are (a) the dyadic OPTION [37] and the SDM-Q-9 [38, 13]; the latter is a 9-point decision-making evaluation questionnaire was developed on a case-by-case basis and measures the extent to which patients are involved in the decision-making process: from the view of the patient (SDM-Q-9) and from the physician's perspective (SDM-Q-Doc). These two tools have been developed for use, both, in research and every-day clinical practice. Both versions can be applied equally for purposes of assessing and improving quality in healthcare.

7. Conclusion

SDM enables the voice of the patient to be heard and considered that his views are significant even at various different stages of the condition. Through this, the patient becomes more autonomous with an active role in his management. By participating in this two-way relationship, the healthcare professionals may interact better with the patient in different situations, with different levels of involvement. By recognizing the importance of patient's involvement process, the healthcare professional confirms that the patient is an important role-player in the process, ie that he is autonomous and equal, transferring the respect and dignity necessary for the balance between power and responsibility. When a healthcare professional encourages their patient's involvement and recognizes the importance of the patient's involvement process, then they are more likely to engage them positively in their own care. Creating a culture of trust is essential to enable the therapeutic environment as a whole to balance the power and responsibility for creating safe care. SDM is considered both, as a philosophy and a process that leads to better-quality care, ensuring that patients receive the 'care they need and no less, and the care they want and no more'. It is believed that many clinicians are already informally engaging patients in SDM without formally recognizing the name or details of the process.

However, more research and evidence are required to ensure that SDM is being routinely used in either primary care or hospital consultations, despite the fact that healthcare professionals believe they are engaging patients in their treatment decisions. Research suggests that SDM does influence the way patients consider treatment decisions and may have a positive impact on outcomes, as it improves compliance and adherence. It is imperative to involve patients as equal partners in healthcare, as part of healthcare professionals' legal and ethical obligation.

Acknowledgements

We would like to help Mr. Sozomenos Hadjivassiliou for his contribution and editing in this work.

Conflict of interest

The authors declare no conflict of interest.

Author details

George Athanasiou[1] and Chris Bachtsetzis[2]*

1 Medical Center, University of Nicosia Medical School, Nicosia, Cyprus

2 University of Nicosia Medical School, Nicosia, Cyprus

*Address all correspondence to: csbachtsetzis@gmail.com

References

[1] General Medical Council. Good Medical Practice. London: General Medical Council; 2006.

[2] Kaba R. and Sooriakumaran P. The evolution of the doctor-patient relationship. International Journal of Surgery. 2007. Elsevier Volume 5. Pages 57-65.

[3] Edelstein L. A history of medicine. Arch Int Med. 1937. 5:201.

[4] Szasz T. and Hollender M. A contribution to the philosophy of medicine: the basic model of the doctor-patient relationship. Arch Int Med 1956. 97:585e92.

[5] Balint M. The doctor, his patient and the illness. London: Pittman Medical. 1964.

[6] Balint E, Courtenay M, Elder A, Hull S, Julian P. The doctor, the patient and the group Balint revisited. London: Rout- ledge; 1993.

[7] Mead N. and Bower P. Patient-centeredness: a conceptual framework and review of the empirical literature. Soc Sci Med. 2000. 51:1087e1.

[8] Balint E. The possibilities of patient centered medicine. J R Coll Gen Pract. 1969. 17:269e76.

[9] Coulter A. and Collins A. Making shared decision-making a reality. No decision about me, without me. London: King's Fund. 2011

[10] Say R, Murtagh M, Thomson R. Patients' preference for involvement in medical decision making: A nar- rative review. Patient Educ Couns. 2006; 60(2): 102-114. https://doi.org/10.1016/j.pec.2005.02.003 PMID: 16442453

[11] Charles C, Gafni A, Whelan T. Shared decision-making in the medical encounter: What does it mean? (or it takes at least two to tango). Soc Sci Med. 1997. 44(5): 681-692. PMID: 9032835.

[12] Rockenbauch K. and Schildmann J. Shared decision making (SDM): A systematic survey of terminology use and concepts. Gesundheitswesen. 2011. 73(7): 399-408. https://doi.org/10.1055/s-0030-1262870 PMID: 20859849

[13] Doherr H, Christalle E, Kriston L, Harter M, Scholl I, Use of the 9-item Shared Decision-Making Questionnaire (SDM-Q-9 and SDM-Q-Doc) in intervention studies—A systematic review PLoS One. 2017. Mar 30;12(3):e0173904. doi: 10.1371/journal.pone.0173904. eCollection 2017.

[14] Chewning B, Bylund CL, Shah B, Arora NK, Gueguen JA, Makoul G. Patient preferences for shared decisions: A systematic review. Patient Educ Couns. 2012. 86(1): 9-18. https://doi.org/10.1016/j.pec. 2011.02.004 PMID: 21474265

[15] Elwyn G, Coulter A, Laitner S, Walker E, Watson P, Thomson R. Implementing shared decision making in the NHS. BMJ. 2010. 341: c5146.

[16] Makoul G. and Clayman ML. An integrative model of shared decision making in medical encounters. Patient Educ Couns. 2006. 60: 301-312.

[17] Lee EO. and Emanuel EJ. Shared decision making to improve care and reduce costs. N Engl J Med. 2013. 368: 6-8.

[18] Legare F, Ratte S, Gravel K, Graham ID. Barriers and facilitators to implementing shared decision-making in clinical practice: update of a systematic review of health professionals' perceptions. Patient Educ Couns. 2008. 73(3):526-35.

[19] Ryan F. and Cunningham S. Shared Decision Making in Healthcare. Faculty Dental Journal. 2014. Volume 5. Issue 3

[20] Department of Health. Equity and Excellence: Liberating the NHS. London: Department of Health. 2010. Available at: https://assets.publishing.service.gov.uk/government/uploads/system/uploads/attachment_data/file/213823/dh_117794.pdf

[21] Department of Health. Health and Social Care Act. London: Department of Health. 2012. Available at: https://www.legislation.gov.uk/ukpga/2012/7/contents/enacted

[22] The NHS Mandate. Available at: https://www.england.nhs.uk/

[23] WHO Europe. Transforming health services delivery towards people centered health systems, 2014. Available at: http://www.euro.who.int/data/assets/pdffile/0016/260710/Transforming-health-services-delivery-towards-people-centred-health-systems.pdf.

[24] Levenstein J. The patient-centred general practice consultation. S Afr Fam Pract. 1984. 5:276-82.

[25] Elwyn G. and Fisher E. Higher integrity health care: Evidence-based shared decision making. Circulation: Cardiovascular Quality and Outcomes. 2014. 7(6), 975-980.

[26] Rise M.B., Westerlund H., Bjorgen D., Steinsbekk, A. Safely cared for or empowered in mental health care? Yes, please. International Journal of Social Psychiatry. 2014. 60(2), 134-138.

[27] Grol R. Wensing M. Mainz J. Jung HP. Ferreira P. Hearnshaw H. Hjortdahl P. Olesen F. Reis S. Ribacke M. Szecsenyi J. and European Task Force on Patient Evaluations of General Practice Care (EUROPEP) Patients in Europe evaluate general practice care: an international comparison. British Journal of General Practice. 2000. 50:882– 887.

[28] Bastiaens H. Van Royen P. Pavlic DR. Raposo V. Baker R. Older people's preferences for involvement in their own care: a qualitative study in primary health care in 11 European countries. Patient Education and Counseling. 2007. 68(1):33-42

[29] Coulter A. and Magee H. The European patient of the future. Maidenhead, Open University Press. 2003.

[30] Stevenson FA. Cox K. Britten N. Dundar Y. A systematic review of the research on communication between patients and health care professionals about medicines: the consequences for concordance. Health Expectations. 2004. 7(3):235-245.

[31] Nicolai J. Moshagen M. Eich W. Bieber C. The OPTION scale for the assessment of shared decision making (SDM): methodological issues. Z Evid Fortbild Qual Gesundhwes. 2012. 106(4): 264-271. https://doi.org/10.1016/j.zefq.2012.03.002 PMID: 22749073

[32] Barr PJ. O'Malley AJ. Tsulukidze M. Gionfriddo MR. Montori V. Elwyn G. The psychometric properties of Observer OPTION(5), an observer measure of shared decision making. Patient Educ Couns. 2015. 98(8): 970-976. https://doi.org/10.1016/j.pec.2015.04.010 PMID: 25956069

[33] Lupton D. Medicine as Culture. Illness, Disease and the Body in Western Societies. Sage: London. 2003

[34] Barr PJ. Thompson R. Walsh T. Grande SW. Ozanne EM. Elwyn G. The psychometric properties of CollaboRATE: a fast and frugal patient-reported measure of the shared decision-making process. J Med Internet

Res. 2014; 16(1): e2. https://doi.org/10.2196/jmir.3085 PMID: 24389354

[35] Elwyn G. Edwards A. Wensing M. Hood K. Atwell Ch. Grol R. Shared decision making: developing the OPTION scale for measuring patient involvement, Quality and Safety in Health Care. 2003. 12: 93-99].

[36] Branda ME. LeBlanc A. Shah ND. Tiedje K. Ruud K. Van Houten H. Pencille L. Kurland M. Yawn B. Montori VM. Shared decision making for patients with type 2 diabetes: a randomized trial in primary care. BMC Health Serv Res. 2013. 13:301.

[37] Melbourne E. Roberts S. Durand MA. Newcombe R. Legare F. Elwyn G. Dyadic OPTION: Measuring perceptions of shared decision-making in practice. Patient Educ Couns. 2011. 83(1): 55-57. https://doi. org/10.1016/j.pec.2010.04.019 PMID: 20537837

[38] Kriston L. Scholl I. Holzel L. Simon D. Loh A. Harter M. The 9-item Shared Decision-Making Questionnaire (SDM-Q-9). Development and psychometric properties in a primary care sample. Patient Educ Couns. 2010. 80(1): 94-99. https://doi.org/10.1016/j.pec.2009.09.034 PMID: 19879711

Chapter 5

Coverage: Measure of Achieving Universal Health Coverage in Nigeria

Habibu Salisu Badamasi

Abstract

This chapter aims to show that extending social health insurance is a possible road to universal health coverage in Nigeria. We suggest that allowing states to set up and operate their own insurance schemes, which presents a unique opportunity to swiftly scale up prepaid coverage for Nigerians. This paper review various healthcare insurance towards achieving universal health coverage in Nigeria. The paper concluded by suggesting other insurance scheme to be covered towards achieving universal coverage.

Keywords: universal health coverage, Coverage, healthcare insurance, health access, and Nigeria

1. Introduction

"Health is the most fundamental human right on which all other rights can be enjoyed. Universal Health Coverage is its guarantee." Dr. Githinji Gitahi [1].

One of the most normal measures of healthcare access is whether an individual has healthcare coverage insurance_ percentage of the population with and without health insurance either by public or private [2]. Health insurance promotes good health by improving access to healthcare. Sufficient access to healthcare encourages individuals to seek health maintenance services more regularly than they otherwise would, thereby prevent potentially serious illnesses. Also, health insurance protects individuals from financial catastrophe that may result from large or unexpected medical bills [3]. In Nigeria, health insurance can be obtained from private organizations or from government agencies [3]. Agencies of the Federal Ministry of Health (FMOH) regulate the National Health Insurance Scheme (NHIS). The NHIS provides health insurance coverage for employees of the federal government. While some state government have adopted social insurance regulated by NHIS because they feel excluded from the scheme [4]. However, only 3% of men and women age 15–49 have health insurance coverage [3]. To achieve universal health coverage expansions have to be made to include other health insurance schemes [4].

2. Structure of Nigeria health system

Nigeria is a lower-middle-income country with a population of 174 million with 36 states, a federal capital territory and a total of 774 local government areas

Health facilities	Tier of government
Tertiary	Federal
secondary	State
Primary	Governmental and non-governmental agencies

Table 1.
An illustration of various healthcare facilities regulate by tiers of government in Nigeria.

(LGAs) across the country. The healthcare system in Nigeria is mainly regulated by public sector, and partly private sector involvement in the provision of health services. There are more than 34,000 health facilities, 66% of which were owned by the three tiers of government (federal, state, and LGAs). The secondary and tertiary level health facilities are mostly found in urban areas, whereas rural areas are predominantly served by primary health care (PHC) facilities. The federal government owns many of the tertiary level health facilities and some secondary health facilities operated by federal agencies. Most of the publicly-owned secondary health facilities are owned by the states. Primary health care is largely led by government departments and agencies, but also by non-governmental organizations. **Table 1** illustrates various health facilities regulate by tiers of government in Nigeria.

3. Health insurance coverage- pathway of achieving universal health coverage

Universal health coverage has being achieved in most countries through some of initiation by their government health financing reforms. These were achieved in many countries by adopting social health insurance scheme [4].

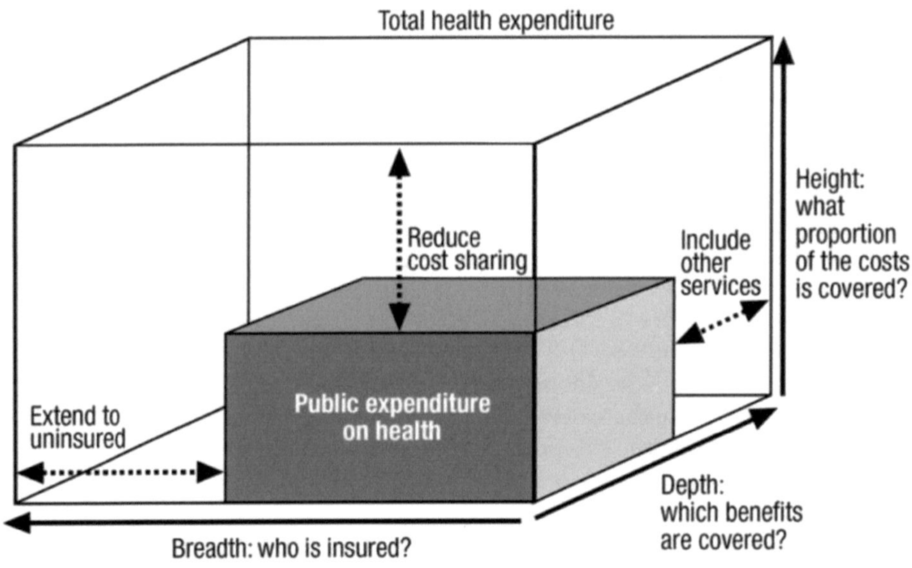

Figure 1.
Three-dimensions to consider when moving towards universal coverage WHO 2010.

The World Health Report 2010 presents a cube in **Figure 1** above to help policy makers think about the potential trade-offs in benefit design for UHC with the following three dimensions:

- Who benefits from pooled resource?
- For what services?
- At what cost at the post of use?

For effective coverage, the depth axis on which benefit are covered (service coverage) must be defined in terms of needed and effective services of good quality. The height axis on cost should reflect relative ability pay in order to assess affordability of care. The breadth axis who is insured, ensure that the needs of the poorest and most vulnerable are effectively covered first and at affordable cost.

4. Scope of health insurance coverage

Health insurance can take the form of private, social, community-based, or tax-based systems [4].

4.1 Tax-based systems

A tax-based system is a State's tax-funded system, in which the State Ministry of Health (SMoH) purchases and provides public health services for the whole state population. The SMoH specifies a minimum package of healthcare services which covers promotive, preventive, and curative care at primary and secondary care levels, and includes services for communicable and non-communicable diseases, child survival, safe motherhood, nutrition, health education, laboratory services and community mobilization, but in some states it's not compulsory. Additionally, SMoH may include other private providers to deliver selected services, such as mortuary and immunization services. However, services that are not on the SMoH's package of services are mostly paid out-of-pocket with user fee required at the point of service utilization. General tax revenue, which the State Government gives to SMoH as part of the State Budget, is the primary source of funding for health services. In service delivery, all government-owned primary and secondary providers are involved. SMoH transfers resources to Primary Health Centers (PHCs) for vertical programs, despite the fact that primary health care is the responsibility of the Local Government Area (LGA) [5].

4.2 Social Health insurance programme

4.2.1 The formal sector health insurance programme (FSSHIP)

4.2.1.1 The Health insurance program for the formal sector (FSSHIP)

The Nigerian National Health Insurance Scheme established the FSSHIP as a Social Health Insurance program (NHIS). Employees in the formal sector are required to participate in FSSHIP. In 2012, about 3% of Nigeria's population was covered. Beneficiary contributions to the plan are calculated as a percentage of earnings and are accompanied by contributions from employer. Through

Formal Sector	Informal Sector	Vulnerable Group
Formal Sector Social Health Insurance Programme	Tertiary Institution Social Health Insurance Programmes	Pregnant Women
Mobile Health	Community Based Social Health Insurance Programmes	Children Under five
Vital Contributors Social Health Insurance Programmes	Public Private Partnership Social Health Insurance Programmes	Prison Inmates
		Retirees
		Aged

Table 2.
Illustration of various NHIS scheme that covered different segment.

the National Health Insurance Fund, the NHIS pools monies at the federal level (NHIF). The National Health Insurance Program (NHIS) hires commercial, for-profit Health Maintenance Organizations (HMOs) to run the purchasing system and distribute funds to providers. Healthcare professionals are paid on a capitation basis for primary care and on a fee-for-service basis for secondary care. A blend of NHIS-accredited public and private healthcare providers are contracted to deliver services under the FSSHIP. High-tech investigations (CT scans, MRIs, etc.) and occupational disorders are excluded from FSSHIP's regular benefit package, which defines primary, secondary, and tertiary treatments. Members of the FSSHIP are assigned to specific HMOs, however they can choose their primary care providers from a list of NHIS-accredited providers [5].

4.2.1.2 National Health Insurance Scheme (NHIS)-MDG-MCH

The MDG-MCH program of the National Health Insurance Scheme (NHIS) was created to address the demand-side problem of financial obstacles to acceptance of prioritized MCH interventions. Its implementation mechanisms, on the other hand, include requiring facilities to use program income to purchase medications, which will improve the provision of PHC services. The Midwives Service Scheme program helps to address the shortage of midwives in frontline PHC facilities, and the Model Primary Health Centers Creation and Upgrading (MPHC) program assists in increasing the number of functional facilities and improving the state of some of those in dilapidated conditions [6].

National Health Insurance Scheme has developed various programmes to cover different segments of the society, In order to ensure that every Nigerian has access to good healthcare services [7], as show in **Table 2**.

5. Conclusion

To fairly include more individuals In line with the goal of UHC, NHIS scheme should prioritize expanding coverage for low-income groups, rural communities, and other groups with limited access to services, health, or both. This is especially critical for services with a high priority. More individuals being fairly included may necessitate specific measures when they are beneficial.

Author details

Habibu Salisu Badamasi
Department of Community Medicine, Bayero University, Kano, Nigeria

*Address all correspondence to: tjhabibulah@yahoo.com

References

[1] Dr. Githinji Gitahi, UHC Day 2018 Global CEO, Amref Health Africa Co-chair, UHC 2030 Steering Committee.

[2] Berk ML, Schur CL. Measuring Access To Care: Improving Information For Policymakers: Even the most thoughtful persons find it difficult to disentangle the research on access. Health Affairs. 1998 Jan;17(1): 180-186.

[3] Demographic N. Health Survey 2013. National Population Commission (NPC)[Nigeria] and ICF International. Abuja, Nigeria, and Rockville, Maryland, USA: NPC and ICF International.

[4] Okpani AI, Abimbola S. Operationalizing universal health coverage in Nigeria through social health insurance. Nigerian medical journal: journal of the Nigeria Medical Association. 2015 Sep;56(5):305.

[5] Ibe O, Honda A, Etiaba E, Ezumah N, Hanson K, Onwujekwe O. Do beneficiaries' views matter in healthcare purchasing decisions? Experiences from the Nigerian tax-funded health system and the formal sector social health insurance program of the National Health Insurance Scheme. International journal for equity in health. 2017 Dec;16(1):1-1.

[6] Atim C, Bhatnagar A. Toward synergy and collaboration to expand the supply of and strengthen Primary Health Care in Nigeria's federal context, with special reference to Ondo State.

[7] Nigeria. Federal minister of Health, National Health insurance scheme [internet]. Formal social Health Insurance Programme (FSSHIP); 2020 (cited 2021 jul 15). Available from https://www.nhis.gov.ng/downloadable-documents/

Chapter 6

Factors Influencing Access to Reliable Healthcare Financing among Elderly Population in Africa

Isaac Akintoyese Oyekola, Oludele Albert Ajani and Eyitayo Joseph Oyeyipo

Abstract

Population is ageing rapidly in all regions of the world and unreliable healthcare financing is capable of hindering older people from seeking competent medical attention which in turn may lead to their suffering, insecurity and/or death. In Africa, lack of access to reliable healthcare financing in old age poses serious development challenges and it is detrimental to healthy ageing, especially because elderly population are known to be facing various health challenges which require huge financial costs. Existing studies have shown that it is not sufficient to provide reliable healthcare financing for older people, it is more important to provide them access to these services. Ensuring that the elderly population has access to reliable healthcare financing in particular as well as other available and possible social support mechanisms that may encourage the provision of and access to reliable healthcare financing in general is a challenge and very key to healthy ageing. Through authors' experiences in the healthcare system, narrative review of existing literature and interactions with some elderly people, this article explores various factors influencing older people's access to reliable healthcare financing. It is believed that understanding of factors influencing access to reliable healthcare financing among older people in Africa will go a long way in directing policies toward the right course.

Keywords: Access to reliable healthcare financing, elderly population in Africa, universal health coverage, healthy ageing, development studies, reduced inequalities, Sociology

1. Introduction

The whole world is ageing. Ageing population has become the experience of many developed countries and is fast reaching the turn of countries in the developing world [1]. People who were 65 years and above in age represented 5.1 per cent of global population in 1950, 9.0 per cent in 2018, and will be 16.0 per cent in 2050 [1, 2]. By that year 2050, 80 per cent of older people (60+ years) globally will be living in low and middle income countries (LMIC) [3]. It is important to note that while this demographic shift is a sign of societal progress which calls for celebration especially for LMIC, it may also pose serious health, security and development challenges if provision of and access to innovative and reliable healthcare financing mechanisms and strategies are not in view. This is because lack of access to reliable healthcare financing is capable of hindering older people from seeking competent medical attention to address their inevitable healthcare needs and challenges, and this in turn may lead to their suffering, insecurity and/or death [4].

In Africa, lack of access to reliable healthcare financing in old age poses serious development challenges and it is detrimental to healthy ageing, especially because older people are known to be facing various health challenges which require huge financial costs. According to World Health Organisation (2010), reliable healthcare financing mechanism is an important factor for healthy ageing [5]. Considering the financial and health vulnerability of many older people especially in developing countries of the world, provision of and access to reliable healthcare financing for this demographic category becomes vitally important and inevitable for healthy ageing [6]. It has been shown that it is not sufficient to provide reliable healthcare financing for older people, it is more important to provide them access to these services [7, 8]. Ensuring that older people have access to reliable healthcare financing in particular as well as other available and possible social support mechanisms that may encourage the provision of and access to reliable healthcare financing in general is a challenge and very key to healthy ageing. What are the factors influencing older people's access to reliable healthcare financing? To answer this question, this article starts by conceptualising key concepts, explains the need for access to reliable healthcare financing among African elderly, provides statistical overview of access to reliable healthcare, and discusses various factors influencing access to reliable healthcare financing. Strategies for providing and accessing reliable healthcare financing are also discussed before providing summary and conclusion.

2. Conceptualising access to reliable healthcare financing: a multi-disciplinary approach

Access to reliable healthcare financing is conceptualised from multi-disciplinary points of view. Generally, ability to have what it takes to finance healthcare services without any constraining factor(s) whatsoever is fundamental in conceptualising access to healthcare financing. Following from this, access to reliable healthcare financing can mean ability to finance healthcare services without financial hardship. To be able to finance healthcare services without resulting in catastrophic or impoverished spending requires that psychological, economic, geographical, political, social, and cultural factors be put into consideration. Psychological point of view describes access to reliable healthcare financing as when an individual or her financial provider is in her right state of mind to finance healthcare services without resulting in catastrophic or impoverished spending [9]. Although financial resources may be physically available to finance healthcare services, it is believed that such resources are not useful if an individual or her representative is not in right state of thinking. From this perspective, a baby or an insane person does not have access to reliable healthcare financing even if she has all the wealth in this world. Hence, older people or their social support providers are considered to have access to reliable healthcare financing when they are in their right state of mind.

From economic perspective, access to reliable healthcare financing is conceptualised as the need for healthcare financing without financial hardship and the availability of such healthcare financing mechanism to meet the need. While the former explains the demand for reliable healthcare financing, the later describes the supply of reliable healthcare financing [10]. Hence, from economic perspective, an older person is said to gain access to reliable healthcare financing when the need for it meets its supply; that is, when there are available scarce resources (especially financial resources) to meet the insatiable need for healthcare services in old age. Again, while it is possible for adequate resources to be available to meet the need for healthcare financing at a given point in time, distance between health seeker and healthcare provider may be an important constraint. This calls for geographical conceptualization of access to reliable healthcare financing.

From geographer's standpoint of view, access to reliable healthcare financing implies ability of healthcare seeker to be physically present at the geography (or location, place, *et cetera*) where healthcare financing services are required and provided [11]. Although an older person may be psychologically fit to finance healthcare services and may eventually have the financial resources (possibly in bank or at the health insurance provider) to meet her healthcare needs and challenges, she still lacks access to reliable healthcare financing if she is unable to physically collect such financial resources from appropriate quarters to finance her healthcare services probably due to physical frailty, lack of mobility or road block.

Political conceptualisation of access to reliable healthcare financing explains the governmental policies and political structures that influence people's access to financial health resources. In every government, there are various healthcare financing mechanisms or models through which healthcare services can be financed [12]. The proportion of these models in total healthcare spending is determined by the political climate of every country. For instance, the proportion of out-of-pocket (OOP) payment in total healthcare expenditure is higher in developing countries than in developed countries [12]. Also, while healthcare providers receive payment for healthcare services more via health insurance in developed countries, the healthcare providers receive payment for healthcare services more via OOP in developing countries [13]. Hence, an older person who has psychological, economic, and geographical ability/advantage to finance her healthcare services may be denied access if such a person is expected to pay via health insurance of which she is not enrolled. Alternatively, an individual who is enrolled for health insurance may be denied access to reliable healthcare financing if payment from health insurance provider is not available probably as a result of workers' strike due to government inability to meet insurance workers' demands.

From social and cultural point of views, access to reliable healthcare financing can be conceived as involving the relationship between agency and structure. Here, agency represents individual ability to finance healthcare services freely and independently with as limited structural constraints as possible. On the other hand, structure entails the broader social, cultural, and structural patterns, arrangement and organisations within which an individual seeks to finance her healthcare services [10]. From these perspectives, an older person with the ability to finance her healthcare services without resulting in catastrophic or impoverished spending can be constrained if the prevailing healthcare system is challenged such as lack of appropriate medical technology or personnel, among many other challenges that may face healthcare system. Sociologists and Anthropologists have debated on whether primacy should be given to agency or structure in the process of analysing a given social system. For examples, Karl Marx, Émile Durkheim, Bronisław Malinowski, Alfred Radcliffe-Brown, and Max Weber gave priorities to either agency or structure in their social analysis. However, recent sociologists such as Anthony Giddens and Pierre Bourdieu have recognised the vitally importance of both agency and structure in altering a given social system. In his notion of structuration, Giddens (1984) stated that just as an agent can alter prevailing structure, the structure can as well change an agent [14]. Also Bourdieu realised the importance of both agency and structure when he used the concepts of 'habitus', 'field', and 'capital' to denotes actors with structured and structuring structure, social space where interaction and activities occur, as well as a symbol for the continual remarking of social order respectively [15]. In other words, Pierre Bourdieu used the concepts to explain an interplay in which the external is internalised, just as the internal becomes externalised [10]. Learning from the works of Giddens and Bourdieu, access to reliable healthcare financing is conceptualised as depending not only on individual, household and/or agency, but also on broader social, cultural and/or structural factors of a given social system. Implicitly, access to reliable healthcare financing not only involves internal forces but also external ones [10].

Older people's access to reliable and sustainable healthcare financing requires that sufficient, uninterrupted and continuing funds are available to meet older people's healthcare needs without compromising or negotiating future generations' ability to achieve same purpose. An important step to achieving reliable healthcare financing for the elderly is to ensure that adequate and satisfactory social support is provided, the elderly have free access to funds or financial resources provided by social support system, and that funding increases consistently over the coming years to meet up with the demand of demographic transition. Raising and accessing reliable fund for healthcare financing of the elderly is the responsibility of household, community, state, and non-state actors of every country. Providing access to reliable healthcare financing is crucial for any country that aims at addressing the inevitable healthcare needs and challenges of the elderly.

3. Need for access to reliable healthcare financing in old age

Everyone desires to reach old age. Old age is the age when many life threatening diseases come up and these health challenges are costly to treat or manage. However, current financial capability of average elderly person in Africa as indicated in the income distribution of African countries shows that many Africans will not be able to afford medical treatment in old age [16, 17]. How can the elderly age gracefully? It is through the provision of and access to reliable (and sustainable) healthcare financing. There is therefore dire and urgent need for the elderly to access reliable healthcare financing in order to save the generation of elderly population in Africa. Older people experience a diversity of health states. While some elderly people in Africa are in relatively good physical and mental health, many more others experience considerable disability, and health and care challenges. Existing studies have established that the health of older people determines their productivity and the roles they play in the society, and that the health status and challenges among the elderly varies between and within countries, across sex, residence, ethnicity, and socio-economic status [18]. As a result, while health across the life-course has a significant impact on ageing experience, many older people are unable to adapt to changes in their health and remain independent and productive into very old age.

Common health challenges among older people include arthritis; heart or cardiovascular disease; cancer or malignancy such as lung, liver, and breast cancers; respiratory diseases; Alzheimer's disease; osteoporosis; and diabetes mellitus, among many others [19]. Hence, the need to access reliable healthcare financing for sustainable healthcare, management and/or cure. Aside common health challenges, the needs of older people vary and are often categorised into physical, intellectual, emotional and social needs [20]. Some of these healthcare needs and challenges require reliable healthcare financing and access to them is crucial for healthy ageing. However, access to reliable healthcare financing are not equitably distributed among elderly population in Africa. While third agers (healthy older people after retirement and are assumed to be productive through a range of activities, reaching from paid work to volunteering, informal care-giving, do-it-yourself and care for oneself) tend to have more access to reliable healthcare financing, fourth agers (older people who are unproductive as a result of poor health after their retirement and they represent the traditional stereotype of older people, who can contribute only little, if any, to the development of a state) seem to have less access to reliable healthcare financing.

4. Access to reliable healthcare financing statistics

Globally, universal access to reliable healthcare financing has not been achieved and the proportion of people who have access to reliable healthcare financing vary from one country to another. Also, the varied rate of access across countries were unequally distributed and disadvantaged or vulnerable people were most denied access, including older people [17, 21]. For example, a study conducted among people aged 50+ years with chronic illness in six middle-income countries showed that access rates were unevenly distributed except in South Africa where primary healthcare was free for all [17]. Specifically, the study demonstrated that the proportion of older people with access to basic chronic care ranged from 20.6 per cent in Mexico to 47.6 per cent in South Africa. In another study among formal sector workers in Ilorin, Nigeria, it was shown that only 13.5 per cent of the respondents had access to reliable healthcare financing [21]. This proportion excluded the elderly population because they were no more members of the federal civil servants considering their retirement status and hence, lacked access to reliable healthcare financing. Ensuring that elderly population are provided with and have access to reliable healthcare financing is therefore crucial especially as the African society experiences demographic change in favour of older people.

Existing studies have not shown consensus on the factors determining access to reliable healthcare services among the elderly. While some agree that education, place of work, residence, income, age, number of general practitioners, sex, social network and social participation determine access to healthcare financing and services, some other scholars disagree to some of these factors. For examples, a study carried out in Ilorin, Nigeria established that respondents who had post-secondary education and who were in the federal civil service were more likely to have access to reliable healthcare financing [21]. This shows that illiterate older people might be denied access to reliable healthcare financing even if exempted from health insurance premium and the elderly who are not in federal civil service might not have the opportunity of being enrolled in health insurance scheme, which provides reliable healthcare financing. Another study conducted among the older Chinese indicated that income group, educational attainment, age-category, marital status, gender, and geographical location influence access to reliable healthcare financing [7]. Inability to access reliable healthcare financing is detrimental to population health and especially to vulnerable older people. Recent statistics in Nigeria showed that only very small proportion of the total population in Nigeria had access to reliable healthcare financing [22]. This is worrisome as it indicates high health inequality. Since pooled resources is the only reliable and sustainable source of healthcare financing [12], provision of, and access to, pooled resources becomes vitally imperative. It is important to note that differential in access to reliable healthcare financing and other social resources is influenced by many factors [23], and these are discussed in next section.

5. Factors influencing access to reliable healthcare financing in old age

Having conceptualised access to reliable healthcare financing, demonstrated the need for access to reliable healthcare financing and shown the statistics of access to reliable healthcare financing, this section discusses various factors influencing access to reliable healthcare financing in old age. The discussions in this section are based on authors' experiences in the healthcare system, narrative review of existing literature and interactions with some elderly people. Specifically, the factors that influence access to reliable healthcare financing in old age, as discussed in this section and depicted in **Figure 1**, include age, sex, availability of health insurance, income level, educational attainment, social capital and geographical factor.

5.1 Age

Age describes how long one has lived on earth. A person's age is considered a critical factor influencing access to reliable healthcare financing. While it is possible for many working class age category not to have any challenge accessing reliable healthcare financing, some retirees may experience more difficulty accessing reliable healthcare financing. This is because the rate of poverty among older people is more than among other age categories due to the fact that many older people are in their economically inactive phase of life [24]. Since older people are less productive (especially the fourth agers), financial resources for healthcare financing tend to be affected. In addition, in some African countries, a person's age determines whether one will have social health protection or not. That is, provisions are made for older people in some African countries such as Ghana, Rwanda, and Senegal to be exempted from paying health insurance premium [25, 26]. This sort of arrangement increases older people's access to reliable healthcare financing. Age factor determining healthcare access was confirmed by a study in Ghana which discovered that enrolment for National Health Insurance Scheme exemption policy in Ghana was higher among the elderly which invariably increases access to healthcare among

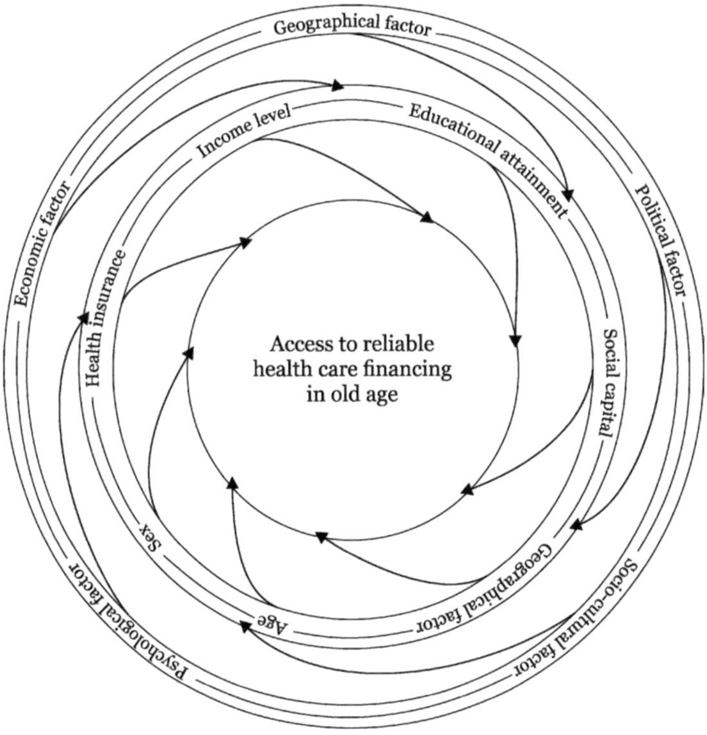

Figure 1.
Factors influencing access to reliable healthcare financing in old age.

older people [26]. Another study conducted among the middle-aged and older Chinese indicated that age-category of the elderly influences their chances of gaining access to reliable healthcare financing [7]. Therefore, as people aged, special consideration must be made in order to ensure that access to reliable healthcare financing is not denied.

5.2 Sex

Sex defines the biological variances between women and men, and these variances are universal and determined at birth. Access to reliable healthcare financing is also influenced by a person's biological composition especially in African setting where patriarchy system dominates. In Africa, men often demonstrate hegemony in virtually all spheres of life including economy, family and religion. By virtue of men's hegemonic position, they have more control over financial resources and this in turn affords them the opportunity to have more access to reliable healthcare financing. According to Mensah (2014), the long-standing patriarchy system on the continent of Africa influences access to healthcare and medicine in favour of males [10]. In addition, some scholars consider women to be in direr need for access to reliable healthcare financing than men considering their healthcare needs as pregnant women, new mothers and widows [7, 27].

5.3 Availability of health insurance

Health insurance refers to a body that provides reliable healthcare financing for enrollees and it aims at ensuring equal access to quality healthcare services without financial hardship. The contribution of (social) health insurance in providing reliable healthcare financing cannot be overemphasised. This is because health insurance performs various benefits that help countries of the world to have access to reliable healthcare financing, and invariably move closer to achieving universal health coverage [12]. Generally, there seem to be consensus among global researchers that health insurance increases access to reliable healthcare financing [7, 16, 17]. Hence, enrolment in health insurance influences older people's access to reliable healthcare financing. Importantly, older people who are excluded from health insurance (as the case is in many African countries) are denied access to reliable healthcare financing. Policies that will ensure that older people are enrolled in health insurance are therefore germane in order to safeguard the healthcare of the elderly and to ensure that their access to reliable healthcare financing are enhanced.

5.4 Income level

This is an important economic factor that influences access to reliable healthcare financing. Income level measures the amount or quantity of money or financial resources that an individual receives over a period of time. Individual income level varies and many factors determine a person's income level [16]. When the income level of an individual is high, such an individual has more access to reliable healthcare financing. That is, there is a direct relationship between income level and access to reliable healthcare financing. In Africa, the income level of many older people is low due to many factors resulting in low access to reliable healthcare financing. To help this demographic category of people, engagement in productive activities for those who are still healthy after retirement, compulsory enrolment in health insurance with exemption of premium payment, and strong social support, among many others, may be the alternative means to increase older people's access to reliable healthcare financing. These alternatives become vitally important because some recent studies confirmed that poverty level or lower income group reduces access to reliable healthcare financing and healthcare utilisation [7, 10].

5.5 Educational attainment

An individual's level of education is another factor that influences reliable healthcare financing. Operations of modern healthcare system requires that one has certain level of formal education such as ability to communicate officially. Those who lack knowledge of how modern healthcare system operate are sometimes deny access to reliable healthcare financing. For example, many people are excluded from social health insurance because awareness level is low or because they lack the knowledge of how it operates. Those affected are mostly those with low educational attainment. In Africa, most people in the informal sector, which more often correlate with those with lower educational attainment, do not have the privilege of being enrolled in health insurance or have the financial resources that can guarantee financial health protection in old age. According to Zhang et al., less-educated older people have a lower chance of accessing reliable healthcare financing [7]. Hence, elderly possible hope lies in strong social support via their social network in order to experience healthy ageing.

5.6 Social capital

Social capital refers to network of relationships between or among people in a social system who share common interest, norms, values, and/or identity and who continue to engage in social interaction for the effective functioning of the social system. While social capital depends largely on extent of one's social network, social network in turn depends on the level of effective and functional relationship one has established over one's lifetime [8]. Hence, access to reliable healthcare financing is influenced by the level of relationship one has established in the life course. Older people need social network for effective and efficient healthcare financing considering their health and financial vulnerability, as well as their inability to engage in full productive activity. This is especially true for majority of older people in African who retired mostly from informal sector and who depend mostly on social capital such as children for their healthcare financing. Every potential older person is therefore encouraged to start building strong social networks in the life course as that can represent a safety net in old age [28]. Social support from social network can be informational, instrumental, emotional, or interactional. In a study conducted in United State of American (USA), it was found that informational support has a positive impact on healthcare access disparity among older people [28]. Another study among the elderly in Taiwan demonstrated that social capital in terms of social participation and social network influences access to reliable healthcare financing which invariably determines access to healthcare services [8].

5.7 Geographical factor

As earlier conceptualised, access to reliable healthcare financing hinges largely on the ability of healthcare seeker to be physically available where healthcare financing services are required and provided. It is important to understand that many older people may have financial wherewithal but may be denied access as a result of their inability to be physically present where they will receive financial health resources or where their healthcare services will be paid for. Access to reliable healthcare financing is therefore influenced by geographical factor of where the health seeker is or where the healthcare services will be financed. In a case study of people living with HIV, 'Mdm. A' was denied access to healthcare financing and services as a result of prohibitive transportation costs [29]. Also, in a cross-sectional study in Sweden, it was found that mobility-related factor was associated with health-related quality of life in old age [11]. The issue of being physically present where healthcare financing is required and provided is crucial for many older people on the continent of Africa for them to experience healthy ageing because many of them rely on public transport that are either costly or unreliable. Also, many health seekers in Africa are very distant from where they will receive and finance their healthcare services because reliable healthcare facilities are often located in cities or urban areas and the ones in rural areas are only for the treatment of mild or minor ailment. Moving from rural areas to urban regions, for instance, poses difficulty for many older people in Africa due to transport mobility challenge [10]. Furthermore, intra-urban, intra-continental, and inter-continental disparities in access to reliable healthcare facilities and financing are usual in this present global society [10].

6. Strategies for providing and accessing reliable healthcare financing

Broadly, to provide and access reliable healthcare financing, three strategies are cogent: Efficient collection of revenue, reprioritisation of government budgets, and engagement of innovative healthcare financing strategies especially through social support [5]. Principally, there are four models of revenue collection and these include compulsory prepayments, voluntary prepayments, external aid and out-of-pocket payment (OOP) [12]. Since OOP is an inequitable, unreliable and unsustainable source of healthcare financing, to provide and access reliable healthcare financing for the elderly therefore requires that countries pay more attention to other revenue collection mechanisms and provide means of accessing these financial resources. While all countries of the world, both poor and rich, can raise more health funding or diversify their funding sources, the number of countries that have any chance of creating sustainable fund from domestic sources alone is very minimal especially in Africa [5]. Hence, the need for global solidarity in order to ensure that many African countries are not denied access to reliable healthcare financing. If countries and international agencies were to fulfil their international pledges, external aid in developing countries will greatly increase and the shortfall in fund to provide reliable healthcare financing especially for the elderly would be virtually eliminated [5].

Given priority to government budgets can also contribute greatly to the provision of and access to reliable healthcare financing. Government budgets in Africa often give health a somewhat low priority. For instance, very infinitesimal number of African countries could reach the target that was agreed to by their Heads of States in the 2001 Abuja Declaration, to spend 15 per cent of their annual budget on health. Currently, only Madagascar allots above the agreed 15 per cent (15.6 per cent) to health [12, 30]. Taken as a group, low- and middle-income countries (LMIC) could raise extra over US$ 15 billion/year for health from local sources by increasing the proportion of health expenditure in total government expenditure to 15 per cent [5]. Many developed countries who are near toward achieving universal health coverage allot considerable share of total government expenditure on health [30]. It is therefore incumbent upon many African countries to follow this path so as to aid the provision of and enhance access to reliable healthcare financing, although, in the long-run, relying solely on government budget to finance healthcare services may not be sustainable.

Generally, reliable healthcare financing can be provided through innovative sources of healthcare financing as well as innovative governance in managing health resources [31], and can be accessed by putting social, political, economic and cultural factors into consideration. Innovative sources of healthcare financing refers to committed funding sources for healthcare services, and these funds come from reserved taxes from health hazardous products such as alcohol, tobacco, sugary and salty foods; contributions from social health insurance or dedicated government budget allocation; taxes on air tickets; diaspora bonds (sold to expatriates); levy on foreign exchange transactions; solidarity levies on a range of products and services such as mobile phone calls; social support from social networks such as spouse, children, siblings, friends, association and community members, among many others [5, 31]. The potential to increase social support exists in many countries. If this is well examined and allocated to health, providing and accessing reliable healthcare financing would be greatly enhanced. On the other hand, innovative governance can be referred to as management of funds for healthcare services such that healthcare seekers have access to such funds [31]. These funds may be managed by a statutory body that is independent of government with its own governing body and represented by multi-stakeholders such as community health partnership [12]. Some countries such as Singapore and Hong Kong, among many others, follow this innovative governance and it is helpful in accessing reliable healthcare financing.

7. Summary and conclusion

This article has conceptualised key concepts from multi-disciplinary stance, explained the need for access to reliable healthcare financing, described access to reliable healthcare financing statistics, discussed various factors influencing reliable healthcare financing and put forward strategies for providing and accessing reliable healthcare financing. One vitally important policy goal in modern healthcare system is equity in access to reliable healthcare financing. Older people require healthcare services more frequently and intensely, but lack of access to reliable healthcare financing in Africa, especially among the vulnerable, poses a challenge. With increasing healthcare costs especially among elderly population in Africa, providing reliable healthcare financing and removing possible barriers to accessing it is crucial for healthy ageing.

Author details

Isaac Akintoyese Oyekola[1,2*], Oludele Albert Ajani[3] and Eyitayo Joseph Oyeyipo[1,2]

1 Department of Sociology, Landmark University, Omu-Aran, Nigeria

2 Landmark University SDG 10 (Reduced Inequalities), Landmark University, Nigeria

3 Department of Sociology and Anthropology, Obafemi Awolowo University, Ile-Ife, Nigeria

*Address all correspondence to: oyekola.isaac@lmu.edu.ng

References

[1] Population Reference Bureau. 2018 World Population Data Sheet with a special focus on changing age structures [Internet]. 2018. p. 1-19. Available from: www.worldpopdata.org

[2] United Nations. World population prospects: the 2015 revision, key findings and advance tables [Internet]. Technical Report, U.N. Department of Economic and Social Affairs, Population Division; 2015. Available from: http://esa.un.org/unpd/wpp/

[3] World Health Organization. Ageing and health [Internet]. 2018 [cited 2019 Dec 2]. Available from: https://www.who.int/news-room/fact-sheets/detail/ageing-and-health

[4] Wang X-Q, Chen P-J. Population ageing challenges health care in China. Lancet. 2014;383(9920):870.

[5] World Health Organization. The World Health Report: Health Systems Financing. Geneva, Switzerland: WHO Press; 2010.

[6] World Health Organization. Global strategy and action plan on ageing and health. Geneva: World Health Organization; 2017. 1-56 p.

[7] Zhang C, Lei X, Strauss J, Zhao Y. Health Insurance and Health Care among the Mid-Aged and Older Chinese: Evidence from the National Baseline Survey of CHARLS. Health Econ. 2017;26:431-449.

[8] Peng Y-I, Lin T-F. Social capital and preventive care use among the elderly under Taiwan's National Health Insurance. Arch Gerontol Geriatr [Internet]. 2018;75:28-36. Available from: http://www.sciencedirect.com/science/article/pii/S016749431730314X

[9] Gyasi RM. Social support, physical activity and psychological distress among community-dwelling older Ghanaians. Arch Gerontol Geriatr [Internet]. 2019;81:142-148. Available from: http://www.sciencedirect.com/science/article/pii/S0167494318302206

[10] Mensah J. The Global Financial Crisis and Access to Health Care in Africa. Afr Today. 2014;60(3):35-54.

[11] Chiatti C, Westerlund Y, Ståhl A. Access to public mobility services and health in old age: A cross-sectional study in three Swedish cities. J Transp Heal [Internet]. 2017;7:218-226. Available from: http://www.sciencedirect.com/science/article/pii/S2214140517300415

[12] Oyekola IA, Ojediran JO, Ajani OA, Oyeyipo EJ, Rasak B. Advancing alternative health care financing through effective community partnership: A necessity for universal health coverage in Nigeria. Cogent Soc Sci [Internet]. 2020;6(1):1776946. Available from: https://www.tandfonline.com/doi/full/10.1080/23311886.2020.1776946

[13] Kutzin J, Witter S, Jowett M, Bayarsaikhan D. Developing a national health financing strategy: A reference guide [Internet]. Health Fin. Switzerland: World Health Organization; 2017. Available from: https://creativecommons.org/licenses/by-nc-sa/ 3.0/igo

[14] Giddens A. The Constitution of Society: Outline of the Theory of Structuration. Berkeley: University of California press; 1984.

[15] Bourdieu P. Outline of a Theory of Practice. Cambridge: Cambridge University press; 1977.

[16] Mulenga A, Ataguba JE. Assessing income redistributive effect of health financing in Zambia. Soc Sci Med

[Internet]. 2017;189(2017):1-10. Available from: http://dx.doi.org/10.1016/j.socscimed.2017.07.017

[17] Goeppel C, Frenz P, Grabenhenrich L, Keil T, Tinnemann P. Assessment of universal health coverage for adults aged 50 years or older with chronic illness in six middle-income countries. Bull World Health Organ. 2016;94(4):276-285.

[18] Olatubi MI, Oyediran OO, Adubi IO, Ogidan OC. Health Care Expenditure in Nigeria and National Productivity: A Review. South Asian J Soc Stud Econ. 2018;1(1):1-7.

[19] World Life Expectancy. World health rankings: Live longer live better [Internet]. World Health Organization. 2019 [cited 2019 Apr 1]. Available from: https://www.worldlifeexpectancy.com/country-health-profile/nigeria

[20] Bruggencate T Ten, Luijkx KG, Sturm J. Social needs of older people: A systematic literature review. Ageing Soc. 2018;38(9):1745-1770.

[21] Adewole DA, Dairo MD, Bolarinwa OA. Awareness and Coverage of the National Health Insurance Scheme among Formal Sector Workers in Ilorin, Nigeria. African J Biomed Res. 2016;19(1):1-10.

[22] World Health Organization. Global Health Expenditure Database [Internet]. 2019 [cited 2019 Jan 30]. Available from: http://apps.who.int/nha/database/ViewData/Indicators/en

[23] Oyekola IA, Oyeyipo EJ. Social Stratification. In: Ogunbameru OA, editor. Introductory Sociology. Ile-Ife, Nigeria: Obafemi Awolowo University Press; 2020. p. 125-138.

[24] Ebimgbo SO, Atumah ON, Okoye UO. Social support, older adults and poverty: Implication for social policy in Nigeria. In: Conferance Paper. 2017.

[25] Parmar D, Williams G, Dkhimi F, Ndiaye A, Ankomah F, Kojo D, et al. Enrolment of older people in social health protection programs in West Africa - Does social exclusion play a part? Soc Sci Med [Internet]. 2014;119:36-44. Available from: http://dx.doi.org/10.1016/j.socscimed.2014.08.011

[26] Duku SKO, Van Dullemen CE, Fenenga C. Does Health Insurance Premium Exemption Policy for Older People Increase Access to Health Care ? Evidence from Ghana. J Aging Soc Policy. 2015;27:331-347.

[27] Laurenzi CA, Skeen S, Coetzee BJ, Gordon S, Notholi V, Tomlinson M. How do pregnant women and new mothers navigate and respond to challenges in accessing health care? Perspectives from rural South Africa. Soc Sci Med [Internet]. 2020 Jun;258:113100. Available from: https://doi.org/10.1016/j.socscimed.2020.113100

[28] Yamada T, Chen C, Murata C, Hirai H, Ojima T, Kondo K, et al. Access Disparity and Health Inequality of the Elderly : Unmet Needs and Delayed Healthcare. Int J Environ Res Public Health. 2015;12:1745-1772.

[29] Clarfield AM, Rosenthal A. Aging in Sub-Saharan Africa: Sub-par? J Am Geriatr Soc. 2017;65(6):1136-1138.

[30] World Health Organization. World Health Statistics 2018- Monitoring Health for the SDG's (Sustainable development goals) [Internet]. 2018. 4, 25 p. Available from: http://apps.who.int/iris/bitstream/handle/10665/272596/9789241565585-eng.pdf?ua=1

[31] Tangcharoensathien V, Sopitarchasak S, Viriyathorn S, Supaka N, Tisayaticom K,

Laptikultham S, et al. Innovative Financing for Health Promotion: A Global Review and Thailand Case Study [Internet]. Second. Vol. 4, International Encyclopedia of Public Health, Second Edition. Elsevier; 2017. 275-287 p. Available from: http://dx.doi.org/10.1016/B978-0-12-803678-5.00234-4

Chapter 7

Medical Hegemony and Healthcare: Centrality in Healthcare

Makoto Takayama

Abstract

Better human healthcare is achieved by increasing the fair use and accessibility of medical information. While this optimism is believed, real-world healthcare can be severely affected by the knowledge and context shared in the healthcare industry and academia. Through the sharing process, the central perception gains consensus in the industry and academic societies and standardized therapies are unified and spread quickly. In this way, mainstreamers' contexts quickly become standardized. Consequently, the mainstream has hegemony and can be strengthened. Mainstreamers neglect any information different from standardized knowledge and therapy. It is universally known that hegemony stabilize its position by undermining the fair use and accessibility of information. The use of patterned knowledge facilitates the utility of medical information. Smart ICT seems to realize the smart use of medical information in our daily lives as well as professional exercises. The method to eliminate such evils and realize true healthcare is required. The fair use and accessibility contribute to the utility of medical knowledge to end-users. The effect and influence of the commons of information are shown as a solution to eliminating adverse events caused by the hegemonic mainstream. As the most effective means in the coming digital healthcare era, this paper shows the following three points. (1) Allow commons of information to enable fair use and search of information. (2) The commons of information release the cognitive bias set by the measure. (3) By creating such a new theory, we will develop a new field called healthcare digital management and/or healthcare digital economics.

Keywords: healthcare, hegemony, centrality, commons of information, network, neutrality

1. Introduction

Achieving wellness and hence well-being is the goal of every human being. On the global scale this is articulated through the Millennium Development Goal and SDGs (Sustainable Development Goals) of the United Nations.

The science of medical and healthcare has transformed the healthcare profession by the extraordinary revolution in information technology. To utilize the true results of science, the use and accessibility of information among different healthcare professionals through network neutrality realize the true human healthcare, bringing the world together as a true global village.

2. Accessibility to medical and healthcare as public goods

It is believed that the better access by ICT will improve information barrier-free, grassroots information dissemination, and information sharing. Better human healthcare will be achieved by increasing the accessibility of healthcare information. While this optimism is believed, real-world healthcare has been severely affected by the shared information among the healthcare industries, professionals, and academia.

If information is not transmitted correctly without distorting the truth, life-threatening situations occur frequently. However, healthcare is usually neglected because it is only demanded when a person becomes unhealthy. Therefore, the supplier can behave to get the best benefit from diseases. What's worse is that the higher the need, the more urgent it is.

Due to the above circumstances, the healthcare provider is likely to take self-interest behavior. To curb such behavior, better access to information does not solve the problem. This is because the information is cleverly rewritten to suit the interest of mainstream in the healthcare industry without being noticed. In this chapter, I'll take a few such mysterious cases and explain why.

2.1 Inclusion of total healthcare by the mainstream in healthcare

According to the Merriam-Webster Dictionary, healthcare is efforts made to maintain or restore physical, mental, or emotional well-being especially by trained and licensed professionals. There are mainstreams and adjuncts among professionals. The mainstream is the most influential actor and is in a privileged position. To maintain privilege, it is common for mainstream people to try to establish a hegemonic position by involving their adjuncts.

In healthcare, medical care is at the center and all other healthcare areas are adjuncts. In medical care, treatment is at the center of the center, and prevention is one of adjuncts. Considering the pursuit of profits and strengthening of the position of medical care providers, it is better to increase the number of patients without prevention even if some patients must die. As a supporting evidence, in the pharmaceutical industry, it is an implicit understanding that the companies should not develop drugs that eliminate diseases, because the market will disappear like smallpox market by its vaccine. That is why RNA vaccine, which works faster and more effective than ordinary protein vaccines, did not take place until it was urgently approved as a corona vaccine. If RNA is used to produce stem cells, iPS cells (induced pluripotent stem cells), pluripotent stem cells, regenerative medicine for diseases including aging care and immunotherapy for the treatment of cancer will advance dramatically. Complete treatment of disease, organ regeneration, and immortal medicine have been hampered by mainstream groups to professionals. Mainstream has denied such a wonderful future as disease-free and immortal medical care.

The medical professionals should be humble about the dignity of life. When new facts are discovered, it is up to the mainstream to spread or not. The mainstream instantly includes new discoveries that can deny the mainstream. However, the mainstream attacks and denies the new discovery which can coexist with the mainstream. The reasons and causes for such absurd things to happen are for the benefit of the mainstream. Various inhumane obstacles occur, so the details are described below,

2.2 The difference in accessibility to medical care between Japan and the US

The openness of medical care is the exact opposite in Japan and the US. In Japan, not only paramedics but the nurses only can watch the patients die until the doctor arrives. Oppositely, in the US, medical practice is open to medical assistants and paramedics. They can take life-saving measures for emergency patients who are clearly likely to die if left untreated.

Why does such a difference between the two countries occur? In short, it depends on whether the market is free or regulated. The American way seeks efficiency through a free and open market. The Japanese government operates policies assuming that medical care is at the center and others are adjuncts. This is derived from the fundamental differences in public policies between the two countries.

The U.S. government and its local agency, the U.S. embassy, have repeatedly demanded the Japanese government to open and liberalize the medical and healthcare market, but with no success, while promoting the reasons for the free-open market. For American businesses to enter the Japanese market, it is essential to deregulate the Japanese market. The U.S., which had been the world's factory until Japan emerged, has attempted to take an initiative to the world's industry by securities financing. Therefore, the US government must protect the domestic market from foreign countries but ask free and open markets to foreign governments for maintaining a global hegemony. Such American diplomacy is well-known as a double standard. The importance of the role of government is strongly asserted by American economists. It is the American way to manage social welfare services such as medical care based on the principle of competition that works in an open market. Consequently, the gap about accessibility to medical care between Japan and the U. S. has been still expanding. **Table 1** shows the accessibilities to medical care by costs for treating appendectomy in major countries.

According to the Japan Medical Association, the US is the country with the widest medical disparity in the world. "Public medical insurance in the US is limited to "Medicare" for the elderly aged 65 and over and persons with disabilities, and "Medicaid" for low-income earners. The active generation, which is not covered by these two, is mainly covered by private medical insurance. The so-called "Obama Care" obliges people who do not have public medical insurance to join a private insurance company, but there are only a limited number of medical institutions available for medical examination. Many people are still uninsured in order not to be able to pay the insurance premium. There is a big disparity in the medical care provided" [1].

Rank	City	Expenses (US$)	Hospitalization Days
1	New York (US)	14,000-40,000$	1–3 days
2	Paris (France)	2,000-8,800	days
3	Madrid (Spain)	4,000-8,350	4 days
4	London (UK)	6,700	2 days
5	Rome (Italy)	6,300-6,650	3 days
6	Geneva (Switzerland)	2,530	3 days
7	Vancouver (Canada)	6,060	3 days
8	Singapore (Singapore)	3,180-3,970	3 days
9	Dusseldorf (Germany)	3,250	3 days
10	(General example) (Japan)	2,730	6–7 days

Cited from Tokio Marine & Nichido Fire Insurance Co., Ltd.
Source: Japan Medical Association Homepage: "World Medical Care and Safety 2010" [1].

Table 1.
Costs for treating appendectomy in major countries (accessibilities to medical care by costs).

In Japan, medicine and healthcare are recognized as public goods. The government has, therefore, an obligation to protect the domestic market from free-competitive destruction. Japan attaches great importance to accessibility that anyone can access anywhere and fair use of medical care as public goods. The Government of Japan is responsible for ensuring that all the people can receive the necessary medical care. Therefore, a fundamental difference between the two countries exists in the medical care and healthcare.

Until around 1955, about 30 million people, mainly farmers, self-employed, and employees of micro enterprises, which is about one-third of the population, were uninsured in Japan, which was a social problem. However, the National Health Insurance Law was enacted in 1958, and the National Health Insurance business began in municipalities nationwide in 1961, establishing a system that allows "anyone," "anywhere," and "anytime" to receive insurance medical care [2].

Japanese Ministry of Health, Labor and Welfare has declared that the role of this system as a safety net is essential as follows:

"Under the universal health insurance system, Japan has realized a medical system that allows anyone to receive medical care securely and has achieved the world's highest average life expectancy and healthcare standards. We will continue to aim for a sustainable public medical insurance system in response to the declining birthrate, increase in the aging population, population, and changes in the economic situation" [3].

2.3 The centralization power by mainstream in the US

From the social side, mainstream blocks the entry of others to strengthen its power. Mainstreamers can get various benefits and others are excluded. Partial optimization for mainstream results in the lack of total optimization as shown in **Table 1**. On the economic side, mainstreams amplify their interests while blocking the entry. This accelerates the centralization by mainstream, that starts to have a gravitational force that attracts various things. Mainstreamers begin to exert hegemonic influence to stakeholders and concessions authorized by the government create a chain of interests.

From the standpoint of the government and the market, initially, everything starts with a good idea for society, but policies act to fix benefits. They compete for the pie of government budgets. Governmental policies will be taken to ensure vested interests. Historically, the economy has set the direction for government. In the US, the globalized economy has gained centrality, set the direction of government, and could therefore gain the hegemony in the healthcare. Thus, as a result, a mechanism has been created in which mainstreamers increase profit and the public does not get the lowest benefits in the world.

2.4 The power of centrality to the publicity in the US

On the publicity in the US, at the center of political economy, the centrality determines everything through funding for politicians, the media, university professors, and researchers. It is well known that every public good is commercialized in the US by the logic, that competition in the market is better than government control.

The situation surrounding the potentially life-threatening medical care is dire and irreversible. A typical example is Medicaid. Medicaid is a government medical benefit system for low-income people who have difficulty in taking out private medical insurances (including persons with disabilities and pregnant women who are recipients of supplementary income security). The cost of Medicaid is increasing from 1980s' when market fundamentalism was applied to medical care, as shown in **Figure 1**.

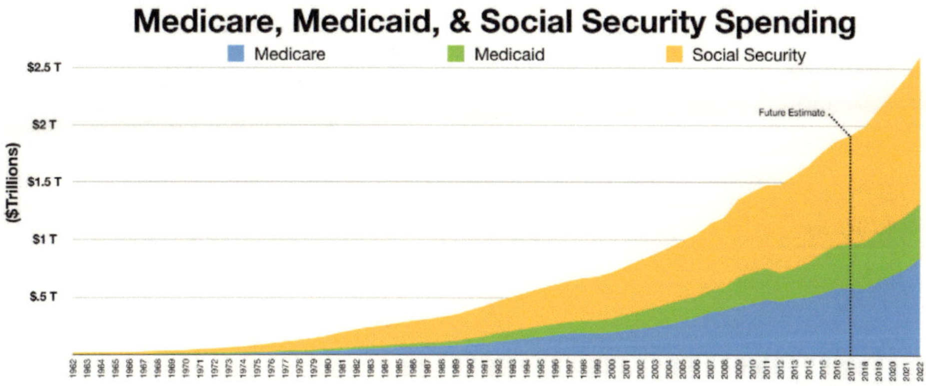

Figure 1.
Public healthcare insurances and social security expenses in the United States (Wikipedia) [Internet]. 2021. Available from: https://commons.wikimedia.org/wiki/File:Medicare,_Medicaid,_and_social_security_spending.png [accessed: 2021-6-7 including citations in the text below].

Regarding medical expenses in the US, according to the Medicare Medicaid Service Center in the US, medical expenses in the US in 2018 totaled $ 3.6 trillion, and $ 11,172 per capita. It accounts for 17.7% of GDP. The medical cost per capita in Japan is $ 2,920 (321,100 yen), which is almost four times higher.

Even though medical expenses and the US government spending on per capita are the highest in the world, it is far from a universal service that allows people to live safely, securely. Only the US and Mexico have failed to achieve universal healthcare in OECD countries [4]. The lack of medical insurance in the US causes 45,000 to 48,000 unnecessary deaths each year [5, 6]. About 25 percent of young citizens have filed for bankruptcy due to high medical costs, and 43 percent of them have sold real estate for that purpose [7].

In the US, the power of centrality introduces market principles to what is in publicity, and businesses succeed in profiting from the people and the government, resulting in poverty and pressure on the government's finances.

3. Accessibility and medical hegemony

3.1 Accessibility to healthcare

As mentioned above, there is a negative correlation between the degree of inequality and accessibility. What makes the difference between Japan and the US? Japan focuses on protecting people. Japan is a country that values dignity for life and ethics. In the US as well, business executives were highly aware of high moral aspirations, wide moral foundation [8] and public institutions [9] for people and society till 1950s'.

Due to the championship of huge securities financing capital, globalization has been progressing in the US. As the securities financing business has played a central role in the US economy, the US have assumed that free competition in the market would solve social problems. Free competition strategy has helped the US securities financing industry rule its economic and political hegemony in the global market.

The US spends the most on healthcare in high-income countries. Total medical expenses per capita has been continuously rising from 1981 [10]. **Table 2** shows the ranking of medical expenses per capita. The total medical expense per capita in the US is 2.22 times that of Japan, 2.60 times that of the United Kingdom, and

Country	Healthcare Rank	Total medical expenses per capita (US$)
United States	1	10,586.08
Switzerland	2	7,316.61
Norway	3	6,186.92
Germany	4	5,986.43
G7 Average		5,539.29
Sweden	5	5,447.11
Austria	6	5,395.11
Denmark	7	5,298.82
Netherlands	8	5,288.44
Luxembourg	9	5,070.17
Australia	10	5,005.32
Canada	11	4,974.33
France	12	4,964.71
Belgium	13	4,943.54
Ireland	14	4,869.36
Japan	15	4,766.07
Oceania Average	16	4,463.98
Iceland	17	4,349.09
Finland	18	4,235.55
United Kingdom	19	4,069.57
OECD Average		3,992.35

Source: OECD Health Data.

Table 2.
Ranking of medical expenses per capita in 2018.

2.65 times that of the OECD average. Total medical expense of the US is the highest, despite the worst medical care for the public.

In Japan, Japan's Big Bang package was done from April 1, 1998 to March 2001. The first liberalization removes barriers for foreign companies to buy or to sell Japanese companies. As a result, shareholders started to ask high dividend on stock. Restructuring was carried out as companies prioritized immediate profits over the future. The unemployment rate in Japan is steadily increasing, and the number of non-regular employees is also increasing, which is a factor of disparity.

Regarding healthcare system, Japanese public opinion and the government have not chosen the policies to widen the inequality, because the right to life is guaranteed by the Constitution as well as the right to live a healthy and cultural life. On the contrary, there is no right-to-life clause in the US Constitution.

3.2 Affordability and timeliness determine the health of people

According to WHO (the World Health Organization), a well-functioning healthcare system requires a steady financing mechanism, a properly-trained and adequately-paid workforce, well-maintained facilities, and access to reliable information to base decisions on. These include the care process (preventative care measures, safe care, coordinated care, and engagement and patient preferences), access (affordability and timeliness), administrative efficiency, equity, and healthcare outcomes (population health, mortality amenable to healthcare, and disease-specific health outcomes) [11]. Based on these five measures, WHO publishes health system rankings "Measuring Overall Health System Performance for 191 Countries" as shown in **Table 3**.

Yet the U.S. population has poorer health than other countries. Life expectancy, after improving for several decades, worsened in recent years for some populations, aggravated by the opioid crisis. In addition, as the baby boom population ages, more people in the US—and all over the world—are living with age-related disabilities and chronic disease, placing pressure on healthcare systems to respond [12].

A study by The Commonwealth Fund [12] used these metrics to rank 11 countries based on their quality of healthcare. The top-ranked countries are the United Kingdom, Australia, and the Netherlands. Regarding care process, the US also performs above the 11-country average on preventive measures like mammography screening and older adult influenza immunization rates. However, the US performs poorly on several coordination measures, including information flows among primary care providers, specialist and social service providers. The US also lags other countries on avoidable hospital admissions.

Among them, the US ranks last on Access. The performance of the U.S. is the worst in all countries on the affordability subdomain, scoring. According to these discussions, there is no dispute that affordability and timeliness are key elements of accessibility. And these factors determine the health of the people in a nation.

3.3 Centralized power of mainstream and innovation

Because of the Japanese strict national licensing system, medical insurance companies lacked the willingness to take on new challenges. Take advantage of the opportunity not to change anything, cancer insurance had come from the US. The typical success case of the US was the monopoly of cancer insurance in the Japanese market by Aflac, a small US insurer, which prevented Japanese insurance companies not to enter the market from1972 to 2001. The US has repeatedly made demands for the US industries, as Japan has always been reluctant and weak against the demands of the US. Japan-US insurance talks held at the same time as the talks to break the trade conflict between Japan and the US. At that time, the original purpose was trade negotiations, but regardless of that, the US securities financing industries, which have economic and political central influence in the US, aimed to enter the Japanese market. It is agreed that cancer insurance and medical insurance cannot be sold by Japanese major life insurance companies and non-life insurance companies in Japan. As a result, Japanese insurance companies have been unable to enter the market for a long time, and Aflac, which entered the Japanese cancer insurance market in 1974, maintains an overwhelming market share.

By this time, the US had already shifted its focus from manufacturing to securities financing. During this period, policy had shifted to increase international influence through the securities financing industries for overwhelming the industrialized nation of Japan. Economists had gotten influential power on federal policymaking since the late 1960s, leading the US in the wrong direction about domestic healthcare system and fostering social disparity. The big problem was that many economists unconditionally believed that free competition and free trade were best. Many economists sacrifice welfare and prioritize efficiency.

It is the American way to manage social welfare services such as medical care based on the principle of competition that works in an open market. This has made the healthcare industry inefficient, as afore mentioned in the former sections. The cost of treatment for common illnesses became unusually high after 1980. Disparity

Country	Healthcare Rank	2021 Population
France	1	65,426,179
Italy	2	60,367,477
San Marino	3	34,017
Andorra	4	77,355
Malta	5	442,784
Singapore	6	5,896,686
Spain	7	46,745,216
Oman	8	5,223,375
Austria	9	9,043,070
Japan	10	126,050,804
Norway	11	5,465,630
Portugal	12	10,167,925
Monaco	13	39,511
Greece	14	10,370,744
Iceland	15	343,353
Luxembourg	16	634,814
Netherlands	17	17,173,099
United Kingdom	18	68,207,116
Ireland	19	4,982,907
Switzerland	20	8,715,494
Belgium	21	11,632,326
Colombia	22	51,265,844
Sweden	23	10,160,169
Cyprus	24	1,215,584
Germany	25	83,900,473
Saudi Arabia	26	35,340,683
United Arab Emirates	27	9,991,089
Israel	28	8,789,774
Morocco	29	37,344,795
Canada	30	38,067,903
Finland	31	5,548,360
Australia	32	25,788,215
Chile	33	19,212,361
Denmark	34	5,813,298
Dominica	35	72,167
Costa Rica	36	5,139,052
United States	37	332,915,073

Table 3.
Ranking of well-functioning national healthcare systems in 2021 (by WHO) [10].

expanded among professionals as well. Low quality doctors go to poor areas. Excellent doctors who can get a high salary gather in the area where rich people live. Medical disparities are further widening due to the phenomenon of cream skimming, which businesses only enter profitable areas. Medical disparity is a detrimental effect of free competition. Therefore, there will be many medical refugees who cannot receive the necessary medical care like developing countries.

On the other hand, Japan attaches great importance to fairness in accessibility that anyone can access anywhere. To give the simplest example, in Japan, anyone can be treated equally by a well-known doctor in any hospital without appointment. As a code of ethics to guarantee the access, doctors are prohibited by law from refusing to see a patient.

It looks like the government is providing good healthcare, but it won't do anything new. Therefore, organizations that should promote innovation can defend themselves. Such a thing was permitted within the authorities, so the approved ranking of anti-corona vaccines was the last among developed countries. In addition to the delay in approval of the vaccine against the anti-cervical cancer virus, which has confirmed clear efficacy and had been approved in advanced countries, it has not been approved for use by men. This is because the head of the vaccine department of the authorities continued to extend approval to the next person in charge for fear of side effects.

The John Maddox Prize is an award given by "Nature" to those who have contributed to the dissemination of science and scientific evidence for the public good. In 2017, it was presented to Riko Muranaka, a medical doctor and journalist who has continued to send out information to verify the safety of the HPV vaccine. Nature described the HPV vaccine as "recognized by the scientific community and medical community as a key to preventing cervical cancer and other cancers and endorsed by the WHO (World Health Organization)." Moreover, in Japan the vaccine has been subject to a national misinformation campaign to discredit its benefits, results in vaccination rates falling from 70% to less than 1%. " Nature evaluated her activities as "spreading science and scientific evidence for the public interest while facing difficulties and hostility," and selected from 100 candidates from 25 countries. Ms. Muranaka said, "I think it's powerless to see that the situation has not changed even though I've written so much." The biggest problem is not being there. The nation must take responsibility for the lives of its people. " Nature severely criticized the situation in Japan, saying that "a false information campaign that undermines the reliability of this vaccine was carried out nationwide" [13]. The data to disseminate false information was deliberately forged by an authoritative university professor who received research funding from the authorities to create fake data to deny.

For public interest, universal services should be obliged by the government to provide benefits to all, regardless of wealth, social class, men and women of all ages, or region. Even in Japan, where bioethics and publicity are the top priorities, the reality is beyond imagination. Professionals try to be central by acting for their own benefit. Once power is centralized, it is a virtue within the mainstream to not change unless it is related to their own interests.

3.4 Lack of accessibility due to medical hegemony

The US government and scholars argue that if regulators decide everything, they will not be able to provide adequate medical care to the public. This is because regulation would make it as if there was only one monopoly and would not try for customers [14]. Mainstream scholars such as Michael Porter have argued that better medical care should be provided in the competition. In fact, the most advanced medical care is being developed and provided in the US. As a result, the most expensive medical ecosystem in the world and the lowest accessibility among developed countries has been created.

Figure 2 shows the annual change in the monopoly of American hospitals. An HHI (Herfindahl–Hirschman Index) score is the sum of the squares of the market share of each player in a market. For example, in a market where there is only one hospital — a monopoly — with 100 percent market share, that market's HHI score is 10,000 (100 squared). A market with only two hospitals, in which one has 60 percent share and the other 40 percent, has an HHI of 5,200 (60 squared plus 40 squared). The Federal Trade Commission considers markets to be "highly concentrated" if their HHI scores are 2,500 or higher. In other industries, such as airlines or cell-phone carriers, the FTC routinely seeks to block mergers that would increase HHI scores above 2,500. In the hospital industry, however, the median market HHI exceeded 2,500 in the year 2000 and reached 2,800 in 2013 [15].

A new wave of hospital mergers is driving market concentration higher. The blue bars denote the number of merger and acquisition transactions in a given year; in the 1990s, penetration of managed-care insurers, with a mandate for more aggressive cost control, led hospitals to merge in response, strengthening their market power over the insurers. The Federal Trade Commission (FTC) and the US. Department of Justice (DOJ) normally consider markets with an HHI above 1,500 as "moderately concentrated" and markets with HHI above 2,500 as "highly concentrated," triggering antitrust litigation. However, consolidated hospital markets have largely avoided antitrust litigation. In 21th century, more than half of the hospital markets in the US have an HHI above 2,500, meaning that the FTC and DOJ would consider them to be "highly concentrated" (Sources: A. Roy/FREOPP analysis and graphics, Robert Wood Johnson Foundation, Martin Gaynor, Irving Levin Associates, HHS ASPE.) [15].

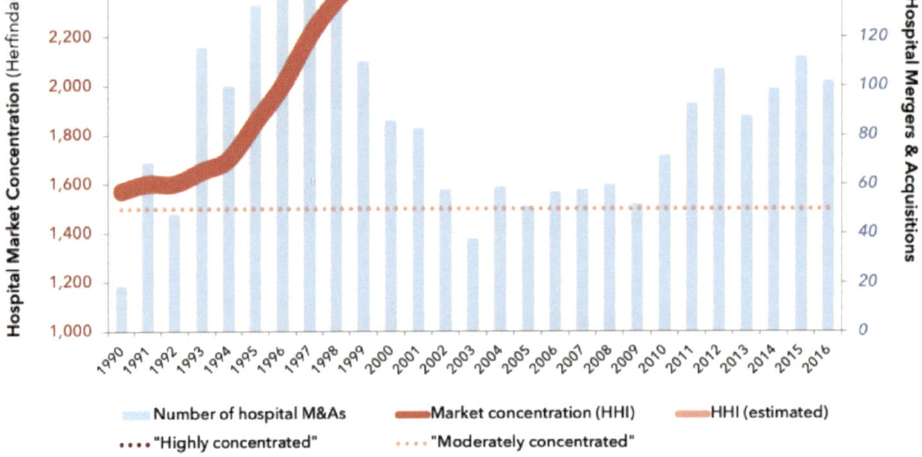

Figure 2.
Annual trends in the degree of monopoly by large hospitals in the US (source: "Avik Roy, The Foundation for Research on Equal Opportunity").

Market concentration contributes to raising the profit margin not only in the medical industry but also in the healthcare industry to get the highest interest rates in the world. In conclusion, the medical industry, which has increased its centrality by concentrating, is the most profitable in the world. The influence of this medical hegemony has resulted in poor accessibility to healthcare in general.

4. Opening medical barriers with digital healthcare

4.1 Barriers built by medical hegemony

The situation in which a hospital becomes huge and has an impact on overall healthcare could be defined as medical hegemony. According to WHO, universal healthcare can be determined by three critical dimensions: who is covered, what services are covered, and how much of the cost is covered [16]. In the US, hospitals, health insurance companies, and pharmaceutical companies have become huge after 1980. Such huge healthcare providers have taken medical hegemonies and guide policies. Eventually, lack of accessibility results in unsatisfactory access to the medical needs of the public. As a result, WHO and the National Academy of Medicine and others have concluded the US is the only wealthy, industrialized nation that does not provide universal healthcare in 2021.

Medical care has its own peculiarities. In the medical and long-term care fields, only the provider has the information. Patients have no choice but to believe and entrust without bargaining even if they lie. Therefore, those who provide low-cost and high-priced medical care services accumulate profits and dominate the market. Once become huge, they can affect various fields and the hegemony has been established.

Even if information is disclosed for the purpose of resolving information asymmetry, it is practically impossible for consumers to have equal bargaining power. Therefore, in free competition, the supply side has an absolute advantage in deciding what to do. In free competition in a state where information is asymmetric and bargaining power is imbalanced, prices rise by the following mechanism, resulting in the exclusion of consumers [17].

1. If the information is completely asymmetric, free competition will bring about market failure. Consumers do not know whether good or bad (lemon), so the bad suppliers survive and the good suppliers disappear. As a result, inferior products (lemon) are on the market. (The market for lemons)

2. If there are essential remedies and treatment methods, the supply side can raise the price as the demand increases. This is the result of price equilibrium when demand increases for limited resources (rents) such as land. (The law of rent)

3. The best management strategy for the supply side is to enter the market with the highest profit margin. Competitors lose if they do not do the same. (Prisoner's dilemma causes bubbles and injustice).

4. The optimization strategy for the supply side causes inefficiency of the entire industry and create barriers that customers cannot get involved with. (Total inefficiency by partial optimization)

In the free competition market, there are many people who cannot receive satisfactory medical care because they cannot pay. On the contrary, those who can afford high treatment can enjoy exclusively top-level medicine. Thus, the barrier between supply and demand remains high. The gap in accessibility from consumers deepens and cannot easily repair once medical hegemony is fixed.

4.2 The source of hegemonic power

Digital healthcare is expected to increase the accessibility of medical information and to remove the medical barrier. Although this optimism is believed, real-world healthcare can be severely affected by the knowledge and context shared in the healthcare industry and academia. The problem is that common knowledge is spread by mainstream people.

The use of patterned knowledge from mainstream facilitates the use of medical information. Further utilization of smart ICT will facilitate to realize the smart use of medical information in our daily lives and therefore improve the accessibility to healthcare information. Through this process, the central perception will quickly gain consensus in the industry and academic societies. Through such a process, practical knowledge is unified and spreads quickly. In this way, mainstream contexts quickly become more and more widespread. In other words, this makes it easier for mainstream to establish hegemony.

Hegemons have become the center of the world and gained centrality by setting a global standard. This strategy allowed hegemony to accumulate economic power and become the center of politics, economy, and society. To maintain centrality, hegemons have no choice but to do rent seeking for themselves, not for the total benefit. **Figure 3** illustrates the transition of hegemonic nations. The hegemonic nation is deprived of the next hegemony by a neighboring country across the sea. By imitating and improving the previous economic system, neighboring countries that do not interact directly have become hegemonic nations one after another [18].

1. Egypt prospered from the fertile land of the Nile and its slave civilization. 2. the Greek police nations become the center of trade, 3. Rome is based on the vast territory that supplies slaves, 4. Islam relays East-west trade, and 5. Spain mined gold and silver in South America and circulated minted coins in Europe. 6. the Netherlands

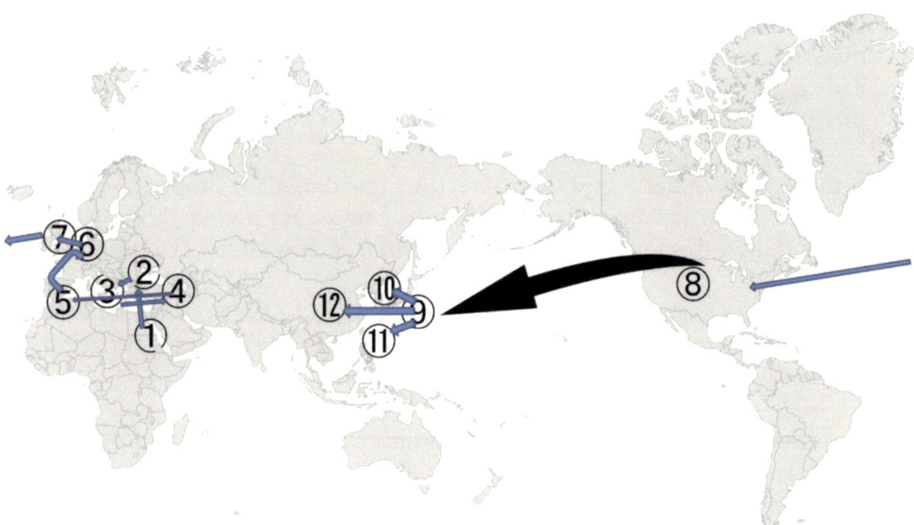

Figure 3.
Transition of hegemonic countries [18].

became the global trade center with currency exchange, 7. the United Kingdom became the financial center (Citi) and the world's factory by Industrial Revolution, 8. the US became the world's factory by the mass production system and then global securities and financial center, 9. Japan realized mixed production system with small-volume plus mass customization and became the world's factory, 10. South Korea, 11. Taiwan, and 13. China acquired the world market with imitation power.

A hegemon could become the center of the world by imitating and surpassing the previous hegemonic power [19].

The reason for the emergence of hegemonic states can be seen from the fact that the source of hegemony is not civilization but economic power.

4.3 Success/failure judgment method for information issued by medical hegemony

Can doctors adhere to justice fairly and selflessly in all situations? Hippocratic oath is an international norm that doctors should comply with. The ethical code attributed to the ancient Greek physician Hippocrates, adopted as a guide to conduct by the medical profession throughout the ages and still used in the graduation ceremonies of many medical schools. The oath dictates the obligations of the physician to students of medicine and the duties of pupil to teacher. In the oath, the physician pledges to prescribe only beneficial treatments, according to his abilities and judgment; to refrain from causing harm or hurt; and to live an exemplary personal and professional life (Encyclopedia Britannica).

In the medical world, the problem is physicians have never accepted novel approaches when treatments does not replace current therapy. Players in the mainstream (stakeholders such as opinion leaders, physicians, pharmaceutical firms, university professors etc.) are not only reluctant to try any noble therapeutic approaches, but they have always denied and attacked.

It is well-known that medical hegemony intends to stabilize its position by undermining the fair use of information. For judging the correctness of medical information, it is possible to check simply whether one piece of simplified information is yes or no. Yes/no methods can clarify responsibility in the event of an error. RNA injection is a typical example that used to be no but became yes. The properties of cells can be altered by introducing RNA instead of genetic engineering. Therefore, the rapid supply of corona RNA vaccine became possible. In addition, RNA injection can be used for in vivo production of pluripotent cells instead of in vitro production of iPS cells.

RNA injection method was denied by mainstreamers. This is explained by inevitable win-lose theory that indirect competitive innovation is neglected by mainstreamers. Surprisingly, in case of direct competition, mainstreamers accept new thing, but in case of indirect competition, they deny the new one [19–22]. The reason is that they will be replaced by challengers if they do not accept directly competitive thing. However, without exception, they deny new things that indirectly compete with. Usually they spread fake information. They choose the immediate stability because they cannot be replaced immediately. It often takes time to be replaced, but the mainstream faction changes. It should be noted that both actions are taken to defend the position of the championship.

Nevertheless, professionals will continue to disseminate the information claimed by the mainstream. This is because expressing disagreement has adverse events. Whenever novel treatments are discovered that do not directly replace traditional one, they are denied without evidence and prevent them from being adopted. **Table 4** shows categorized patterns of disinformation deliberately created by the mainstreamers [23].

Therapy	Traditional	Novel therapeutics
1) Few targeted patients		
CV in Japan (Cardiovascular)	Ca blocker	ARB (Angiotensin receptor blocker)
2) Slow onset of effect		
GI in Japan (Gastrointestinal)	H2 blocker	PPI (Proton pump inhibitor) Helicobacter pylori extermination
3) Not immediate effect		
Anti-cancer drug	Chemotherapy	Antibody drug, cancer vaccine
4) High satisfaction		
RA (Rheumatoid Arthritis)	Symptomatic treatment (MTX: methotrexate)	Antibody drug (anti-TNF)
5) Evaluation criterions are unknow		
Transfusion alternative	Red blood cells transfusion	EPO (Erythropoietin, red blood substitute)
6) Biopharmaceuticals	Small compounds	G-CSF
7) Regeneration	No way	iPS cells, RNA drugs
8) Oligonucleotide Therapeutics	Oligonucleotide does not enter the cell. Anxiety of possible genetic mutations, without evidence	RNA or DNA injection, Speed-up approval for in vivo antibody production against coronavirus Autologous cell therapy by pluripotent cell proliferation

Table 4.
Disinformation on novel therapy created by the mainstream [23].

1. CV (Cardiovascular) was the most major therapeutic area in the world. Ca blocker has created a market with a particularly high share in Japan. Authorities in the CV area were respected as representatives of physicians. This therapeutic area covers not only hypertension, but also all over the lifestyle-related disease. In this type of prioritized therapeutic area, companies create mainstream by writing treatises and giving research achievements to company-nominated opinion leaders, young doctors, and supporters based on each strategy. Therefore, major physicians in the CV field have kept a tight relationship with pharmaceutical firms and have received financial support especially as research fund. Pharmaceutical companies have also set up programs to train prominent young doctors for next new product developments and marketing purposes.

According to major Japanese pharmaceutical firms, fast onset was the key point of Ca blockers. Therefore, common opinion was that there were few cases to be targeted by a new ARB (Angiotensin receptor blocker) therapy because ARB is not fast-acting. However, the fact was exactly the opposite. Only amlodipine, which had a slow onset and a long half-life just like ARB, was increasing sales.

In Japan, all opinion leaders and major journals did not support ARB, even after ARB became the first choice among all other countries. By author's effort, a Japanese firm could get a license of ARB from a German big Ca player despite company-wide opposition.

Despite such industry-wide dissenting opinions, the share of the new therapy reached over 70% of the patients once the first ARB was launched. Although the overall evidence approved lifestyle-related diseases, professionals ignored the merit of organ-protective effect of ARB. Mainstream companionship is not evidence-based.

2. GI (Gastrointestinal) area is the largest market in the world till around 2010. A world-top share H2 (Histamine 2 receptor) blocker was originated by a Japanese firm. It was well recognized among Japanese firms and mainstream professors that extermination of *H. pylori*, the causative bacterium, would completely cure the gastric ulcer and prevent stomach cancer.

Mainstream professors and physicians received financial supports. Running out of money is a problem. The world top share product, which is originated by a Japanese firm, suppresses the immune elimination of cancer cells by NK cell inactivation since histamine is essential to activate NK cells.

Japanese pharmaceutical firms advertised that new PPI (Proton pump inhibitor) therapy did not cure the symptoms. Eradication of gastric ulcer and gastric cancer causative bacteria, Helicobacter pylori, by PPI was a standard therapy in Europe and the US. Approval in Japan delayed more than 10 years. PPI became the first choice once the patent for top-seller H2 blocker expired. This witnesses the strength of dominance.

Table 5 shows that the ratio of deaths by stomach cancer is the highest among other countries in 2005 (before the PPI era). The death rate of stomach cancer in Japan is 10 times higher than that of Americas. It is known in the pharmaceutical industry that this is due to the widespread of a top-seller H2 blocker in Japan.

3. Anti-cancer therapy is mainly by drug therapy in combination with surgery or radiation. Anticancer drugs control the growth of cancerous cells by toxicity.

When antibodies that suppress the growth factors of breast cancer cells had been developed, firms, professors and physicians have denied every time. As proof of lack of intension, they do not conduct in-hospital trials for applicants like toxic drug candidates. The drug delay has happened all over the world.

All professionals have denied the effectiveness of antibody drugs and the anti-cervical cancer vaccine mentioned above. HTLV (Human T) was first discovered as a causative virus of adult T-cell lymphoma (ATL) by Dr. Hinuma at Kyoto University in 1977. A negative campaign against cancer viruses' existence was held through the 20th century. Many scholars, who have been associated with the prestigious professors of the mainstream, have been openly, unfounded, and emotional, and have continued to deny until very recently. It has been proved that more than 30 percent of cancers have been caused by cancer viruses, which are increasing year by year.

4. Rheumatoid arthritis destroys joints due to autoimmunity, and eventually the organs are gradually destroyed, resulting in multiple organ failure and death. MTX (methotrexate), which have an immunosuppressive effect on symptomatic treatment, is widely used. New antibody therapy (anti-TNF antibody),

	Cancer Death	Overall Stomach Cancer	Lung Cancer
Japan	303.3	52.2	67.6
Americas	207.2	5.3	65.5
UK	279.2	13.7	70.0
France	303.2	11.0	72.0

Source: Cancer Statistics, National Cancer Center Japan.

Table 5.
The ratio of deaths by stomach cancer per 100,000 men in 2005.

which blocked immune cells from killing patients' bodies, were neglected, despite mainstreamers watched an evidence that patients with difficulty of walking started walking quickly after injection. If they are cured completely, they do not need to visit doctors.

MTX therapy is practiced as a standard treatment all over the world and satisfied doctors. MTX is mildly toxic but are popular as a first choice, so the conclusion was there was no need to change treatments.

5. EPO(Erythropoietin) stimulates red blood cell proliferation (erythropoiesis) in the bone marrow. EPO is an alternative to blood transfusions, but it was denied that red blood cell transfusion is cheap.

EPO is now used in treating anemia resulting from chronic kidney disease, chemotherapy induced anemia in patients with cancer, inflammatory bowel disease (Crohn's disease and ulcerative colitis) and myelodysplasia caused by cancer chemotherapy or radiation.

The risk of viral infection is greatly reduced. If a cancer patient can be operated on without blood transfusion, the rate of recurrence and metastasis of cancer is greatly reduced because immune disturbance is not caused without blood transfusion.

6. Biopharmaceuticals are categorized 5 major classes; extracts from living systems, recombinant products, vaccines, gene therapy, RNA or DNA drugs (nucleic acid drugs).

G-CSF (Granulocyte Colony-stimulating Factor) is a type of growth factor. Patients might have G-CSF after chemotherapy to help their white blood cells recover after treatment.

It was rejected by mainstreamers except bio-venture firm, because of different treatment criteria. Mainstreamers and larger pharmaceutical firms resisted and opposed the new treatment to stimulate granulocyte proliferation.

Total market size of Biopharmaceuticals is beyond the half. This means the utility of biopharmaceuticals has been neglected by mainstreamers and professionals. According to IQVIA World Review Analyst 2020 forecast [24], the pharmaceutical market in 2019 was $ 1.2624 trillion, up 3.3% from last year. The market share of the top 100 pharmaceutical sales items (hereinafter referred to as the top items) was about 32%. Total sales of top items in 2019 were $ 401.3 billion, up 6.4% from last year. According to the technical classification of active ingredients (chemically synthesized drugs and biopharmaceuticals), there are 55 items of chemically synthesized drugs and 45 items of biopharmaceuticals, which is higher than the 2018 survey (59 items and 41 items, respectively). biopharmaceuticals increased by 4 items. Among the top items, 10 items have been replaced since 2018, of which 5 items have been replaced by 9 items and biopharmaceuticals items have been replaced by 5 items and 1 item has been replaced year by year. In addition, biopharmaceuticals sales accounted for $ 209.7 billion, 52% of top item sales, and although synthetic drugs accounted for more items, biopharmaceuticals accounted for more than half of sales for the first time in previous surveys.

7. Regeneration

Regenerative medicine will be the ultimate medical treatment aiming at immortalization and complete cure. Drug companies and mainstreamers do not develop complete cures that will eliminate the need for drug administration and shrink the market.

Around 1988, the author applied to MHW (the Ministry of Health and Welfare), Japan Health Sciences Foundation, major firms and JPMA (Japan Pharmaceutical Manufacturers Association) a research project on the generation of pluripotent cells by gene transfer as an innovative research theme. The proposal was neglected to adopt as a research theme because complete cures eliminate the market.

All doctors have still denied that the cells were reprogrammed. This is incompatible with a basic principle of embryology, the developmental process of higher organisms repeats evolutionary process (the law of developmental repetition, Haeckel's Law). For biologists, regeneration overturns their basic assumptions.

That is why mainstreamers at Kyoto University still underestimate the possibility of iPS cells and overstate that the risk. Since the mutation rate of cells is higher in liquid culture than in vivo, they should develop a culture system like in the body. The creation of iPS cells or pluripotent cells by direct injection of RNA into the human body would reduce the risk of genetic mutation.

8. Oligonucleotide therapeutics uses basically RNA or DNA. Oligonucleotides are nucleic acid polymers with the potential to treat or manage a wide range of diseases and can be used to modulate gene expression via a range of processes including RNAi (RNA interference), target degradation by RNase H-mediated cleavage, splicing modulation, non-coding RNA inhibition, gene activation and programmed gene editing. As such, these molecules have potential therapeutic applications for myriad indications, with several oligonucleotide drugs recently gaining approval [25]. As shown in the above Nature Review [25], although the majority of oligonucleotide therapeutics have focused on gene silencing, other strategies are being delayed or neglected by mainstreamers.

Oligonucleotide drugs such as RNA or DNA injection for producing antibodies was supposed to be ineffective and risky without evidence. Well-known mainstream scholars slandered the developers. As a matter of fact, only venture companies were developing quietly.

Suddenly in early 2020, rapid vaccine development and urgent supply were needed to prevent the spread of coronavirus. Speed-up approval of RNA or DNA vaccines against coronavirus was given worldwide, but Japan was the lowest in the world.

As a matter of life and death, the clinical trials were urged to conduct development of coronavirus vaccine. Similarly, immunotherapy for cancer should be as safe and effective as vaccines in post-infection adverse effects. However, almost professionals and drug companies are still not willing to admit.

RNA produces iPS cells therapeutics will repair complete body and will pave the way for spontaneous healing with their own cells. There is some evidence that such treatments are effective. As an example, in our brains, 50,000 nascent neural stem cells are born every day. Even at the age of 80, the same amount of regeneration as young people happens. Full-function recovery therapeutics by oligonucleotide will become the ultimate complete cure treatment. Complete healing of aging or diseases is unacceptable to mainstreamers. They do not intend to contribute to human healthcare, because they will definitely lose the hegemony in the current system. How to solve the problem is the next issue to be discussed.

4.4 Freedom from the centrality of hegemony by setting network neutrality through commons of information

Through the discussions so far, author has analyzed the actions taken by mainstream people in medical care and healthcare, which deal with life and health. The mainstreamers always win any new product developments that directly competes with and therefore replace the mainstream [19–22].

In case of indirect competition, mainstreamers inevitably lose any new product developments. As far as a new does not directly compete with the mainstream, they deny the fact until the mainstream is replaced. Even if treatments begin to be adopted, mainstreamers always deny and criticize the use of alternative treatments. For example, the evidence is that the discovery of the presence of a cancer virus, the ability to artificially generate pluripotent stem cells, and the fact that RNA can be used for treatment are not acknowledged and criticized.

Mainstreamers do not approve such facts until they understand that they will be replaced soon. Due to the dominant structure of the mainstream, novel therapeutics such as desensitization therapy using oral immunity for pollinosis and cervical cancer virus vaccination for men many innovative approaches delayed approvals by the Authorities. Many have been sacrificed by mainstreamers.

The method to eliminate such evils and realize truly useful healthcare is required. The effect and influence of the commons of information will become a solution to eliminating adverse events caused by the hegemonic mainstream. As the most effective means in the coming digital healthcare era, commons of information is now under construction. In July of 2020, Japanese Ministry of Health, Labor and Welfare confirmed its policy of intensively working over the next two years to operate a system that allows medical institutions and pharmacies nationwide to share medical information of patients online and use it for patient treatment and health promotion. Customers and service providers such as doctors pharmacists, health instructors, nurses in charge can check the treatment history. In these ways, the information that the doctor has kept secret is inevitably made public and reviewed, which can lead to criticism in some cases. Even if that patient can find a provider, the existing healthcare system is likely to create a lot of unnecessary impediment and expense in the US. Digital pharmacy expands access to professional healthcare. It would be a great start to access and utilize such kind of commons of information.

With the rapid penetration of the mobile Internet into everyday life, the ruler of the information is changing. Innovative ideas are realized instantly on the mobile and advanced media, according to instant innovation [26–28].

As various media are put to practical use in general life, the media affects not only on everything in our society and life. As a result of the widespread use of mobile terminals, advanced media has being breaking down the barriers built by the mainstream with hegemony by setting net neutrality in the instant communication through mobile.

Mobiles process various information in parallel and multiple parallel worlds exist at the same time. Information selection has made it possible for users to create necessary information from the side that creates information, and users have come to directly experiment and implement it. This kind of instant communication leads instant innovation [26].

Already, some app platforms for disclosure and use of medical information have been developed. Open information will be searchable in Information Commons, a platform for sharing information. There is no doubt that patients and end users who need information will become aware of everything from daily healthcare to disease information.

Instant innovation that happens on mobile is the opposite of traditional innovation, because end users choose their best. Moreover, the product is evaluated immediately. Therefore, the adjustment is performed so that it is easy to use from the customer side. A platform that is open and can bring the best solution survives automatically [26].

The effect and influence of the commons of information eliminate adverse events caused by the hegemonic mainstream. As the most effective means in the coming digital healthcare era, the commons of information has instantly created network neutrality on the mobiles. The network neutrality is independent of the mainstream. Therefore, only the commons of information, which is a platform with the following three points, survive:

1. Allow commons of information to enable fair use and fair search of information.

2. The commons of information release the cognitive bias set by mainstream.

3. The platform with fair use develop fairness of digital management and digital economics in the healthcare.

Author details

Makoto Takayama
Taisho University, Tokyo, Japan

*Address all correspondence to: takayama-makoto@arion.ocn.ne.jp

References

[1] Japan Medical Association. Medical standards and medical expenses in Japan and other countries [Internet]. 2021. Available from: https://www.med.or.jp/people/info/kaifo/compare/ [Accessed: 2021-5-24]

[2] Kenporen (Health Insurance Federation, Japan) home page. In fact, we are blessed! Japan's universal health insurance system [Internet]. 2021. Available from: https://www.kenporen.com/health-insurance/basic/01.shtml [Accessed: 2021-5-24]

[3] Ministry of Health, Labor and Welfare home page. Aiming for long-term stability of the medical insurance system [Internet] 2021. Available from: https://www.mhlw.go.jp/stf/seisakunitsuite/bunya/kenkou_iryou/iryouhoken/index.html [Accessed: 2021-5-24]

[4] OECD. Health at a Glance 2013 (Report) [Internet]. 2021. Available from: https://www.oecd.org/els/health-systems/Health-at-a-Glance-2013.pdf [Accessed: 2021-5-24]

[5] Cecere D. New study finds 45,000 deaths annually linked to lack of health coverage. Harvard Gazette [Internet]. 17 September 2009. Available from: https://news.harvard.edu/gazette/story/2009/09/new-study-finds-45000-deaths-annually-linked-to-lack-of-health-coverage/ [Accessed: 2021-5-24]

[6] Woolhandler, S. Despite slight drop in uninsured, last year's figure points to 48,000 preventable deaths. in Physicians for a National Health Program [Internet]. 9 December 2012. Available from: https://pnhp.org/news/despite-slight-drop-in-uninsured-last-years-figure-points-to-48000-preventable-deaths-health-expert/ [Accessed: 2021-5-24]

[7] Kelley A S, McGarry K, Fahle S, Marshall S M, Du Q, Skinner J S: Out-of-Pocket Spending in the Last Five Years of Life. Journal of General Internal Medicine. 2012; 28 (2): 304-309. doi:10.1007/s11606-012-2199-x.

[8] Barnard C I. The Function of the Ex ecutive. Harvard University Press; 1938.

[9] Drucker P F. The Practice of Management. Harvard University Press; 1954.

[10] OECD: OECD Health Statics [Internet]. 2020. Available from: https://www.oecd.org/els/health-systems/health-data.htm [Accessed: 2021-5-24]

[11] WHO. Measuring Overall Health System Performance For 191 Countries [Internet]. 2020. Available from: https://www.who.int/healthinfo/paper30.pdf [Accessed: 2021-5-24]

[12] Eric C S, Dana O S, David S, Arnav S, Michelle M D. The Commonwealth Fund. The US Health System Falls Short [Internet]. 2021. Available from: https://interactives.commonwealthfund.org/2017/july/mirror-mirror/ [Accessed: 2021-5-24]

[13] BuzzFeedNews. Riko Muranaka: A doctor and journalist who has verified the safety of the HPV vaccine, is commended by the leading overseas scientific journal Nature [Internet]. 2017. Available from: https://www.buzzfeed.com/jp/naokoiwanaga/rikomuranakajohnmaddoxprize?utm_term=.ieMJdOwV7#.gaoQYkO8B [Accessed: 2021-5-24]

[14] Porter M, Teisberg E, Olmsted T. Redefining Health Care: Creating Value-based Competition on Results. Boston: Harvard Business Press; 2006.

[15] The Foundation for Research on Equal Opportunity. Improving Hospital Competition: A Key to Affordable

Health Care —— Reversing a decades-long trend towards hospital consolidation will reduce health costs for patients [Internet]. 2017. Available from: https://freopp.org/improving-hospital-competition-a-key-to-affordable-medicine-343e9b5c70f [Accessed: 2021-5-24]

[16] World Health Organization (November 22, 2010). The world health report: health systems financing: the path to universal coverage. Geneva: World Health Organization. ISBN 978-92-4-156402-1. [Internet]. 2010. Available from: https://www.who.int/home/cms-decommissioning [Accessed: 2021-5-24]

[17] Takayama Makoto, Umeda M. Particularities and strategic management of healthcare business. Office Automation,. 2003: Vol. 24, No. 3, pp.11-16,

[18] Takayama, Makoto: Management in Strategic Space: Dynamics of Center-Periphery Relationships. Journal of Information and Management, 2020. Vol. 40, No.3, pp. 96-106.

[19] Takayama Makoto, Watanabe C, Griffin C: Myth of Market Needs and Technology Seeds as a Source of Product Innovation--- An Analysis of Pharmaceutical New Product Development in an Anti-hypertensive Product Innovation. Techonovation, Elsevier, 2001; Vol. 22, pp.353-362.

[20] Takayama Makoto: Win without Fail and Fail without Win in Bio-Management: Revenge of Success, Office Automation. 2005. Vol. 25, pp.15-21.

[21] Takayama Makoto. Law of win without fail and lose without win in Japan Society for the Study of Business Administration ed. Innovation of Japanese firms, Japan Society for the Study of Business Administration: 2009; pp. 62-67.

[22] Takayama Makoto. Law of Success or Failure in the High Tech Driven Market - 'Revenge of Success' in the Biotech, Nanotech, and ICT Industry. In Igor Furstner ed. Products and Services from R&D to Final Solutions: SCIYO, 2010, p. 15-36. DOI: 10.5772/10402. Available from: https://www.intechopen.com/books/products-and-services--from-r-d-to-final-solutions/law-of-success-or-failure-in-the-high-tech-driven-market-and-bio-industry [Accessed: 2021-7-1]

[23] Takayama Makoto. Points for cooperation and unification of intentions between departments when selecting KOL. in Tips for selecting accurate personnel and building good relationships with KOL doctors Technical Information Institute.

[24] Global Use of Medicines in 2020. Report by the IMS Institute for Healthcare Informatics. IMS [Internet]. 2015. Available from: https://www.iqvia.com/-/media/iqvia/pdfs/institute-reports/global-medicines-use-in-2020 [Accessed: 2021-5-24]

[25] Thomas C R, Robert L, Matthew J A W: Advances in oligonucleotide drug delivery, Nature Reviews Drug Discovery: 2020; volume 19, pp. 673-694.

[26] Takayama Makoto: Open and integral innovation on tablet PC by popularized advanced media as industrial cradle: In Constantin Volosencu ed. New Technology: InTech; 2012. pp. 379-396. DOI: 10.5772/32764. Available from: https://www.semanticscholar.org/paper/Open-and-Integral-Innovation-on-Tablet-PC-by-Media-Takayama/c58e0e86f7689770f916b02005798e7f2a157d67 [Accessed: 2021-7-1]

[27] Takayama Makoto, Fukushima M: Instant Innovation from Experiment to Implementing New Technology. Journal of Japan Society for Information and

Management. 2014: Vol. 34, Number 3, pp.86-102.

[28] Fujita M, Takayama Makoto: The Osmosis of instant innovation by mobile devices. Journal of Japan Society for Information and Management. 2015: Vol. 35, Number 4, pp. 72-80.

Chapter 8

The Implications of Health Financing for Health Access and Equity in Nigeria

Adelakun Edward Odunyemi

Abstract

The Nigeria health system has performed woefully against all vital health indices, trailing behind many African countries despite its enormous potentials. The reason for this is mainly due to the financial risk Nigerians face in accessing healthcare. This study addresses the implications of the current healthcare financing in Nigeria on access and equity. It shows the imperativeness of an alternative healthcare financing in line with best practices, from comparable Low- and Middle-Income Countries (LMICs), apart from the current National Health Insurance Scheme (NHIS). The findings from this study recommend that the NHIS should be strengthened through the policy reform to embrace fund pooling/risk-sharing, subsidisation for the poor and the vulnerable, mandatory enrolment, and fragmentation of NHIS. Other considerations include increasing domestic fiscal space for health and utilising a tax-based financing mechanism that has been progressive in all LMICs, thereby preventing the need for unsustainable reliance on external funding. A comprehensive package of health at the point of care is also necessary. However, all these recommendations require the government to show a commitment to improve the country's healthcare system through its health spending.

Keywords: universal health coverage, out-of-pocket expenditure, health insurance, health financing, health reform

1. Introduction

1.1 Universal health coverage in Nigeria

In 2005, the pervading global inequality in access to healthcare prompted the World Health Assembly to pronounce a resolution on Universal Health Coverage (UHC) [1]. UCH rests on two essential bedrocks: equitable access to quality healthcare and protection from financial risk. UHC forms target 8 of the United Nation's Sustainable Development Goal 3 (SDG 3). It also plays a crucial role in achieving other important SDGs, such as poverty reduction (SDG 1), gender equality (SDG 5), inclusive economic growth (SDG 8) and reduced general inequalities (SDG 10) [2–5].

The prevailing poor health indices and extreme poverty in the sub-Sahara African region, especially in Nigeria, have been attributed to inequality in access and financial protection in healthcare utilisation [4, 6, 7]. In 2000, Nigeria was ranked by the WHO as the fourth country with the worst health system, only

IntechOpen

topping three war-torn nations [8]. After two decades, Nigeria still has one of the worst health indices in Africa (see **Tables 1–3**), despite being Africa's largest economy in terms of Gross Domestic Product (GDP) and most populous country with an abundance of both human and material resources [5, 9–11]. For instance, while Nigeria's infant mortality rate in 2015 was 69 deaths in every 1,000 live births, the respective figures for neighbouring Africa countries like Ghana, Niger and Cameroon were 43, 57 and 57 per 1,000 live births [12]. The maternal mortality ratio of 814 per 100,000 live births in Nigeria exceeds only those of three countries in Africa [5, 12]. Moreover, the country has the highest number of extremely poor people worldwide after India [13]. Although these abysmal indices were derived from multiple factors, the issue of poor equitable access and exposure to financial hardship arising from catastrophic healthcare costs is the most significant.

A proven mechanism for achieving the objectives of UHC is the institution of a suitable mechanism of health financing [14]. Health Financing is a mechanism by which funds are generated, mobilised and utilise for healthcare [1, 15]. An effective healthcare financing mechanism gives people adequate financial protection from impoverishment arising from health services utilisation [14]. In Nigeria, health financing has been predominantly through out-of-pocket (OOP) spending - a regressive form of health financing. OOP payment accounts for about 69% of total healthcare expenditures in Nigeria [16]. As a result, poor households in Nigeria are either unable to access quality healthcare or face financial hardship from healthcare spending [1, 2]. More often than not, OOP payment makes people refrain from utilising health services, present late to health facilities, or patronise sub-standard healthcare facilities. OOP expenditure produces inequity because quality healthcare is only available to those who can pay and not those who need it. In most instances,

Country Name	1975	1980	1985	1990	1995	2000	2005	2010	2015
Ghana	50.811	52.277	54.127	56.776	57.528	57.002	58.719	61.03	62.772
Nigeria	43.187	45.333	46.127	45.9	45.854	46.267	48.252	50.896	53.112
Rwanda	45.315	48.527	51.685	33.413	31.037	48.649	55.254	63.433	67.45
South Africa	55.428	58.107	60.946	63.307	61.561	56.048	53.447	57.669	62.649
Cote d'Ivoire	48.147	51.072	52.922	53.254	51.569	49.635	50.12	52.964	56.065

Table 1.
Life expectancy at birth (total) (in years) in Nigeria compare with selected African countries (composed from world development indicators 2021).

Country Name	1975	1980	1985	1990	1995	2000	2005	2010	2015
Ghana	186.5	166.8	154.7	127.2	114	99.4	82.9	69.1	54.6
Nigeria	241.5	211.8	206.9	209.5	204.1	183.1	155.5	136	126.8
Rwanda	246.2	218.4	159.6	149.8	249.7	178.7	109.3	63.7	41.5
South Africa	121.7	92.2	71.1	57.3	59.4	71.1	79.1	51.2	37.1
Cote d'Ivoire	202.6	168.2	154.1	152.3	152	142.3	125.3	106.4	90.6

Table 2.
Mortality rate, under-5 (per 1,000 live births) in Nigeria compare with selected African countries (composed from world development indicators 2021).

Country	Demographic Indicators		Health Indicators			Health Expenditure Indicators	
	Population (total)	GDP per capita (US$)	Life expectancy at birth (years)	Infant mortality rate (per 1,000 live births)	Under-5 mortality rate, (per 1,000 live births)	General government health expenditure (% of GDP)	Out-of-pocket expenditure (% of current health expenditure)
Ghana (2016)	28,481,946	1931.389	63.124	37.4	52.2	1.327	37.823
Nigeria (2016)	185,960,289	2176.002	53.541	78.5	125	0.475	75.187
Thailand (2016)	68,971,331	5994.231	76.403	8.9	10.3	2.858	11.345
Ghana (2017)	29,121,471	2025.932	63.463	36.1	50	1.087	41.212
Nigeria (2017)	190,873,311	1968.564	53.95	77.3	122.8	0.532	77.224
Thailand (2017)	69,209,858	6592.914	76.683	8.4	9.9	2.934	10.898

Table 3.
Key demographic, health and economic indicators- Nigeria, Ghana and Thailand (2016–2017).

the poor and vulnerable groups, most in need of the services, have to sell their valuables, incur debts, or spend the family savings to access healthcare, resulting in further impoverishment. This phenomenon is referred to as catastrophic health spending [1, 17–20].

A household is usually classified as having incurred catastrophic expenditure "if it spends 40% or more of its discretionary (non-food), or 10% or more of its total expenditure on healthcare" [21]. Catastrophic health expenditures arise not only from direct spending on transportation to health facilities, treatment, investigations, medication and hospitalisation, but also from indirect costs resulting from depreciating health status and a resulting reduction in productivity [16]. Consequently, a household is caught up in a cycle of perpetual poverty (**Figure 1**). Ilesanmi et al. show an increase in poverty of 66.2% due to OOP spending on healthcare, especially among households in the rural communities in Nigeria [23]. Since more than 50% of Nigerians, representing more than 100 million people, live below the poverty line, catastrophic health expenditure is endemic [16, 20, 24]. This situation, therefore, calls for an urgent need to break this cycle of poverty and health-related misery by eliminating OOP payments.

1.2 Nigeria health system financing and relevant policies

Healthcare in Nigeria is financed through government budgetary allocation, donor funding, NHIS and private funding. The Nigeria 1999 Constitution empowers all the three tiers of government (federal, state and local) to mobilise and deploy resources to provide healthcare in their jurisdiction [24, 25]. The Nigerian government expenditure on health is less than nearly those of any country in the world (see **Figures 2–5**) [27, 28]. For example, only 4% of the federal budget was allocated to health in 2018 (below the 15% commitment of the 2005 Abuja Declaration). The situation is worse in the states and local government, where even less is allocated to health [1, 3]. This reflects the value the government places on health and it is the most significant challenge faced in achieving UHC by Nigeria [15, 25].

Even though Nigeria is the leading recipient of Developmental Assistance for Health (DAH) in Sub-Sahara Africa, the fund constitutes only about 4% of the

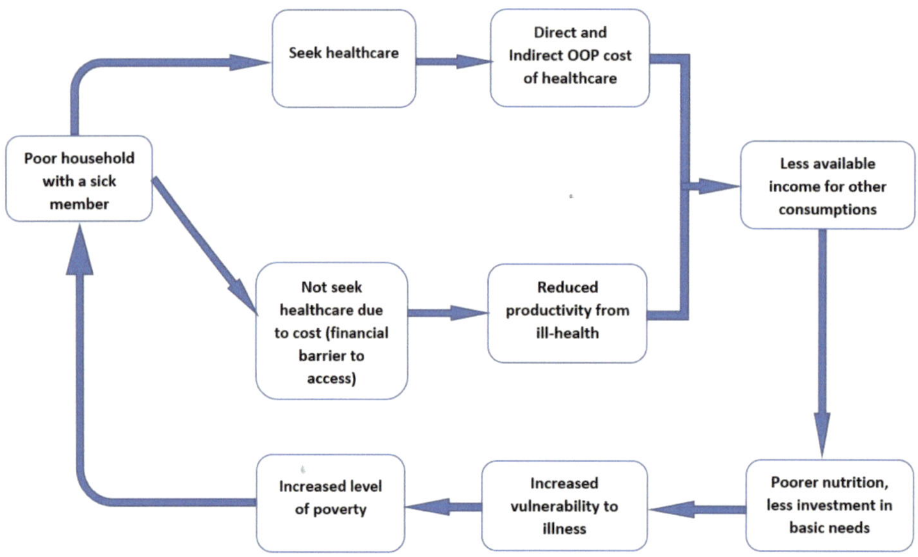

Figure 1.
Cycle of impoverishment due to out-of-pocket (OOP) health spending by poor households. (Adapted from Han [22]).

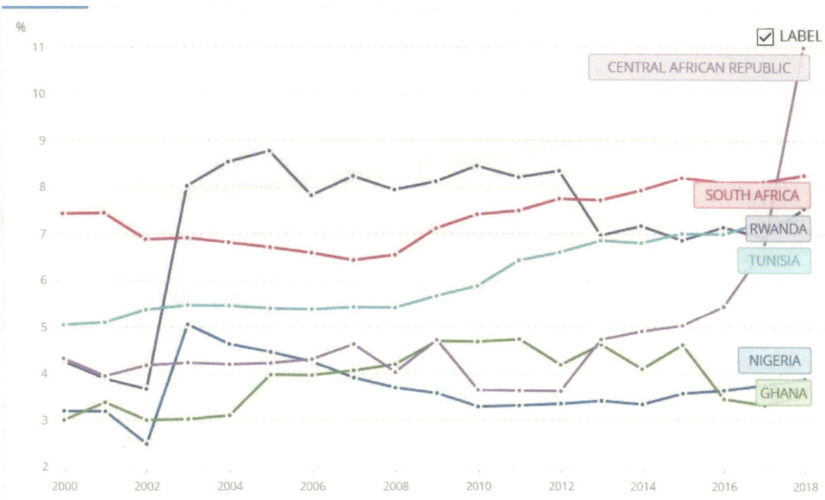

Figure 2.
Public health expenditure (% of total expenditures) in selected African countries. (Source: World Development Indicators).

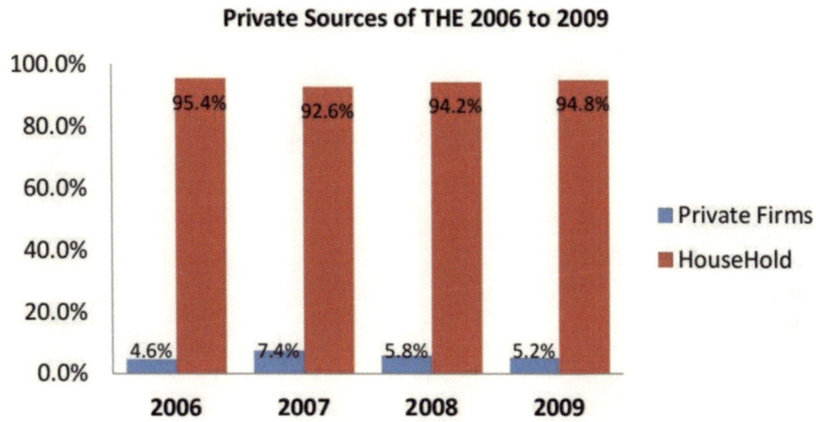

Figure 3.
Breakdown of THE by private financing sources, 2006, 2007, 2008 and 2009. (Source: National Health Accounts 2006-2009).

county's total health spending [18, 29]. Moreover, the funding administration is bedevilled with numerous challenges such as a high technical assistance cost, unevenness in sponsored activities, poor fund tracking, and counterpart funding issues [18]. In essence, DAH is not a reliable mechanism of healthcare financing in the country.

To achieve UHC, Nigeria adopted a social health insurance scheme known as the National Health Insurance Scheme (NHIS) in 2005 through an Act of Parliament. This is now known as Cap N42 Laws of the Federation of Nigeria, 2004 [11, 30]. However, after more than a decade, this scheme has not covered more than 4% of Nigerians [3, 16]. Despite its enormous potential in Africa, Nigeria's NHIS has performed worse than many countries on the continent [4, 5, 31]. This poor performance can be attributed to several policy deficiencies. First, the scheme is fragmented, being divided into Formal Sector, Informal Sector and Vulnerable Group categories and other sub-categories [32]. Second, despite commencing operation with the formal sector, it has not moved beyond the federal civil servants (constituting only 4% of the country's population). These federal employees have refused to

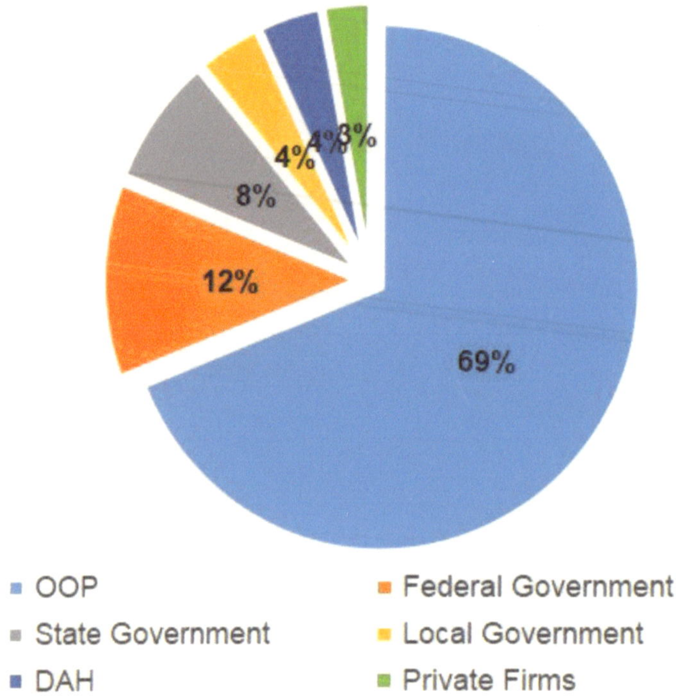

Figure 4.
Health Funding in Nigeria. (Source: National Health Account 2006-2009).

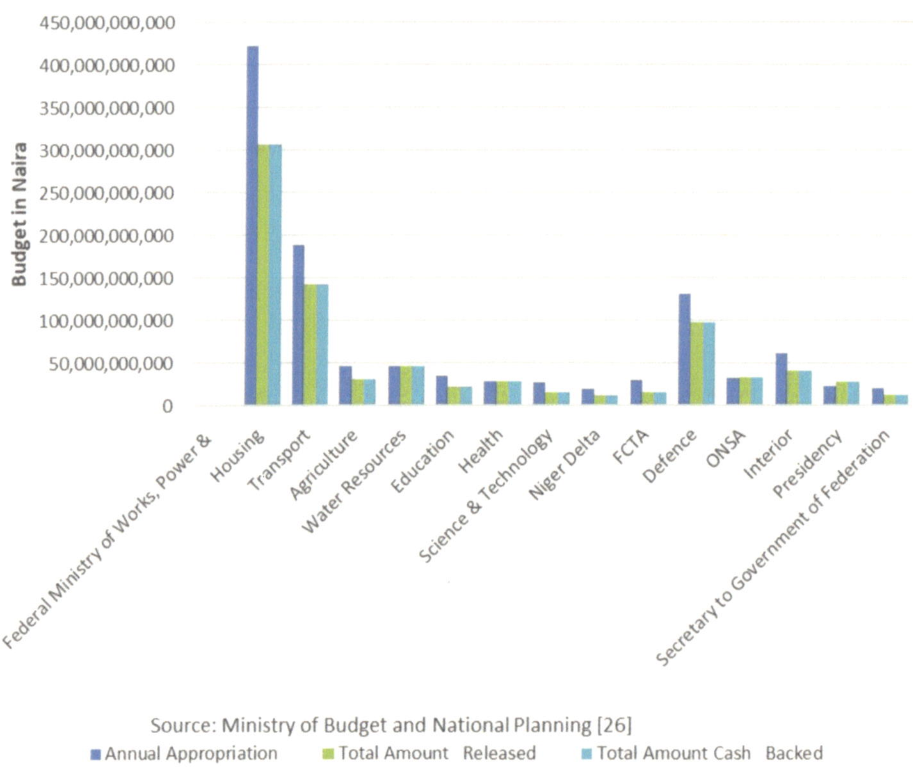

Figure 5.
Capital budget implementation across selected Ministries Departments and Agencies (MDas), 2016 [26].

contribute their 5% counterpart share of the 15% required. Therefore, the federal government is subsidising the health of a more affluent segment of the population by 10% at the expense of the poor and vulnerable people, the informal sector and the state employees, worsening the inequality situation [16, 17, 33]. Third, many states have not embraced the NHIS because the Act that set up the scheme did not capture the states in its operation [3, 14]. Even the Community Based Health Insurance (CBHI) that was recently inaugurated to cover the rural population and the informal sector has fared poorly with less than 3% enrolment. This insufficient enrolment has been attributed to unaffordable premiums, lack of trust, and poor quality of health [14, 34, 35]. Fourth, the Act that established NHIS made it voluntary for enrollees. It stripped the NHIS of the power to enforce the regulation guiding its operations, thereby causing poor participation and ineffective functioning of NHIS [33]. Fifth, the vulnerable group has not yet been covered. For example, Raji et al. discovered that retirees were not covered [36]. Sixth, the scheme's fragmentation has prevented it from having adequate resource pooling [3]. Therefore, these problems are possibly responsible for the failure of NHIS to fulfil its goal of saving Nigerians from regressive OOP health spending, which stands at 95% of the private health expenditures and 69% of the Total Health Expenditures (THE) (see **Figure 4**).

2. Healthcare financing mechanisms

Substantial evidence has proven that OPP health expenditures, rampant in LMICs, are the most regressive, inefficient and inequitable healthcare financing method [2, 24, 37]. While there is a concession that LMICs need to discard OPP expenditure, the debate is about which of the pre-payment health financial mechanisms will be the best. There is no silver bullet mechanism since each country's challenges are different [38, 39]. Moreover, each country is unique in its socio-demographic, economic and political structure. However, a health finance mechanism that can produce equitable access in LMICs must be based on compulsory pre-payment, fund pooling/risk-sharing and subsidisation, for those who cannot afford to pay [39–41]. Fund pooling and risk-sharing involves aggregating funds and redistributing them equitably between the rich and the poor, the employed and the unemployed, and the healthy and the sick [6, 14, 41]. Therefore, an exploration of different health financing mechanism follows in the next section.

2.1 Developmental assistance for health (DAH)

External funding in the form of DAH is becoming a vital funding mechanism in LMICs, especially in SSA [42]. As pointed out earlier, it is an unreliable mechanism of funding. Although DAH has decreased in the last two decades, there has not been a commensurate increase in SSA domestic financing [29]. This development could worsen the existing access, equity and financial risk problem in those countries [42]. However, DAH may be required, in the short to medium term, as complementary or supplementary funding for UHC in LMICs [40].

2.2 Community-based health insurance (CBHI)

CBHI is a form of private health insurance in which a group of people in a community contributes to financing their healthcare. It is used in LMIC to cater for the rural population and the informal workers usually not covered by other health insurance. CBHI suffers adverse selection and low participation and retention, resulting in low fund pooling and risk-sharing like any voluntary insurance scheme.

The poor resource pooled also produces high administrative costs and sustainability issues. Moreover, no matter how small, the premium may be unaffordable for the poorest members of the community [18, 42]. Although CBHI can potentially protect the enrollee from OOP spending, the very poor, who are not covered suffer financial risk, poor access and inequity. Therefore, CBHI is only helpful as a short-term measure against OOP spending [35, 42].

2.3 Social health insurance

Most developed countries have protected people from financial risk using social health insurance (SHI) or a tax-based funding mechanism [37]. SHI is a scheme in which the government mandates people to contribute to financing their health. It is usually funded jointly by the employees and their employers. The government pays for those who cannot pay, such as the poor, unemployed and vulnerable. SHI became the predominant health financing method in LMICs having been adopted by the African Union Conference of health ministers in 2007 [1, 37, 42]. While some countries such as Kenya, Tanzania and Nigeria introduced their SHI beginning with the formal sector and planned to expand it later, others like Ghana, Rwanda and Mali began with the entire population. Generally, countries in the latter group have successfully covered a more significant population, while the former has been unable to move beyond the formal sector. This issue has generated a severe equity problem of leaving behind the poor community of informal employees [42]. Consequently, a bottom-up approach, starting with the poor and vulnerable group and then the informal sector, has been suggested if this scaling-up approach is adopted [43].

SHI's success story in high-income countries like Germany has not been replicated in LMICs because of the mostly poor, unemployed and informal population. Moreover, LMICs cannot wait the length of time usually required for SHI to achieve UHC. Germany had to wait for 127 years [40]. Ghana and Rwanda's success stories with SHI have been made possible by subsidising mandatory enrolment for the poor and vulnerable group, a large percentage of their population, through tax revenue and donor funds [42].

2.4 Domestic government funding through taxation

A mechanism in which government funds healthcare mainly from its revenue or general taxation is called tax-based health financing [1, 18]. by Wagstaff et al. in their study of thirteen OECD countries, proved that direct taxes are progressive and indirect taxes are regressive in all the countries. It, however, shows that SHI is only progressive in eleven countries [44]. In contrast, a global review by Aurelio Mejía shows that direct and, even, indirect tax-funded systems are generally more progressive than SHI in LMICs [45].

A growing body of evidence has shown that tax-generated revenue is a significant potential source for expanding domestic fiscal space for health (DFSH) [42, 46]. Some consumption taxes on products (such as tobacco, alcohol and sugar) that are harmful to health (the so-called "sin tax") could be earmarked for healthcare financing as has been carried out in Thailand [42, 47]. Mobile phone usage tax is another revenue source for healthcare, considering the sizeable mobile phone subscriber base in Nigeria [48]. Subsidy from petroleum products can also be used to fund healthcare as is done in Indonesia [49]. It has been established that an increase in health expenditure can increase the economic growth of LMIC by 0.4 [10]. However, governments in LMIC must prioritise health financing following the example of countries like China, Cuba and South Korea [29, 50].

Two approaches to healthcare financing have shown consistent results in LMICs. First, the adoption of a tax-based health financing mechanism for population coverage as used with great success in Sri Lanka, Malaysia and Brazil. Second, SHI and general tax use to target the formal sector and the rest of the country, respectively. This approach was employed to achieve UHC in Thailand, Mexico and Kyrgyzstan [40].

3. Healthcare financing in Nigeria compared with selected countries

3.1 Ghana social health insurance Scheme

Ghana is a middle-income country in West Africa with a total population of 28,207,000 in 2015 and gross national income per capita of $3,880 in 2013 [51]. It is noteworthy that Ghana and Nigeria operate SHI (both known as National Health Insurance Scheme. Ghana began its SHI in 2004, just a year before Nigeria. Although Ghana has not achieved the recommended 90% UHC, it has become a success story in Africa within two decades of commencing the scheme, having covered about 64% of its total population. It has gone through different phases and challenges to reach this pedestal [6, 40]. Therefore, Nigeria can learn from Ghana how it was able to achieve this success, despite limited economic and human capital resources compared to Nigeria [11, 17]. Although, Ghana has not reached the targeted UCH goal, but it prides itself on achieving better health outcomes than Nigeria (see **Table 4**). This is not unrelated to its achievement so far with universal health coverage [33, 52]. While Nigeria's NHIS coverage stands at less than 5%, Ghana's rose exponentially from 6.5% in 2005 to 36% in 2010, then 40% at the close of 2015, and about 64% in 2018 [5, 6, 31]. In 2012, the previous National Insurance Act 2003 that established Ghana's NHIS was amended to accommodate some efficient changes, including merging all previously existing schemes into a unifying scheme under NHIS [5]. This 'umbrella' mechanism contrasts with the mostly fragmented NHIS in Nigeria, as discussed earlier.

One approach that helped Ghana to scale up coverage within a short time is the level of awareness and advocacy in the mass and electronic media [5]. Oni et al. has shown that the level of awareness of and access to NHIS has significant impact on service delivery [6]. The compulsory enrollment into NHIS by all residents of Ghana is another important reason why the scheme has been able to cover the country widely. This is in sharp contrast to Nigeria, where it is statutorily voluntary. Although Ghana's implementation of NHIS is faced with the problem of poverty like Nigeria, it has exempted the poor and other vulnerable groups from paying an insurance premium. This exemption resulted in increasing access and equity in healthcare. Although Nigeria NHIS made provision for the vulnerable group to include the physically and mentally challenged, prisoners, pregnant women, under-five children, and the aged, the reality in Nigeria is that no such exception is provided [5, 31, 52].

Moreover, enrollees of Nigeria NHIS still pay some hidden charges, co-payments and deductibles at the point of care, in contrast to Ghana, where no additional payment is required from their counterparts. Besides, there is a variable benefits package offered by Nigeria NHIS depending on the membership category. This is not the case in Ghana, where all benefit packages are uniform across the board using the diagnosis-related group (DRG). The most important factor contributing to the achievement recorded by Ghana is the fact that there has been an increase in total health expenditure as a percentage of total government expenditure to meet the 15% Abuja target. Moreover, Ghana finances 70% of its NHIS from taxation, used mainly for those exempted from paying the premium. The situation in Nigeria is the

Country	Demographic indicators				Hearth indicators				Health expenditure indicators			
	Population (millions)	GDP (p.cap)	LE (Male)	LE (Female)	IMR	U-5 year MR	p-HIV (% pop)	i-TB (cases)	THE (*p*.cap)	THE (% GDP)	Public HE (%THE)	OOP HE (% private)
Nigeria 2000	123.7	371	48	47	116	186	3.9	172	17	4.7	33	93
Ghana 2000	192	260	58	59	64	99	2.3	152	19	7.2	41	80
Nigeria 2002	129.8	455	47	48	107	177	3.8	182	18	4.0	26	90
Ghana 2002	20.1	306	58	60	61	94	2.2	138	20	6.5	36	80
Nigeria 2004	136.4	644	48	49	102	168	3.7	180	44	7.0	32	95
Ghana 2004	21.1	420	60	61	58	88	2.1	125	26	6.3	35	80
Nigeria 2006	143.3	1,014	49	50	97	159	3.6	168	59	5.7	34	96
Ghana 2006	21.1	920	61	63	55	83	1.9	112	48	44	57	65
Nigeria 2008	150.7	1,374	50	51	93	151	3.6	145	80	5.7	41	95
Ghana 2008	233	1,226	62	64	53	79	1.8	99	68	5.6	58	67
Nigeria 2010	158.4	1,278	51	52	88	143	3.6	133	63	5.1	38	95
Ghana 2010	24.4	1,325	63	65	50	74	1.8	86	67	5.2	60	66
OECD 2010	**N/A**	**34,774**	**77**	**82**	**6.8**	**8.2**	**0.3**	**N/A**	**4,365**	**12.6**	**65**	**67**

***Notes: OECD**, Organisation for Economic Co-operation and Development; **LE**, life expectancy at birth; **IMR**, infant mortality rate per 1,000 live births; **U-5 year MR** is per 1,000 live births; **p-HIV**, prevalence of HIV % of population aged 15–49; **i-TB**, incidence of TB per 100,000; **GDP**, Gross Domestic Product (in 2012 USS); **THE**, total healthcare expenditure; **p.cap**, per capita; **OOP**, Out of pocket.*

***Source:** World Bank [15]. (Adapted from Odeyemi and Nixon [52]).*

Table 4.
Key demographic, health and economic indicators - Nigeria, Ghana and OECD mean 2000–2010.

opposite [4, 5, 31, 52]. All these benefits offered by Ghana NHIS have contributed to expanding equity in access and provision of healthcare. Recently, Ghana is proposing a one-time payment for healthcare services known as the "One-time Premium Payment Policy" to mainly serve those in the informal sector [14, 15]. This step has the potential of boosting NHIS coverage and in turn, reducing OOP.

3.2 Thailand health insurance Scheme

Thailand is a middle-income country in South-East Asia, with a population of 69 million and a GDP per capita of $7,792. About 56% of its population is in rural area [51]. Thailand's health financing is worthy of consideration because of its long history of challenges similar to Nigeria, and its eventual rapid success which has become a global reference [53, 54]. The quest of Thailand toward achieving UHC began as early as 1975. After several trials with several health insurance mechanisms, Thailand achieved UHC in 2002 after commencing its Universal Coverage Scheme (UCS) the previous year [55]. By 2015, Thailand had been able to provide health coverage for 98% of its population [54]. Before 2001, the formation of different health insurance types to cater for various risk pool resulted in the fragmentation and failure of those schemes. When UCS was introduced, against all the odds, other fragments were collapsed into UCS except the Civil Servant Benefit Scheme (CMBS) and the Social Security Scheme (SSS). CMBS is a tax-funded health insurance that provides coverage for the formal sector, while SSS is a form of SHI for the private sector, covering about 12.3 million people.

Three essential factors contributed to the success of UCS within just a year. First, it is funded exclusively through government tax except at the beginning of the scheme when patients were required to pay 30 Baht ($0.75) co-payment. Excise tax on alcohol and tobacco were earmarked to fund the scheme [43, 56]. Evidence has proven that tax-funded (especially direct-tax) health insurance is less regressive compared to SHI [45, 57]. Second, contrary to what operates in Nigeria, UCS uses a comprehensive medical package with only very few diseases not covered. This saw improvement in access and equity. Third, there is a purchase-provider split in the payment for health services. Capitations are paid for outpatient service, while DRG is used to pay for inpatient care [57]. Since UCS was introduced, there has been an improvement in health outcomes of the population reflected in Thailand's positive health indices. Moreover, the number of households suffering from catastrophic health spending became insignificant [47, 53]. Thailand's success story will not be complete without pointing out that the resilient political determination, community engagement, evidence-based research, and regular monitoring and evaluation employed by the Thai government were instrumental to achieving the feat [58].

4. Conclusion and recommendations

This study has shown that about 70% of Nigerians pay for healthcare through OOP, hindering their access to quality healthcare. While the trend continues, many households in the country have been impoverished through catastrophic health expenditure. This has culminated in the poor health-seeking and consequent poor health indices. Therefore,

However, the country has the potential to reverse the trend by learning from other countries all over the globe which have achieved UHC by adopting either a tax-based insurance scheme or an SHI scheme. Consequent to this, it is recommended the scheme is overhauled and repositioned to promote equity and access to healthcare. This can be done using an excise tax or "sin tax". The revenue generated could be used to finance the health of the entire country in combination with the existing NHIS. Moreover, this study recommends that the law that established the NHIS should be amended to make insurance mandatory to increase participation. However, adequate awareness should be created for the same reason. The currently fragmented NHIS should be amalgamated for efficiency, risk sharing and fund pooling. The benefits package should also be reviewed to be more comprehensive to attract and encourage enrollees. Enrolment could also be boosted by providing free healthcare to the poor and the vulnerable group, thereby removing inequality and inaccessibility. Finally, in line with the 15% Abuja declaration, there is a need for the government to demonstrate political commitment toward UHC by increasing budgetary allocation to health.

Acknowledgements

I would like to take this opportunity to express my immense gratitude to the many wonderful people who have given their invaluable support and assistance during the preparation of this work.

First and foremost, I am profoundly indebted to my supervisor and mentor, A/ Prof Khurshid Alam who has provided unalloyed support and guide for me during my study at Murdoch University. His enthusiasm and encouragement are instrumental to the success of this work.

I am deeply grateful to Ms. Sandra Crewes for painstakingly reviewing and editing this work, even at a very short notice.

I owe a special debt of gratitude to my darling wife, Abimbola Odunyemi and my daughters, Adebola Odunyemi and Adebusola Odunyemi for being always there for me through thick and thin.

I would like to thank the Australian Government, the Department of Foreign Affair and Trade that provided me the scholarship that allowed me to obtain this lifetime opportunity to acquire first-class learning experience in Australia.

Finally, my profound gratitude goes to God Almighty who is the ultimate source of wisdom and knowledge.

Conflict of interest

The author declares no conflict of interest.

Author details

Adelakun Edward Odunyemi
Murdoch University, Perth, Western Australia, Australia

*Address all correspondence to: drodunyemi@yahoo.com; drlarkay@gmail.com

References

[1] Michael, G., I. Aliyu, and B. Grema, Health financing mechanisms and extension of health coverage to the poor and vulnerable groups: What options are available in the Nigerian context? Journal of Health Research and Reviews, 2019. 6(3).

[2] Qin, V.M., et al., The impact of user charges on health outcomes in low-income and middle-income countries: a systematic review. BMJ Glob Health, 2018. 3(Suppl 3): p. e001087.

[3] Enabulele, O., Achieving Universal Health Coverage in Nigeria: Moving Beyond Annual Celebrations to Concrete Address of the Challenges. World Medical & Health Policy, 2020. 12(1): p. 47-59.

[4] Umeh, C.A., Challenges toward achieving universal health coverage in Ghana, Kenya, Nigeria, and Tanzania. Int J Health Plann Manage, 2018. 33(4): p. 794-805.

[5] Nnamuchi, O., et al., Successes and Failures of Social Health Insurance Schemes in Africa-Nigeria versus Ghana and Rwanda: A Comparative Analysis. Annals of health law / Loyola University Chicago, School of Law, Institute for Health Law, 2019. 28: p. 127 – 148.

[6] Oni, M. Abiodun, and B. Olayinka. Awareness of and Access to National Health Insurance Scheme in Nigeria and Ghana. 2019.

[7] Asante, A., et al., Equity in Health Care Financing in Low- and Middle-Income Countries: A Systematic Review of Evidence from Studies Using Benefit and Financing Incidence Analyses. PLoS One, 2016. 11(4): p. e0152866.

[8] Tandon, A., et al., Measuring overall health system performance for 191 countries. Geneva: World Health Organization, 2000.

[9] Aregbeshola, B.S., A Tax-based, Noncontributory, Health-Financing System Can Accelerate Progress toward Universal Health Coverage in Nigeria. MEDICC review, 2018. 20: p. 40-45.

[10] Edeme, R.K. and O. Olisakwe, Public Health Expenditure, Economic Growth and Health Outcomes in Nigeria. International Journal of Public Policy and Administration Research, 2019. 6(1): p. 23-32.

[11] Adebisi, S.A., J.M. Odiachi, and N.A. Chikere, The National Health Insurance Scheme (NHIS) in Nigeria: Has the Policy Achieved its Intended Objectives? Academic Journal of Economic Studies, 2019. 5: p. 97+.

[12] Oladayo Timothy, P., Needs for Restructuring the Health Sector Financing in Nigeria: An Exploratory Comparative Study. International Journal of Economics & Management Sciences, 2018. 07(03).

[13] Katayama, R. and D. Wadhwa. Half of the world's poor live in just 5 countries. 2019; Available from: https://blogs.worldbank.org/opendata/half-world-s-poor-live-just-5-countries.

[14] Uzochukwu, B.S., et al., Health care financing in Nigeria: Implications for achieving universal health coverage. Niger J Clin Pract, 2015. 18(4): p. 437-444.

[15] Onisanwa, I.D., B.S.-I. Sunday, and M.O. Adaji, Healthcare Financing and Health Status Analysis in Nigeria. Amity Journal of Healthcare Management, 2018. 3 (2): p. 31-42.

[16] Olaniyan, O. and C. Oburota, Equitable Health Care Financing and Universal Health Care Coverage in Nigeria. 2019. 8: p. 25-31.

[17] Adewole, D., A. Adebayo, and K. Osungbade, A qualitative survey of

pre-payment scheme for healthcare services in a rural Nigerian community. African Journal of Biomedical Research, 2017. 20(1): p. 17-24.

[18] Olakunde, B., Public health care financing in Nigeria: Which way forward? Annals of Nigerian Medicine, 2012. 6(1).

[19] Aregbeshola, B.S. and S.M. Khan, Out-of-pocket health-care spending and its determinants among households in Nigeria: a national study. Journal of Public Health, 2020.

[20] Aregbeshola, B.S. and S.M. Khan, Determinants of impoverishment due to out of pocket payments in Nigeria. Journal of Ayub Medical College Abbottabad, 2017. 29(2): p. 194-199.

[21] Amakom, U. and U. Ezenekwe, Implications of households catastrophic out of pocket (OOP) healthcare spending in Nigeria. Journal of Research in Economics and International Finance (JREIF) Vol, 2012. 1(5).

[22] Han, W., Health care system reforms in developing countries. Journal of public health research, 2012. 1(3): p. 199.

[23] Ilesanmi, O.S., A.O. Adebiyi, and A.A. Fatiregun, Contribution of household health care expenditure to poverty in Oyo State, South West Nigeria: A rural and urban comparison. Journal of Health Management & Informatics, 2017. 4(3): p. 64-70.

[24] Onwujekwe, O., et al., Exploring effectiveness of different health financing mechanisms in Nigeria; what needs to change and how can it happen? BMC health services research, 2019. 19(1): p. 661.

[25] Hafez, R., Nigeria Health Financing System Assessment. 2018: World Bank.

[26] Ministry of Budget and National Planning. 2016 Fourth Quarter and Consolidated Budget Implementation Report, Abuja. 2016.

[27] World Bank. World Development Indicators. 2021; Available from: https://data.worldbank.org/indicator/SH.XPD.CHEX.GD.ZS?end=2018&start=2000&view=chart.

[28] Federal Ministry of Health, National Health Accounts 2006-2009. 2009.

[29] Chang, A.Y., et al., Past, present, and future of global health financing: a review of development assistance, government, out-of-pocket, and other private spending on health for 195 countries, 1995-2050. The Lancet, 2019. 393(10187): p. 2233-2260.

[30] Ogaboh, A., N. Osuchukwu, and E. Ushie, National Health Insurance Scheme (NHIS) and Employees' Access to Healthcare Services in Cross River State, Nigeria. Global journal of health science, 2010. 10: p. 9-16.

[31] Amu, H., et al., Understanding variations in health insurance coverage in Ghana, Kenya, Nigeria, and Tanzania: Evidence from demographic and health surveys. PLoS One, 2018. 13(8): p. e0201833.

[32] National Health Insurance Scheme. Programmes. 2020; Available from: https://www.nhis.gov.ng/our-services/#.

[33] Adewole, D. and K. Osungbade, Nigeria National Health Insurance Scheme: A Highly Subsidized Health Care Program for a Privileged Few. International Journal of TROPICAL DISEASE & Health, 2016. 19(3): p. 1-11.

[34] Odeyemi, I.A., Community-based health insurance programmes and the national health insurance scheme of Nigeria: challenges to uptake and integration. International journal for equity in health, 2014. 13(1): p. 20.

[35] Adebayo, E.F., et al., A systematic review of factors that affect uptake of community-based health insurance in low-income and middle-income countries. BMC Health Serv Res, 2015. 15: p. 543.

[36] Raji, B.A., et al., Health status of senior citizens vis-à-vis the National Health Insurance Scheme in Nigeria. Nnamdi Azikiwe University Journal of International Law and Jurisprudence, 2019. 10(1): p. 176-182.

[37] Ezat Wan Puteh, S. and Y. Almualm, Catastrophic Health Expenditure among Developing Countries. Health Systems and Policy Research, 2017. 04(01).

[38] Sakha, M.A., et al., Health financing assessment and policy analysis toward universal health coverage: a systematic review of qualitative research. Global J Health Sci, 2017. 9(5): p. 131-142.

[39] Kutzin, J., W. Yip, and C. Cashin, Alternative Financing Strategies for Universal Health Coverage. 2019.

[40] Averill, C. and A. Marriott, Universal health coverage: why health insurance schemes are leaving the poor behind. 2013: Oxfam International.

[41] Ahangar, A., et al., The Role of Risk-sharing Mechanisms in Finance Health Care and Towards Universal Health Coverage in Low-and Middle-income Countries of World Health Organization Regions. Journal of Preventive Medicine and Public Health, 2018. 51: p. 59-61.

[42] McIntyre, D., et al., Challenges in Financing Universal Health Coverage in Sub-Saharan Africa, in Oxford Research Encyclopedia of Economics and Finance. 2018.

[43] Cotlear, D., et al., Going universal: how 24 developing countries are implementing universal health coverage from the bottom up. 2015: The World Bank.

[44] Wagstaff, A., et al., Equity in the finance of health care: some further international comparisons. J Health Econ, 1999. 18(3): p. 263-290.

[45] Mejía Mejía, A., Is tax funding of health care more likely to be regressive than systems based on social insurance in low-and middle-income countries? Lecturas de Economía, 2013(78): p. 229-239.

[46] Barroy, H., et al., Can Low- and Middle-Income Countries Increase Domestic Fiscal Space for Health: A Mixed-Methods Approach to Assess Possible Sources of Expansion. Health Syst Reform, 2018. 4(3): p. 214-226.

[47] Sumriddetchkajorn, K., et al., Universal health coverage and primary care, Thailand. Bulletin of the World Health Organization, 2019. 97(6): p. 415.

[48] Brown, O., FIXING HEALTHCARE IN NIGERIA. 2018: Flying Doctors Nigeria.

[49] Gupta, V., R. Dhillon, and R. Yates, financing universal health coverage by cutting fossil fuel subsidies. The Lancet Global Health, 2015. 3(6): p. e306-e307.

[50] Doherty, J., et al., Does expanding fiscal space lead to improved funding of the health sector in developing countries? lessons from Kenya, Lagos State (Nigeria) and South Africa. Glob Health Action, 2018. 11(1): p. 1461338.

[51] World Health Organization. Countries. 2020; Available from: https://www.who.int/countries/.

[52] Odeyemi, I.A. and J. Nixon, Assessing equity in health care through the national health insurance schemes of Nigeria and Ghana: a review-based comparative analysis. Int J Equity Health, 2013. 12: p. 9.

[53] Hanvoravongchai, P., Health financing reform in Thailand: toward universal coverage under fiscal constraints. 2013.

[54] Tangcharoensathien, V., et al., The Political Economy of UHC Reform in Thailand: Lessons for Low- and Middle-Income Countries. Health Syst Reform, 2019. 5(3): p. 195-208.

[55] Tangcharoensathien, V., et al., Health systems development in Thailand: a solid platform for successful implementation of universal health coverage. The Lancet, 2018. 391(10126): p. 1205-1223.

[56] Coady, D., B. Clements, and S. Gupta, The Economics of Public Health Care Reform in Advanced and Emerging Economies, in CHAPTER 16: Evidence-Based Health Financing Reform in Thailand. 2012, INTERNATIONAL MONETARY FUND.

[57] Paek, S.C., N. Meemon, and T.T.H. Wan, Thailand's universal coverage scheme and its impact on health-seeking behavior. SpringerPlus, 2016. 5(1): p. 1952-1952.

[58] Dutta, A. and C. Hongoro, Scaling up national health insurance in Nigeria: learning from case studies of India, Colombia, and Thailand. 2013.

Section 2

Healthcare Services

Chapter 9

Screening for Antenatal Depression by Midwives in Low Resource Settings in Primary Care Settings in Malawi

Genesis Chorwe-Sungani

Abstract

Depression significantly contributes to the disease burden of pregnant women. However, depression is often under diagnosed by health professionals especially in antenatal clinics. This is the situation in Malawi where there is no routine screening for depression in antenatal clinics. Nonetheless, screening can enable the effective management of pregnant women with depression at antenatal clinics. There is therefore a need to integrate screening for depression into routine antenatal services to enhance the early identification of antenatal depression and intervention to improve and maintain the well-being of pregnant women and contribute towards achieving the efforts of the Government of Malawi in scaling up the treatment of depression.

Keywords: depression, antenatal, screening, midwives, pregnancy

1. Introduction

Depression affects pregnant women during all stages of their pregnancy [1]. Currently, there is no reliable comprehensive epidemiological statistics about the prevalence of depressive disorders during pregnancy in Malawi, though one study in a rural district reported prevalence of depression as 10.7% (major depression) and 21.1% (minor depression) [2]. These figures fall within prevalence range of depressive disorders during pregnancy (8.3–41%) reported in sub-Saharan Africa [3] with highest prevalence (47%) registered in rural parts of South Africa [4]. There are numerous risk factors which are linked to antenatal depression. In Malawi, a previous study found that lower social support and intimate partner violence were linked with antenatal depression [2]. Similarly, another study revealed that being single, poverty, stressful life events, unplanned pregnancy, childhood trauma, and intimate partner violence predicted antenatal depression [5].

Evidence indicates that antenatal depression and its associated risk factors may be addressed through psychosocial interventions including screening to reduce burden they may cause on an individual [2, 6]. Depression is often under diagnosed by treating health professionals [7] which leads to poorer prognosis of co-morbid physical health conditions in primary healthcare settings [8]. This is likely to put pressure on the poor resources available in antenatal clinics in low resource settings and add an additional burden to pregnant women themselves. The lack of routine screening can also delay identification and treatment of women who are affected by antenatal depression. Delayed diagnosis and treatment of antenatal depression may lead to the early disruption of mother-infant relationships and prolong distress for a mother [6].

Antenatal depression thus causes adverse effects on the mother, family, and community which necessitate interventions of health professionals. Screening for depression can help in timely detection of pregnant women with depression [9]. Currently, there are many instruments for the screening of antenatal depression that are validated in low resource settings [10–12]. Some of these instruments were not specifically developed for use during pregnancy but have been used in these settings. Nevertheless, screening instruments for depression must be accurate (be sensitive and specific) in identifying individuals who have a condition [sensitivity (Se)] and those without a condition [specificity (Sp)] [13].

Currently, pregnant women are not routinely screened for depression in antenatal clinics in Malawi. However, mental health is integrated in general healthcare system at policy level in Malawi [14], so that people could have increased access to mental health services. This means that pregnant women should also receive mental healthcare at antenatal clinics along with the usual antenatal care as needed. Services at antenatal clinics in Malawi include history taking, physical and laboratory examination, antenatal drugs and vaccines and antenatal education [15]. This is similar to what happens in South Africa where antenatal care generally focuses on physical examinations [16].

Integrating mental health with antenatal care requires midwives to assess and deal with mental health problems affecting pregnant women in antenatal care settings in Malawi. Nonetheless, some policy makers fear that mental health interventions may deter midwives from concentrating on other 'priority' interventions [9]. Furthermore, many general healthcare workers, including midwives, in Malawi are not confident and competent enough deal with mental health problems [17]. Research studies have asserted that midwives may lack skills and confidence in screening and treating antenatal depression [18]. This is corroborated by Mathibe-Neke, Rothberg [19] who asserted that midwives from sub-Saharan Africa are not skilled enough to assess and treat common perinatal mental disorders even though they encounter many pregnant women with psychosocial problems. Nonetheless, there is evidence that nurses and midwives can effectively intervene to reduce depressive symptoms during pregnancy [6].

Dealing with antenatal depression can assist in achieving the 17 Sustainable Development Goals (SDGs), particularly, goal number three which focuses on ensuring healthy lives and promoting well-being for all ages [20]. The government of Malawi is already making efforts to achieve SDG 3 (good health and well-being) through the Essential Health Package (EHP) [21] which includes mental disorders as priority conditions for the first time. The government has gone a step further in the Malawi Health Sector Strategic Plan II 2017–2022 to emphasise the first line treatment of depression for the entire population at community, primary and secondary levels of care [22]. It is estimated that there are 847 767 people who are in need of treatment for depression, and the Government has targeted providing access to treatment for 27 822 people by 2022 [22]. In this regard, the Government of Malawi has prioritised research on mental health in the National Health Research Agenda for Malawi (2012–2016) to promote the development of innovative and appropriate treatment strategies for mental health problems affecting the population [23].

1.1 Antenatal care

Antenatal care includes the health assessment of pregnant women, encouraging good health habits, addressing pregnancy related complications and providing social and psychological support [24]. The World Health Organisation (WHO) recommends the implementation of new focused antenatal care which consists of a minimum of eight contacts between the pregnant woman and the healthcare providers with their first contact during the first 12 weeks' gestation, then following contacts taking place at 20, 26, 30, 34, 36, 38 and 40 weeks' gestation [25]. Malawi adopted focused antenatal care more than a decade ago [15, 26] with the aim of helping women to maintain normal pregnancies through identification of pre-existing health conditions, early detection of complications arising during pregnancy, health promotion, disease prevention, birth preparedness and complication readiness planning [27]. It encourages careful identification of pregnant women with special health conditions or risk factors for complications [28]. As described in literature, detection and treatment of diseases, is one of the essential elements of care during pregnancy [29].

In Malawi midwives are frequently the first health professionals who could identify antenatal depression, or to whom a pregnant woman with antenatal depression or any other common perinatal mental disorders may go to seek for help. The country has low mental health specialists to patients ratios (0.01 psychiatrists per 100 000 and 0.22 psychiatric nurses per 100 000) [30] for more than16 million people. This shows that pregnant women attending antenatal clinics may have limited access to mental health specialists. Despite a gross shortage of mental health specialists in the country, midwives therefore could participate in the detection of pregnant women with depression when providing antenatal care.

1.2 Clinical and public health significance of antenatal depression

The lancet series on maternal mental health have established the clinical and public health importance of antenatal depression [31–34]. There is evidence that antepartum depression is highly prevalent in low resource settings [31]. Literature show that antenatal depression is associated with increased rates of adverse child outcomes in low resource settings where pregnant women have increased exposure to risk factors for depression [35]. The adverse mental health outcomes for the child include an increased risk of anxiety, depression, attention deficit hyperactivity disorder, and conduct disorder [35]. It is documented that pregnant women with untreated depression have a higher likelihood of obstetric complications, premature deliveries, and low birthweight infants [34].

Antenatal depression and HIV infection form a vicious cycle, whereby the symptoms of each disease worsen the status of the other, and each needs to be sufficiently treated for the pregnant woman to become healthy [32]. It is of public health concern that pregnant women with co-morbidity of depression and HIV infection are less likely to adhere to antiretroviral therapy, which is critical for her survival and prevention of HIV transmission to the child [33]. Stringer, Meltzer-Brody [32] recommended integration depression-screening technique in antenatal services that could identify a large proportion of affected women to break the cycle of depression and HIV infection interaction. It is documented that integrating mental health services into primary care may be the most viable way of closing treatment gap for mental health in low resource settings [31]. An important step in this direction is the incorporation of the capacity to prevent, recognise, and treat depression within antenatal care [36]. This may help to meet the immediate mental health needs of a pregnant woman, ensure better maternal and child outcomes, and contribute towards success of HIV/AIDS services [32].

Integrated antenatal services aimed at identifying and treating women with antenatal depression are needed because antenatal care is typically the first and only time of interaction with the healthcare system for many women in low resource settings [31]. As such, antenatal care visits provide critically important opportunities for mental health interventions to occur. There is a need to develop protocols for early identification, treatment and preventing the adverse effects of antenatal depression in low resource settings because they do not exist [31]. There is also a need to develop, refine and rigorously evaluate the predictive validity and reliability of instruments for screening of antenatal depression in low resource settings [31].

2. Screening for depression

Screening is the application of an instrument to identify people at risk of a specific condition among people who have not sought medical attention because of symptoms of that condition to warrant further investigation or direct prevention [37]. Literature suggests that it is reasonable to consider screening when the condition in question is significant and prevalent, can be effectively treated and cannot be readily detected without screening [38]. Screening for depression encompasses the use of instruments for measuring symptoms of depression to identify patients who may have depression but who have not sought treatment and whose depression has not already been detected by clinicians [38].

For screening to be successful, it must detect a substantial number of individuals with undiagnosed depression and provide treatment to obtain sufficiently positive results to justify the costs and potential harms associated with screening [38]. It is documented that screening for depression in primary care requires the availability of a lot of resources [9]. In low resource settings, allocation of resources to screening activities could lead to a decline in the quality of care received by patients with more severe depression and who are more clearly in need [38]. More importantly, it is recommended that the WHO minimum criteria for screening should be met before screening is implemented [39].

According to Andermann et al. [39], the following is the aforementioned recommended minimum criteria for screening: [1] the screening programme should respond to a recognised need; [2] the objectives of screening should be defined at the outset; [3] there should be a defined target population; [4] there should be scientific evidence of screening programme effectiveness; [5] the programme should integrate education, testing, clinical services and programme management; [6] there should be quality assurance, with mechanisms to minimise potential risks of screening; [7] the programme should ensure informed choice, confidentiality and respect for autonomy; [8]; the programme should promote equity and access to screening for the entire target population; [9]; programme evaluation should be planned from the outset; and [10] the overall benefits of screening should outweigh the harm. This criteria clearly focuses at improving clinical outcomes of individuals who participate in screening programmes, including pregnant women.

This study complied with the minimum criteria for implementing screening in many ways. Firstly, the aim of this study to develope a screening protocol was response to a need for detecting antenatal depression and associated risk factors. Secondly, the study clearly indicated that pregnant women attending antenatal clinic as target population for the screening of depression. Thirdly, the evidence about effectiveness of the proposed screening protocol for antenatal depression was locally generated by this study some of it was gathered from literature. Fourthly, this study minimised harm and ensured quality by submitting the proposal for review to two research and ethics committees, allowing participants to give consent for their voluntary participation in the study and ensuring privacy by not collecting personal details that could identify them during data collection. Pregnant women who were diagnosed as having depression were refered to a psychiatric unit. Finaly the protocol will be piloted to assess its clinical application and benefits and cost before it is adopted for clinical use. It is hoped that the proposed screening protocol will be used for screening depression in all pregnant women after its adoption.

Screening for depression is useful if it improves patient outcomes beyond those of standard care [38]. However, the Canadian Task Force on Preventive Health Care asserted that there is insufficient evidence about the benefits of screening to recommend routine screening of depression in adults in primary care settings [40]. The fact that there is insufficient evidence to recommend routine screening of depression does not change the importance of depression as a condition that negatively affects quality of life [41]. As such, clinicians in primary care settings should be alert to the possibility of depression in patients with characteristics that may increase their risk of depression [40, 41]. The American College of Preventive Medicine upholds the United States Preventive Services Task Force (USPSTF) proposal that all adults should be screened for depression in primary care settings and that there should be collaboration between primary care providers and mental health specialists to ensure accurate diagnosis and treatment of depression [42].

2.1 Screening for depression in antenatal clinics

During antenatal care, midwives have a duty to screen pregnant women for various conditions [15]. Midwives are expected to routinely screen depression in all pregnant women [43] to improve detection of antenatal depression [44]. There is evidence that screening for depression during pregnancy may reduce depressive symptoms among these women [45]. The American College of Obstetricians and Gynaecologists recommended that pregnant women should be screened for antenatal depression using a standardised and validated instrument [46].

For the routine screening for depression in antenatal care to occur, there is a need for standardised instruments for screening of depression to be designated for use in antenatal clinics in Malawi. Internationally there is evidence that midwives can effectively use instruments for screening of depression during antenatal care [16]. Currently, there are reports which show that EPDS and SRQ are used in research to screen depression during antenatal care in low resource settings [10]. However, screening instruments such as EPDS and SRQ are considered to be too long and time consuming for routine screening [47]. This could present a problem in busy antenatal clinics. In Malawi, antenatal clinics are usually staffed by one or two midwives who attend to a multitude of pregnant women. Literature indicates that antenatal clinics in low resource settings are understaffed, lack infrastructure and do not have adequate instruments for assessing antenatal depression [19]. Screening protocols for antenatal depression could help midwives to implement effective interventions systematically without adding to their workload [9] in these busy antenatal clinics. Routine antenatal visits by pregnant women could provide an appropriate time for antenatal depression screening [48]. Protocols for screening antenatal depression which include instruments that are accurate, acceptable and easy to use in busy, low resource settings therefore are needed [49].

However, midwives may consider screening for antenatal depression to be too demanding and requiring too much effort and this may result in a decreased frequency of screening [50]. The ideal timing and interval for screening for depression is not known [51]. However, Wisconsin Association for Perinatal Care recommends that screening of depression should be done at first antenatal visit and the third trimester of pregnancy [52].

2.2 Treatment for depression

Literature indicates that treatment for antenatal depression exists [53, 54]. A systematic review found that drug therapy, acupuncture, the use of morning light, individual psychotherapy, cognitive behavioural therapy, counselling and end psychodynamic therapy are forms of depression treatment that are used during pregnancy [55]. In addition, systematic reviews and controlled clinical trials found that various forms of psychotherapy [45, 54, 56–62], massage therapy [54, 61], exercise [63, 64], and drug therapy [55] may be effective in treating depression during pregnancy. This is supported by Whooley [65] who asserted that exercise and other self-management strategies, behavioural activation, structured psychotherapy, and/or pharmacotherapy are effective treatments for depression.

However, some authors of systematic reviews have argued that there is no conclusive evidence on the effectiveness of these treatments for depression during pregnancy [54–56]. All in all one can argue that the lack of evidence on effectiveness of some treatments for depression during pregnancy does not mean that antenatal depression cannot be treated but simply means that evidence is not available.

2.3 Instruments for screening of depression

Screening for depression during pregnancy can be done using various instruments such as EPDS [66], Hopkins Symptoms Checklist 15 (HSCL-15) [67], SRQ [68] and Whooley's Questions [69]. Most of these screening instruments were not specifically developed for use during antenatal periods [66–68]. However, there are also numerous instruments for screening antenatal depression that were also validated for use in low resource settings [70] (**Table 1**).

Screening instruments which were validated in specific settings have a high likelihood of generating accurate results [71] and may reduce the under-detection of depression in those settings. However, screening instruments are generally limited in their accuracy [72] and their performance varies with populations or settings [73]. For instance, previous studies found that EPDS had different levels of accuracy and validity in antenatal clinics in various countries [10, 70, 74–76].

2.4 Validity of screening instruments

The performance of screening instruments may vary with settings [73]. A concern is that most instruments for the screening of depression were validated in high

S.No	Screening Instrument	AUC	Se	Sp
1	Beck Depression Index	.87	.87	.74
2	Centre for Epidemiologic Studies Depression Scale 20	.82	.73	.79
3	Edinburgh Postnatal Depression Scale	.97	.87	.92
4	Hamilton Rating Scale for Depression	.86	.88	.75
5	Hopkins Symptoms Checklist 25	.86	.89	.8
6	Kessler Psychological Distress Scale 10	.95	1	.81
7	Self-Reporting Questionnaire	.83	.76	.81

Source: Chorwe-Sungani and Chipps [70].

Table 1
Summary of screening instruments that were validated in low resource settings.

income countries (HICs) whose contexts are dissimilar from those of low resource settings [77]. For example, there is evidence that the Edinburgh Postnatal Depression Scale's (EPDS) discriminant ability in detecting antenatal depression varies according to settings [74–76]. The two most commonly used instruments in low resource settings, namely the EPDS and the Self Reporting Questionnaire (SRQ), were reported to be easy to administer to pregnant women by interviewers in Malawi [10]. However, evidence is emerging that some health professionals may find screening instruments which have 5 or more items as long, cumbersome and time consuming for routine screening [47]. Ultra-brief screening instruments (having 4 or less items) can promote screening for depression in busy antenatal clinics [78] and screening instruments with binary questions such as Whooley's questions are less time consuming and easy to score [49].

It is documented that screening instruments which require individuals to choose more than 2 responses for each question may not be easy to apply among illiterate pregnant women in Malawi [10]. These screening instruments should be valid to assist health professionals to effectively detect antenatal depression [38, 79]. A validation process through the application of a gold standard (a clinical diagnostic assessment) is required to confirm a diagnosis of depression among pregnant women who test positive on a screening instrument.

Midwives should use valid screening instruments for them to effectively detect pregnant women with antenatal depression. A valid instrument should have an ability to measure what it is supposed to measure [80] and this is determined by its Se, Sp, PPV and NPV [81]. The sensitivity of a screening instrument refers to the proportion of people with disease that are correctly identified (true positives) by the instrument while specificity is the proportion of people without the disease who will have a negative result (true negatives) [71]. Sensitivity and specificity of a screening instrument are determined by comparing the results of the instrument against the outcomes of a gold standard. A gold standard is the single instrument (or a combination of instruments) that is considered the current preferred method of diagnosing a particular condition [82]. A good screening instrument should have both high sensitivity and specificity [83]. Nevertheless, sensitivity and specificity of a screening instrument are often in balance (trade off) and can vary with optimum cut off scores which are determined through using a Youden index [84, 85].

Both sensitivity and specificity are equally important although a screening instrument can be very specific without being sensitive, or it can be very sensitive without being specific [83]. It is recommended that a suitable screening instrument should have a minimum acceptable balance of Se/Sp (.8/.7) [86]. However, the sensitivity and specificity of a screening instrument has limited use in clinical practice when compared to PPV and NPV because they do not help clinicians to estimate the probability of disease in individual patients [71]. PPV and NPV measure the likelihood that a positive or negative screening result is accurate for an individual [53]. PPV and NPV of a screening instrument depend on the prevalence of disease in a population so that PPV increases with increasing prevalence of disease and NPV decreases with increasing prevalence [82].

These predictive values are more useful measures of diagnostic accuracy in routine clinical practice because they assist a clinician to know the probability of a correct diagnosis being made [71]. An instrument which has high sensitivity and NPV 'rules OUT' the disease while the one with high specificity and PPV 'rules IN' the disease [82]. Thus a highly sensitive screening instrument is most helpful to the clinician when the result is negative because an individual who screens negative is very unlikely to have the disease [71]. Similarly, a screening instrument with high specificity is also most helpful to the clinician when the result is positive because an individual who screens positive is likely to have the disease. Literature indicates that a screening instrument cannot be valid without it reliably and consistently measuring what it is supposed to measure [87]. This suggests that for effective screening of depression in antenatal clinics, clinicians must utilise accurate screening instruments. Screening for antenatal depression using valid instruments can assist health professionals to accurately identify pregnant women who need mental health interventions [79].

Accuracy refers to the degree to which a measurement represents the true value of the attribute being measured, and can be determined by comparing results from a screening instrument with results generated by a gold standard using scores for area under curve (AUC) [88], sensitivity and specificity [89]. In this context validity and accuracy may be used synonymously. AUC scores are used to categorise the accuracy of a screening instrument as low (0.5–0.7), moderate (>0.7–0.9) and high (>0.9) [90]. The higher the AUC score, the more accurate a screening instrument is in detecting individuals with or without the condition being tested [83]. As such, highly accurate instruments are necessary for the screening of depression in antenatal clinics [70]. In addition, these screening instruments should be quick and easy to use in low resource settings [8, 78].

3. Ethics of screening

Health professionals, including midwives, are required to deal with diverse ethical issues when new intervention strategies are developed because they may be unfamiliar with the ethical standards associated with the new practice [91]. It is documented that screening may do more harm than good and it is ethical for clinicians to ensure that the benefits from the screening of each individual must outweigh the harm [39]. Potential harms from routine screening for depression include the treatment of depression in individuals who are incorrectly identified as having the condition, and the treatment of mild symptoms that would often resolve without intervention [38]. As such, clinicians must be open and honest in telling their clients about the accuracy of screening instruments [91] in detecting antenatal depression. According to Sjögren [72], screening instruments are generally limited in their accuracy and interpretation of their results may lead to incorrect conclusions such that if the result is falsely negative, the individuals will consider themselves healthy, when they are actually ill, or if the result is falsely positive, a healthy individual will leave the practice with a false diagnosis.

3.1 Ethics of screening for depression

Screening for depression should include the provision of depression care support apart from those targeted at improving the effectiveness of treatment [92]. It should also ensure that an individuals' rights to informed choice, confidentiality and autonomy are respected by clinicians [39]. It is important that individuals should provide fully informed consent and be assured of confidentiality before they are screened for [91] depression. Literature suggests that screening and referral for depression within the clinical settings makes it difficult for clinicians to maintain confidentiality [93] about a client's information. Clinicians have an ethical responsibility to ensure that the findings of screenings are not misunderstood or misused in manner that is detrimental to their client's well-being by the clients themselves, their families, community, other clinicians or policymakers [91].

3.2 Ethics of screening for depression in antenatal clinics

Screening for depression during pregnancy may evoke a lot of ethical questions that need to be answered before midwives start implementing screening programmes. For instance, false positives may be of ethical concern because they may add a burden to pregnant women and to clinical services. Screening may result in the use of medications, many of which can cause adverse effects [94] in pregnant women who are falsely detected as having depression. As such, a screening programme must be socially acceptable and must be at an acceptable cost [95] to pregnant women and their families. It is possible that some pregnant women may be placed on anti-depressant medications unnecessarily and will consequently be exposed to the negative side effects associated with these drugs [38]. However, when screening for antenatal depression, a higher level of false positives may be considered acceptable as, ethically, it would seem better not to miss a pregnant woman who needs treatment and support. As described in literature, it is possible for clinicians to exclude false positives from unnecessary treatment by conducting a further diagnostic assessment (gold standard) on all individuals, who screened positive, to confirm the presence of the disorder [94, 96, 97]. This is corroborated by Thombs, Coyne [38] who asserted that individuals who screen positive for depression need further assessment and, if confirmed, should be offered treatment.

A drawback is that the infrastructure and human resources required to implement an effective screening programme can be so costly that allocation of scarce resources demand the appropriate application of ethical principles of justice and equity [39]. It is documented that it is unethical to screen individuals without providing them with relevant interventions because it deprives them of rights to control their own lives and access to treatment [91]. Pregnant women who are diagnosed with depression may be discriminated or socially rejected by society [98]. It is an ethical concern that after screening, a substantial proportion of women diagnosed with false positives may experience discrimination, self-stigma, and stress for unjustifiable reasons [91]. Although little is known about the possible "nocebo effect" of telling individuals who are otherwise not specifically concerned about their mental health that they have depression [38], a label of antenatal depression may negatively affect personal identity, relationships and the self-esteem of pregnant women [91]. The "nocebo effect" occurs when verbal suggestions of an adverse outcome can lead to the onset or exacerbation of symptoms [99].

The new label of having antenatal depression may influence the future goals of individuals and the type of support they may receive from significant others [91]. It is documented that individuals labelled with mental illness may lose their sense of entitlement to participation in community activities [98]. It is possible that pregnant women, who screen positive for depression, may start distancing themselves from others, in anticipation of the associated stigma of depression, and this may negatively impact on their utilisation of antenatal and other social services. There is evidence which shows that stigmas due to a diagnosis of depression is one of the barriers to treatment among women [100]. However, opposing evidence showed that pregnant women who participated in screening for antenatal depression did not feel stigmatised, labelled or distressed by the screening process [101]. This is corroborated by Siu, Bibbins-Domingo [51] who asserted that the negative effects of screening for depression in adults is small or sometimes non-existent.

4. Cultural aspects of depression and treatment in Malawi

In Malawi, all communities have their own explanations for illness. It is believed that mental disorders such as depression is caused by witchcraft, possession by spirits and 'evil eye' (punishment directed at a person by another person or a supernatural being) [102]. In addition, 'Chauta' (God) may punish wrongdoers who violate taboos [102]. Mental disorders may be caused by parents performing culturally disapproved forms of sexual intercourse such as not abstaining from sexual activity from seventh month of pregnancy until six months after delivery to prevent the child from suffering from mental disorder [103]. This shows that cultural beliefs should be considered as one of important factors which influence mental health interventions [104].

People may have negative cultural beliefs about mental disorders embedded in their community. Cultural beliefs related to mental disorders may affect the way the mentally ill person is handled locally [102]. Explanations of mental disorders, be it witchcraft, angry ancestors, will of God determine the acceptance of affected person's condition [103]. People who believe in witchcraft as a cause of mental disorders may have no hope about recovery in the absence of traditional medicine [104]. It is believed that pregnant women should avoid conflict with others because they may bewitch her to cause delay and complications in labour [105]. It is documented that people who fear witchcraft avoid offending other people who might use magical charms to retaliate [102]. Stewart, Umar [105] found that witchcraft was considered as a very real danger that makes a pregnant woman and her unborn baby vulnerable to illness.

Traditional healers use charms, herbs or mental suggestions to treat mental disorders [102]. However, stigma towards mental disorders exists in Malawi [106] such that treatment may not be sought for an individual with depression who is not causing any trouble [102]. Furthermore, when people are sick, they want to know cultural explanations of their sickness such that they consult traditional healers before going for western medicine, or use both to be on the safe side [102]. This may suggest the need for developing culturally appropriate mental health interventions [106] for screening and treating of depression in pregnant women and other populations in the country.

There is evidence that the pathway to psychiatric care for patients with psychological problems in Malawi is comparable to other developing countries whereby traditional healers and paramedics play a significant role [107]. However, many cultural beliefs related to mental disorders are being challenged [102] and there is high utilisation of health services for people with common mental disorders in the local Primary Health Care settings [108]. This may suggest that screening for depression in local antenatal clinics may be feasible despite the prevailing cultural beliefs on mental disorders. In Malawi, mental health services are provides in all health centres, district hospitals and central hospitals across the country [17].

5. Task shifting in screening of antenatal depression in low resource settings

Mental disorders are underdiagnosed by primary care health workers in low resource settings, where mental health specialists are scarce [31]. This poses a challenge to integration of screening of depression into antenatal care. However, literature suggests task shifting approaches could be used to effectively deliver mental healthcare in primary health care settings [109]. Task shifting refers to the rational redistribution of tasks among health workforce teams, with specific tasks moved from highly qualified health workers to health workers with shorter training and fewer qualifications in order to make efficient use of the available human resources [110]. In task shifting, tasks are shifted from health workers with more general training to workers with specific training for a particular task [111]. For instance, non-specialist health professionals or lay workers able to detect, diagnose, treat, and monitor individuals with mental disorders after receiving brief training and appropriate supervision by mental health specialists [109]. This may help to mitigate the impact of health worker shortages an may provide an opportunity for establishing equitable and sustainable health systems in low resource settings [110].

Task shifting aims at increasing the number of healthcare services provided at a given quality and cost, or providing the same level of healthcare services at a given quality at a lower cost [111]. As such, task shifting may be of essence in this study because it proposes the inclusion of screening of depression in antenatal services which requires midwives to take up new tasks of detecting and treating of antenatal depression. In Uganda, nurses who run health centres diagnose and prescribe in addition to their usual nursing and midwifery duties [110]. Similarly, anecdote reports indicate that task shifting makes nurses/midwives in Malawi, especially those deployed in health centres, to operate beyond their scope of practice because circumstances demand that they do patient assessment, diagnosis and prescribing. This underscores the importance of having relevant policies and legislations to regulate the implementation of task shifting without compromising quality of care [110] in antenatal clinics.

In line with task shifting, the WHO recommended that the provision of mental health services in primary care should be the responsibility of primary care workers such as nurses and midwives who must receive ongoing training and supervision from specialist mental health specialists [112]. This is corroborated by Honikman, van Heyningen [16] who found that midwives were able to screen for depression and refer pregnant women appropriately after receiving some training in South Africa. Non-specialist health workers can effectively detect, diagnose, treat, and prevent common and severe mental disorders [109]. It is documented that task-shifting mental health interventions from specialised to non-specialised health workers to treat common mental disorders could expanding access to mental healthcare [112]. Furthermore, task shifting can substantially reduce the expected number of healthcare providers otherwise needed to close mental health service gaps at primary health care level in low resource settings [113].

However, task-sharing should not be viewed as an “outright solution” to the human resource crisis in low resource settings because specialist services will always be required regardless of the innovativeness and effectiveness of task shifting approaches in reducing the mental health treatment gap [112]. Considering that midwives in antenatal clinics in low resource settings are overburdened with increased workload [19], there is a need to ensure that task shifting happens in a team, based on which cadres are available, which tasks need to be undertaken and who has which competencies [110]. This study proposed that midwives who are readily available in antenatal clinics and mental health specialists-though scarce-should collaborate when screening for antenatal depression.

In Malawi task sharing initiative which involved lay health workers in providing mental health services led to the establishment of a new service within the community which increased access to mental health services [114]. The lay health workers received mental health training and were supervised by health professionals. There was increase in detection of people with severe mental illness by lay health workers. Lay health workers were also able to treat or refer patients with distress based on their assessment. However, the decision to refer patients to a district hospital was made by professional health workers. This is a local mental health initiative on which may inform successful implementation of the proposed screening protocol for antenatal depression in the country.

Best-buy interventions may be another approach of implementing mental health services in antenatal clinics. These interventions emphasise cost effectiveness, feasibility, affordability and scalability [115]. Implementation of buy-in interventions depends on appropriateness of setting, capacity of system to deliver a given intervention to a targeted group of people, technical complexity of intervention and acceptability. It is hoped that screening of depression using the proposed screening protocol would be best-buy interventions because it will be integrated in usual antenatal care provided by midwives. However, mental health specialists remain key in screening of antenatal depression due to complexity of its diagnostic assessments and treatments. This may suggest the importance of utilising task sharing when providing best buy-interventions.

Mantal health services have traditionally been offered in psychiatric institutions. Nonetheless, the proposed screening protocol for antenatal depression suggests provision of mental healthcare to pregnant women in unconventional settings of care. Interventions in unconventional settings model focuses on expanding care beyond traditional locales of service into settings where individuals attend [115]. Provision of care in unconventional settings open multiple opportunities to reach out to individuals or populations not otherwise served. However, implementation of this approach in local antenatal clinics may increase workload for midwives who are already burdened.

6. Screening algorithm

This section present a screening algorithm that can facilitate provision of maternal mental healthcare that is not readily accessible to pregnant women in Malawi [116]. It is underpinned by the proposition that routine screening in antenatal clinics improves detection of pregnant women with depression and that midwives can be trained to effectively screen for antenatal depression, offer psychoeducation and, make appropriate referrals. The aim of the algorithm is to improve the health of pregnant women and the child they are expecting. The algorithm includes aim, rationale, scope, objectives, principles underpinning algorithm, and components of algorithm.

6.1 Rationale for the algorithm

The algorithm will ensure a standardised and quality assured approach for detecting and dealing with pregnant women who have or are at risk of developing depression. It will make it possible for midwives to detect pregnant women with depression at an early stage and be able to put in place appropriate support systems for these women. In addition, the algorithm allows for the involvement of the pregnant women and their families in discussions about their care and treatment options. Furthermore, it ensures that information about pregnant women with depression is documented and shared appropriately with all relevant practitioners providing care. Collaborative care for adults with depression which produces substantial clinical improvements and has a high prospect of long-term cost savings is recommended. Collaborative care of depression includes a systematic, multicomponent, and team-based approach that strengthens and supports self-care, while assuring that effective medical, preventive, and health maintenance interventions take place to improve the quality and outcome of patient care. Therefore, the Algorithm recommends effective collaboration of antenatal services and mental health services for effective screening of antenatal depression.

6.2 Scope of the algorithm

The Algorithm is specifically designed for pregnant women with depression and it is not intended to cover the whole spectrum of pregnant women with other mental disorders. It focuses on improving the quality and accessibility of maternal mental healthcare by integrating routine screening for depression into antenatal services so that pregnant women with, or at risk of, depression are timeously detected, and the appropriate treatment can commence. The Algorithm is intended to reflect optimum practice in routine screening for depression and the management of pregnant women at risk or with depression in antenatal clinics in Malawi.

6.3 Objectives of the algorithm

The objectives of the Algorithm are to:

1. Detect pregnant women who have or are at risk of depression in local antenatal clinics;

2. Refer pregnant women, who have been detected with depression, to the relevant mental health services.

6.4 The principles underpinning algorithm

The following principles will enable the Algorithm to be useful in the context of antenatal clinics in Malawi:

1. The Algorithm should facilitate human rights based screening for depression which will ensure early identification and treatment.

2. The Algorithm should be based on the clinical needs of pregnant women and clinicians involved in the provision of health services in antenatal clinics.

3. The Algorithm should be owned by the midwifery profession which should take a leading role in lobbying for the integration of routine screening for depression into antenatal services and policy.

4. An implementation plan for the Algorithm need to be developed.

6.5 Algorithm for screening

The Algorithm, to ensure an effective and multidisciplinary approach to routine screening of depression in antenatal clinics, is diagrammatically presented in **Figure 1**.

6.6 Components of the algorithm

The components of the Algorithm include: antenatal services and antenatal care assessment; midwives' functions, screening instruments and mental health assessment.

6.6.1 Antenatal services and antenatal assessment

Midwives provide antenatal services to the majority of women in Malawi. These services include antenatal assessment, encouraging good health habits, addressing pregnancy related complications and provision of psychosocial support. The World Health Organisation (WHO) recommends that antenatal care should consists of four visits for normal pregnancies with the first visit in the first trimester (before 12 weeks but not later than16 weeks) and subsequently at 24–28 weeks, 32 weeks and 36 weeks. An antenatal assessment includes taking a psychosocial, medical and

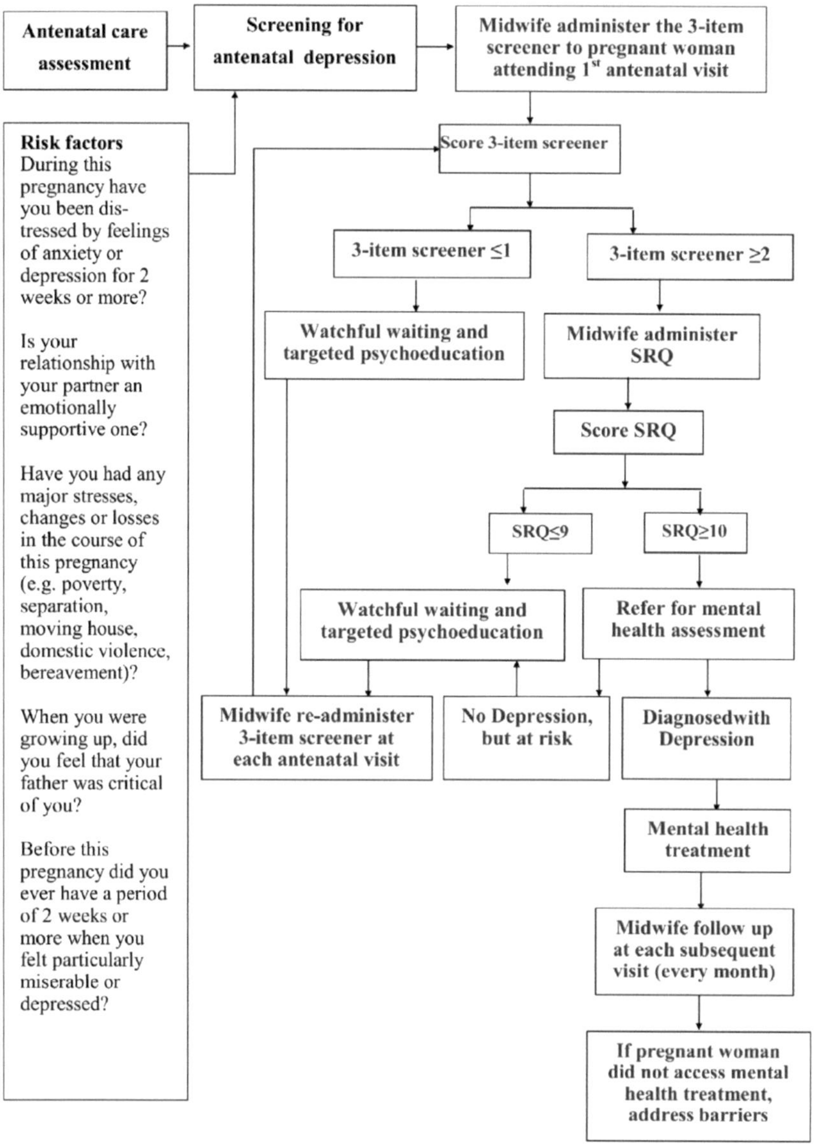

Figure 1.
Algorithm for screening of antenatal depression.

obstetric history; a complete general and obstetrical examination; screening for HIV and Syphilis; and testing for proteinuria, blood/rhesus group and bacteriuria. History taking provides the midwife with an opportunity to screen for depression during the antenatal assessment.

6.6.2 Midwives functions

The functions of a midwife in screening for antenatal depression include:

Screening for depression of all pregnant women attending antenatal clinics and to facilitate the management of those detected with depression;

- Appropriately referring pregnant women with probable depression for mental health assessment using Algorithm pathway;

- To be a resource person for other healthcare professionals in the care of pregnant women undergoing screening for antenatal depression;
- To provide information about the screening for antenatal depression and available specialist support services to pregnant women and their families;
- To liaise with the relevant members of the multidisciplinary team to facilitate the effective screening for depression; and provision of appropriate care and support for pregnant women with depression in antenatal clinics;
- To maintain a knowledge base in screening for antenatal depression by attending in-service training, undergoing continuous professional development sessions and attending relevant conferences;
- To provide education and training related to screening for depression to all staff in antenatal clinics;
- To maintain a register of results, of the screening for depression done, in antenatal clinics and produce reports to relevant authorities;
- To participate in the development of policies, procedures and guidelines related to screening for depression in antenatal clinics; and
- To monitor quality and effectiveness of screening for depression inantenatal and take effective action to address issues and promote quality.

6.6.3 1Screening instruments

Algorithm recommends the use of the 3-item screener and the SRQ to screen for antenatal depression in the local setting.

6.6.3.1 The 3-item screener

6.6.3.1.1 Instructions

Remember - The 3-item screener is a screening instrument and should never override clinical judgement. A Self Reporting Questionnaire (SRQ) should be administered to confirm caseness of pregnant women who screen positive on the 3-item screener.

6.6.3.1.2 Administration

1. Administer either Chichewa or English versions of the 3-item screener depending on the language which a client can easily understand.
2. Read the questions aloud to the pregnant woman and ask her to respond 'Yes' or 'No' depending on how she is feeling now or has been feeling in the **past month**.
3. Circle the response given by a woman against the corresponding question
4. All the 3 items in the 3-item screener must be completed.
5. Care should be taken to avoid the possibility of the pregnant woman discussing her answers with others. (Answers should come directly from the pregnant woman)

6.6.3.1.3 Scoring

1. Each question is scored with a 0 for 'No' (AYI) or 1 for 'Yes' (EYA).
2. The higher a score is, the more likely the woman is experiencing some level of antenatal depression.
3. When validating the 3-item screener in antenatal clinics in the Blantyre district, optimum cut off score of greater than 1 was used.
4. Administer SRQ to all pregnant women who score 2 or more on the 3- item screener. If the 3-item screener score is 1 or less, stop.

Please circle the response that comes closest to how a client has been feeling. *Please answer all questions*

Here is an EXAMPLE already completed

	No	Yes	
Are you tired?	0	(1)	This would mean: 'Client is feeling tired'. Please complete the other questions in the same way

English version

	NO	YES
During the past month, have you been bothered by feeling down depressed or hopeless?	0	1
During the past month, have you been bothered by little interest or pleasure in doing things?	0	1
Are you depressed?	0	1

Chichewa version

	AYI	EYA
Kodi mmwezi wapitawu mwakhala mukuvutika mumtima mwanu chifukwa chakukhumudwa kapena kukhala opanda chiyembekezo?	0	1
Kodi mmwezi wapitawu mwakhala mukuvutika mumtima mwanu chifukwa chokhala opanda chidwi kapena kusasangalatsidwa pochita zinthu?	0	1
Kodi mumtima mwanu mukumva kuti ndinu okhumudwa?	0	1

For official use only	**Screened on**	**Score**
Name of Client:______________________	Date: __________	Total: _____
Administered by: ______________________		

Sources: Whooley, M. A., Avins, A. L., Miranda, J., & Browner, W. S. (1997). Case-finding instruments for depression. *Journal of general internal medicine, 12* (7), 439-445.

Vahter, L., Kreegipuu, M., Talvik, T., & Gross-Paju, K. (2007). One question as a screening instrument for depression in people with multiple sclerosis. *Clinical rehabilitation, 21*(5), 460-464.

6.6.3.2 Self-Reporting Questionnaire (SRQ)

6.6.3.2.1 Instructions

Remember - The SRQ is a screening instrument and should never override clinical judgement. A diagnostic mental health assessment should be done to confirm presence or absence of depression.

6.6.3.2.2 Administration

1. Administer either Chichewa or English versions of the SRQ depending on the language which a client can easily understand.

2. Read the questions aloud to the pregnant woman with low literacy and ask her to respond 'Yes' or 'No' depending on how she has been feeling in the previous 4 weeks.

3. Circle the response given by a woman against the corresponding question

4. All the 20 items in the SRQ must be completed.

5. Care should be taken to avoid the possibility of the pregnant woman discussing her answers with others. (Answers should come directly from the pregnant woman)

6.6.3.2.3 Scoring

1. Each question is scored with a 0 for 'No' or 1 for 'Yes'.

2. The higher a score is, the more likely the woman is experiencing some level of antenatal depression.

3. Standard cut off score of 10 or greater is recommended as an indicator of possible depression [117]

4. When validating SRQ in antenatal clinics in the Blantyre district, optimum cut off score of greater than 9 was used.

5. Refer for diagnostic mental health assessment all pregnant women who score 10 or more on SRQ.

6. If a pregnant woman scores 1 specifically on questions 16 or 17, immediate action is needed. An immediate emergency referral to a mental health professional may be the most appropriate next step if a patient has suicidal ideation.

Self-Reporting Questionnaire (SRQ)

Instructions

Please circle the response that comes closest to how you have been feeling **IN THE PAST 4 WEEKS**. Please answer all questions

---

Here is an EXAMPLE already completed

	NO	YES	
Do you feel restless?	0	(1)	This would mean: 'I have felt restless in the past 4 weeks' Please complete the other questions in the same way

---

Please answer all questions below:
(Circle one answer in each question)

With reference to the past 4 weeks:

	NO	YES
1. Do you often have headaches?	0	1
2. Is your appetite poor?	0	1
3. Do you sleep badly?	0	1
4. Are you easily frightened?	0	1
5. Do your hands shakes?	0	1
6. Do you feel nervous, tense or worried?	0	1
7. Is your digestion poor?	0	1
8. Do you have trouble thinking clearly?	0	1
9. Do you feel unhappy?	0	1
10. Do you cry more than usual?	0	1
11. Do you find it difficult to enjoy your daily activities?	0	1
12. Do you find it difficult to make decisions?	0	1
13. Is your daily work suffering?	0	1
14. Are you unable to play a useful part in life?	0	1
15. Have you lost interest in things?	0	1
16. Do you feel that you are a worthless person?	0	1
17. Has the thought of ending your life been on your mind?	0	1
18. Do you feel tired all the time?	0	1
19. Do you have uncomfortable feelings in your stomach?	0	1
20. Are you easily tired?	0	1

For official use only	**Screened on**	**Score**
Name of Client:______________________________	Date: ____________	Total: ______
Administered by: ____________________________	Scores for #16 and / or 17 ________	

Sources: Beusenberg, M., Orley, J. H., & World Health Organization. (1994). A User's guide to the self reporting questionnaire (SRQ). Geneva: World Health Organisation.

Kumbhar, U. T., Dhumale, G. B., & Kumbhar, U. P. (2012). Self Reporting Questionnaire as a tool to diagnose psychiatric morbidity. *Natl J Med Res, 2*, 51-54.

Self-Reporting Questionnaire (SRQ)-Chichewa version

Malangizo

Chondezungulizaniyankholomwelikufananirandimomwemwakhalamukumvera ma **SABATA ANAYI APITAWA.**Chondeyankhanimafunsoonse

Ichindi CHITSANZO choyankha kale

	AYI	EYA	
Kodi mumakhala osakhazikika?	0	1 (circled)	Tanthauzo: 'Mumakhala osakhazikika mmasabata anayiapitawa'

Chonde yankhani mafunso enawanso chimodzimodzi

Chondeyankhanimafunsoonsealimmunsiwa:

(Zungulizaniyankholimodzi pa funsolirilonse)

	AYI	EYA
1. M'masabata anayi apitawa, kodi mumamvakupweteka mutu pafupipafupi?	0	1
2. M'masabata anayi apitawa, kodi simumakhala ndichilakolako cha chakudya?	0	1
3. M'masabata anayi apitawa, kodi mumavutika kugona usiku?	0	1
4. M'masabata anayi apitawa, kodi manja anu amanjenjemera?	0	1
5. M'masabata anayi apitawa, kodi mumakhala ndinkhawa, mantha kapena madandaulo?	0	1
6. M'masabata anayi apitawa, kodi simumachedwa kututumutsidwa?	0	1
7. M'masabata anayi apitawa, kodi mumadzimbidwa dzimbidwa?	0	1
8. M'masabata anayi apitawa, kodi mumakhala ndivuto kuganiza bwinobwino?	0	1
9. M'masabata anayi apitawa, kodi mumakhala osasangalala kapena osakondwa?	0	1
10. M'masabata anayi apitawa, kodi mumaliralira pafupipafupi ndipo koposera muyeso?	0	1
11. M'masabata anayi apitawa, kodi mumaona ngati ndichinthu chokuvutani kusangalatsidwa ndizinthu zimene mumapanga tsiku ndi tsiku?	0	1
12. M'masabata anayi apitawa, kodi mumakhala ndivuto kupanga maganizo Kapena kumangamfundo?	0	1
13. M'masabataanayiapitawa, kodintchitozanuzatsikunditsikusizimayenda bwino?	0	1
14. M'masabataanayiapitawa, kodimumalepherakupangazinthuzaphindu kapenazofunikiram'moyowanu?	0	1
15. M'masabataanayiapitawa, kodimunasiyakukhalandichidwi mu zinthu zosiyanasiyana?	0	1
16. M'masabata anayi apitawa, kodi mumaziona ngati ndinu munthu wopanda ntchito kapena wosafunikira?	0	1
17. M'masabataanayiapitawa, kodimaganizoodziphaanayambaakubwereranipo?	0	1
18. M'masabata anayi apitawa, kodi mumamva kapena kukhala otopatopa nthawi zonse?	0	1
19. M'masabata anayi apitawa, kodi mumakhala ndi vuto losamva bwino m'mimba?	0	1
20. M'masabata anayi apitawa, kodi simumachedwa kutopa?	0	1

For official use only	**Screened on**	**Score**
Name of Client: ____________	Date: ________	Total: _____
Administered by: ____________	Scores for #16 and / or 17 _______	

Sources:Beusenberg, M., Orley, J. H., & World Health Organization. (1994). A User's guide to the self reporting questionnaire (SRQ). Geneva: World Health Organisation.

Kumbhar, U. T., Dhumale, G. B., & Kumbhar, U. P. (2012). Self Reporting Questionnaire as a tool to diagnose psychiatric morbidity. *Natl J Med Res, 2*, 51-54.

7. Conclusion

Depression significantly affects women during pregnancy and may lead to adverse outcomes. Screening for depression does not usually form part of antenatal care in low resource settings. Midwives in these settings may often have limited consultation time to screen for depression due to inadequate human and material resources. Antenatal depression is highly prevalent among pregnant women living with HIV. Antenatal depression also remains an important condition which negatively affects pregnant women's quality of life, but one that may respond to treatment. Numerous instruments are validated for screening antenatal depression in low resource settings although they were developed in high income countries. When screening, a short screening instrument can be used for initial screening with only positives screens being referred for more detailed screening. This would allow for a distributed workload in busy antenatal clinics. For effective screening for depression to be achieved in antenatal clinics, screening protocols for depression should be integrated into standard antenatal care. Successful implementation of the proposed screening would require implementation of relevant task shifting approaches that to effectively deliver mental healthcare in local settings. Ethical questions may arise around screening for depression during pregnancy as there is the potential that it may cause harm. However, the extent of harm from screening for depression is negligible or at times non-existent. Despite the prevailing cultural beliefs on mental disorders, screening for depression in local antenatal clinics may be feasible. Antenatal care contacts provide opportunities for screening depression and there is a need to develop protocols for early detection, treatment and preventing the adverse effects of antenatal depression in low resource settings.

Conflict of interest

None.

Notes/thanks/other declarations

Not applicable.

Author details

Genesis Chorwe-Sungani
Kamuzu College of Nursing, University of Malawi, Blantyre, Malawi

*Address all correspondence to: genesischorwe@kcn.unima.mw

References

[1] Kaaya S, Mbwambo J, Fawzi MS, Van Den Borne H, Schaalma H, Leshabari M. Understanding women's experiences of distress during pregnancy in Dar es Salaam, Tanzania. Tanzania journal of health research. 2010;12(1):36–46.

[2] Stewart RC, Umar E, Tomenson B, Creed F. A cross-sectional study of antenatal depression and associated factors in Malawi. Arch Women's Ment Health. 2014;17(2):145–154.

[3] Stewart RC, Kauye F, Umar E, Vokhiwa M, Bunn J, Fitzgerald M, et al. Validation of a Chichewa version of the self-reporting questionnaire (SRQ) as a brief screening measure for maternal depressive disorder in Malawi, Africa. Journal of Affective Disorders. 2009;112 (1):126–134.

[4] Rochat TJ, Tomlinson M, Bärnighausen T, Newell M-L, Stein A. The prevalence and clinical presentation of antenatal depression in rural South Africa. Journal of Affective Disorders. 2011;135(1):362–373.

[5] Brittain K, Myer L, Koen N, Koopowitz S, Donald KA, Barnett W, et al. Risk factors for antenatal depression and associations with infant birth outcomes: Results from a South African birth cohort study. Paediatric and Perinatal Epidemiology. 2015;29(6):505–514.

[6] Clarke K, King M, Prost A. Psychosocial interventions for perinatal common mental disorders delivered by providers who are not mental health specialists in low-and middle-income countries: a systematic review and meta-analysis. PLoS Med. 2013;10(10): e1001541.

[7] Vahter L, Kreegipuu M, Talvik T, Gross-Paju K. One question as a screening instrument for depression in people with multiple sclerosis. Clin Rehabil. 2007;21(5):460–464.

[8] Hanlon C, Medhin G, Selamu M, Breuer E, Worku B, Hailemariam M, et al. Validity of brief screening questionnaires to detect depression in primary care in Ethiopia. Journal of Affective Disorders. 2015;186:32–39.

[9] Rahman A, Surkan PJ, Cayetano CE, Rwagatare P, Dickson KE. Grand challenges: Integrating maternal mental health into maternal and child health programmes. PLoS Med. 2013;10(5): e1001442.

[10] Stewart RC, Umar E, Tomenson B, Creed F. Validation of screening tools for antenatal depression in Malawi-A comparison of the Edinburgh Postnatal Depression Scale and Self Reporting Questionnaire. Journal of Affective Disorders. 2013;150(3): 1041–1047.

[11] Natamba BK, Achan J, Arbach A, Oyok TO, Ghosh S, Mehta S, et al. Reliability and validity of the center for epidemiologic studies-depression scale in screening for depression among HIV-infected and-uninfected pregnant women attending antenatal services in northern Uganda: a cross-sectional study. BMC psychiatry. 2014;14(1):1.

[12] Fernandes MC, Srinivasan K, Stein AL, Menezes G, Sumithra R, Ramchandani PG. Assessing prenatal depression in the rural developing world: A comparison of two screening measures. Archives of women's mental health. 2011;14(3):209–216.

[13] Pilowsky DJ, Wu LT. Screening instruments for substance use and brief interventions targeting adolescents in primary care: A literature review. Addict Behav. 2013;38(5):2146–2153.

[14] MOH. Malawi National Mental Health Policy. In: Health Mo, editor. Lilongwe: Ministry of Health; 2020.

[15] Mgawadere FM. Assessing the Quality of Antenatal Care at Lungwena Health Centre in Rural Malawi. Blantyre: University of Malawi; 2009.

[16] Honikman S, van Heyningen T, Field S, Baron E, Tomlinson M. Stepped care for maternal mental health: A case study of the perinatal mental health project in South Africa. PLoS Med. 2012; 9(5):e1001222.

[17] Kauye F. Management of mental health services in Malawi. Int Psychiatry. 2008;5:29–31.

[18] Rollans M, Schmied V, Kemp L, Meade T. 'We just ask some questions ... ' the process of antenatal psychosocial assessment by midwives. Midwifery. 2013;29(8):935–942.

[19] Mathibe-Neke JM, Rothberg A, Langley G. The perception of midwives regarding psychosocial risk assessment during antenatal care. Health SA Gesondheid (Online). 2014;19(1): 01–09.

[20] Izutsu T, Tsutsumi A, Minas H, Thornicroft G, Patel V, Ito A. Mental health and wellbeing in the Sustainable Development Goals. The Lancet Psychiatry. 2015;2(12):1052–1054.

[21] MOH. Malawi Health Sector Strategic Plan 2011–2016: Moving Towards Equity and Quality. In: Health Mo, editor. Lilongwe: Ministry of Health; 2011.

[22] MOH. Health Sector Strategic Plan II 2017-2022: Towards Universal Health Coverage. Lilongwe: Ministry of Health; 2017.

[23] MOH. National Health Research Agenda 2012-2016. In: Health Mo, editor. Lilongwe: Ministry of Health; 2012.

[24] Akhund S, Avan BI. Development and pretesting of an information, education and communication (IEC) focused antenatal care handbook in Pakistan. BMC Research Notes. 2011;4 (1):91.

[25] Tunçalp Ö, Pena-Rosas JP, Lawrie T, Bucagu M, Oladapo OT, Portela A, et al. WHO recommendations on antenatal care for a positive pregnancy experience —going beyond survival. BJOG: An International Journal of Obstetrics & Gynaecology. 2017;124(6):860–862.

[26] Banda C. Barriers to Utilization of Focused Antenatal Care Among Pregnant Women in Ntchisi District in Malawi. Tampere: University of Tampere; 2013.

[27] Ejigu T, Woldie M, Kifle Y. Quality of antenatal care services at public health facilities of Bahir-Dar special zone, Northwest Ethiopia. BMC Health Services Research. 2013;13(1):443.

[28] Villar J, Bergsjo P, World Health Organization. WHO Antenatal Care Randomized Trial: Manual for the Implementation of the New Model. Geneva: World Health Organisation; 2002.

[29] WHO. Provision of effective antenatal care: Integrated management of pregnancy and childbirth (IMPAC). Geneva: Department of making pregnancy safer; 2006.

[30] WHO. Mental Health Atlas 2011. Geneva: World Health Organization; 2011.

[31] Gelaye B, Rondon M, Araya R, Williams MA. Epidemiology of maternal depression, risk factors, and child outcomes in low-income and middle-income countries. The Lancet Psychiatry. 2016;3(10):973–982.

[32] Stringer EM, Meltzer-Brody S, Kasaro M, Stuebe AM, Wiegand S, Paul R, et al. Depression, pregnancy, and HIV: the case to strengthen mental

health services for pregnant and postpartum women in sub-Saharan Africa. The Lancet Psychiatry. 2014;1(2):159–162.

[33] Howard LM, Piot P, Stein A. No health without perinatal mental health. The Lancet. 2014;384(9956):1723–1724.

[34] Rondon MB, Stewart DE. Disentangling the heterogeneity of perinatal depression. The Lancet Psychiatry. 2017;4(6):432–433.

[35] Herba CM, Glover V, Ramchandani PG, Rondon MB. Maternal depression and mental health in early childhood: an examination of underlying mechanisms in low-income and middle-income countries. The Lancet Psychiatry. 2017;3(10):983–992.

[36] Herrman H. Protecting the mental health of women in the perinatal period. The Lancet Psychiatry. 2015;2(2):116–118.

[37] Wald NJ. Guidance on terminology. J Med Screen. 2008;15(1):50.

[38] Thombs BD, Coyne JC, Cuijpers P, De Jonge P, Gilbody S, Ioannidis JP, et al. Rethinking recommendations for screening for depression in primary care. Canadian Medical Association Journal. 2012;184(4):413–418.

[39] Andermann A, Blancquaert I, Beauchamp S, Déry V. Revisiting Wilson and Jungner in the genomic age: A review of screening criteria over the past 40 years. Bulletin of the World Health Organization. 2008;86(4):317–319.

[40] Joffres M, Jaramillo A, Dickinson J, Lewin G, Pottie K, Shaw E, et al. Recommendations on screening for depression in adults. Canadian Medical Association Journal. 2013;185(9): 775–782.

[41] Thombs BD, Ziegelstein RC. Does depression screening improve depression outcomes in primary care? BMJ: British Medical Journal (Online). 2014;348.

[42] Nimalasuriya K, Compton MT, Guillory VJ. Screening adults for depression in primary care: A position statement of the American College of Preventive Medicine. Journal of Family Practice. 2009;58(10):535–539.

[43] Choi SK, Kim JJ, Park YG, Ko HS, Park IY, Shin JC. The simplified Edinburgh Postnatal Depression Scale (EPDS) for antenatal depression: Is it a valid measure for pre-screening? International journal of medical sciences. 2012;9(1):40.

[44] Jones CJ, Creedy DK, Gamble JA. Australian midwives' awareness and management of antenatal and postpartum depression. Women and Birth. 2012;25(1):23–28.

[45] O'Connor E, Rossom RC, Henninger M, Groom HC, Burda BU. Primary care screening for and treatment of depression in pregnant and postpartum women: Evidence report and systematic review for the US Preventive Services Task Force. JAMA. 2016;315(4):388–406.

[46] Committee on Obstetric Practice. The American College of Obstetricians and Gynecologists Committee Opinion no. 630. Screening for perinatal depression. Obstetrics and Gynecology. 2015;125(5):1268.

[47] Lombardo P, Vaucher P, Haftgoli N, Burnand B, Favrat B, Verdon F, et al. The 'help' question doesn't help when screening for major depression: external validation of the three-question screening test for primary care patients managed for physical complaints. BMC medicine. 2011;9:114.

[48] Lancaster CA, Gold KJ, Flynn HA, Yoo H, Marcus SM, Davis MM. Risk factors for depressive symptoms during pregnancy: A systematic review.

American journal of obstetrics and gynecology. 2010;202(1):5–14.

[49] van Heyningen T, Baron E, Field S, Lund C, Myer L, Tomlinson M, et al. Screening for common perinatal mental disorders in low-resource, primary care, antenatal settings in South Africa. CPMH Policy Brief. Cape Town: Centre for Public Mental Health; 2014.

[50] Mitchell A, Coyne J. Screening for postnatal depression: Barriers to success. BJOG: An International Journal of Obstetrics & Gynaecology. 2009;116(1): 11–14.

[51] Siu AL, Bibbins-Domingo K, Grossman DC, Baumann LC, Davidson KW, Ebell M, et al. Screening for depression in adults: US Preventive Services Task Force recommendation statement. JAMA. 2016;315(4):380–387.

[52] Wisconsin Association for Perinatal Care. Position statement: Screening for prenatal and postpartum depression 2016 [Available from: http://www.perinatalweb.org/assets/cms/uploads/files/PPD%20Position%20Statement_FINAL.pdf.

[53] Vanderheyden AM. Technical adequacy of response to intervention decisions. Exceptional Children. 2011;77 (3):335–350.

[54] Dennis CL, Dowswell T. Interventions (other than pharmacological, psychosocial or psychological) for treating antenatal depression. The Cochrane Library, . 2013(7).

[55] Syka A. Depression in pregnancy and ways of dealing. International Journal of Caring Sciences. 2015;8(1): 231.

[56] Dennis CL, Ross LE, Grigoriadis S. Psychosocial and psychological interventions for treating antenatal depression. The Cochrane Library, . 2007(3).

[57] Sockol LE, Epperson CN, Barber JP. A meta-analysis of treatments for perinatal depression. Clinical Psychology Review. 2011;31(5):839–849.

[58] Spinelli MG, Endicott J. Controlled clinical trial of interpersonal psychotherapy versus parenting education program for depressed pregnant women. American Journal of Psychiatry. 2003;160(3):555–562.

[59] van Ravesteyn LM, Lambregtse-van den Berg MP, Hoogendijk WJ, Kamperman AM. Interventions to treat mental disorders during pregnancy: A systematic review and multiple treatment meta-analysis. PLoS One. 2017;12(3):e0173397.

[60] Sockol LE. A systematic review of the efficacy of cognitive behavioral therapy for treating and preventing perinatal depression. Journal of Affective Disorders. 2015;177:7–21.

[61] Field T, Diego M, Hernandez-Reif M. Prenatal depression effects and interventions: A review. Infant behavior & development. 2010;33(4):409–418.

[62] Lavender TJ, Ebert L, Jones D. An evaluation of perinatal mental health interventions: An integrative literature review. Women and Birth. 2016;29(5): 399–406.

[63] Daley A, Foster L, Long G, Palmer C, Robinson O, Walmsley H, et al. The effectiveness of exercise for the prevention and treatment of antenatal depression: systematic review with meta-analysis. BJOG: An International Journal of Obstetrics & Gynaecology. 2015;122(1):57–62.

[64] Robledo-Colonia AF, Sandoval-Restrepo N, Mosquera-Valderrama YF, Escobar-Hurtado C, Ramirez-Velez R.

Aerobic exercise training during pregnancy reduces depressive symptoms in nulliparous women: A randomised trial. Journal of physiotherapy. 2012;58(1):9–15.

[65] Whooley MA. Screening for depression-A tale of two questions. JAMA Intern Med. 2016;176(4):436–438.

[66] Cox JL, Holden JM, Sagovsky R. Detection of postnatal depression: Development of the 10-item Edinburgh Postnatal Depression Scale. British Journal of Psychiatry. 1987;150(6):782–786.

[67] Derogatis LR, Lipman RS, Rickels K, Uhlenhuth EH, Covi L. The Hopkins Symptom Checklist (HSCL): A self-report symptom inventory. Systems Research and Behavioral Science. 1974; 19(1):1–15.

[68] Beusenberg M, Orley JH, World Health Organization. A User's Guide to the Self Reporting Questionnaire (SRQ). Geneva: World Health Organisation; 1994.

[69] Whooley MA, Avins AL, Miranda J, Browner WS. Case-finding instruments for depression. J Gen Intern Med. 1997; 12(7):439–445.

[70] Chorwe-Sungani G, Chipps J. A systematic review of screening instruments for depression for use in antenatal services in low resource settings. BMC Psychiatry. 2017;17(1): 112.

[71] Akobeng AK. Understanding diagnostic tests 1: Sensitivity, specificity and predictive values. Acta Paediatrica. 2007;96(3):338–341.

[72] Sjögren P. Ethics of health screening. BDJ. 2012;213(9):434.

[73] Bossuyt PM, Reitsma JB, Bruns DE, Gatsonis CA, Glasziou PP, Irwig L, et al. STARD 2015: An updated list of essential items for reporting diagnostic accuracy studies. Radiology. 2015;277 (3):826–832.

[74] Martins CdSR, Motta JVdS, Quevedo LA, de Matos MB, Pinheiro KAT, Souza LDdM, et al. Comparison of two instruments to track depression symptoms during pregnancy in a sample of pregnant teenagers in Southern Brazil. Journal of Affective Disorders. 2015;177:95–100.

[75] Rubertsson C, Börjesson K, Berglund A, Josefsson A, Sydsjö G. The Swedish validation of Edinburgh Postnatal Depression Scale (EPDS) during pregnancy. Nord J Psychiatry. 2011;65(6):414–418.

[76] e Couto TC, Brancaglion MYM, Cardoso MN, Protzner AB, Garcia FD, Nicolato R, et al. What is the best tool for screening antenatal depression? Journal of affective disorders. 2015;178: 12–7.

[77] Akena D, Joska J, Obuku EA, Amos T, Musisi S, Stein DJ. Comparing the accuracy of brief versus long depression screening instruments which have been validated in low and middle income countries: A systematic review. BMC Psychiatry. 2012;12(1):1.

[78] Tsai AC, Scott JA, Hung KJ, Zhu JQ, Matthews LT, Psaros C, et al. Reliability and validity of instruments for assessing perinatal depression in African settings: systematic review and meta-analysis. PLoS One. 2013;8(12):e82521.

[79] Ajinkya S, Jadhav PR, Srivastava NN. Depression during pregnancy: Prevalence and obstetric risk factors among pregnant women attending a tertiary care hospital in Navi Mumbai. Industrial psychiatry journal. 2013;22(1):37.

[80] Bannigan K, Watson R. Reliability and validity in a nutshell. Journal of

Clinical Nursing. 2009;18(23):3237–3243.

[81] Wong HB, Lim GH. Measures of diagnostic accuracy: Sensitivity, specificity, PPV and NPV. Proc Singapore Healthcare. 2011;20(4):316–318.

[82] Parikh R, Mathai A, Parikh S, Sekhar GC, Thomas R. Understanding and using sensitivity, specificity and predictive values. Indian J Ophthalmol. 2008;56(1):45.

[83] Zhu W, Zeng N, Wang N. Sensitivity, specificity, accuracy, associated confidence interval and ROC analysis with practical SAS implementations. NESUG 2010: Health care and life sciences; 27th May 2015; Baltimore2010. p. 1–9.

[84] Fluss R, Faraggi D, Reiser B. Estimation of the Youden Index and its associated cutoff point. Biom J. 2005;47 (4):458–472.

[85] Youden WJ. Index for rating diagnostic tests. Cancer. 1950;3(1): 32–35.

[86] Pettersson A, Boström KB, Gustavsson P, Ekselius L. Which instruments to support diagnosis of depression have sufficient accuracy? A systematic review. Nordic Journal of Psychiatry. 2015;69(7):497–508.

[87] Tavakol M, Dennick R. Making sense of Cronbach's alpha. Int J Med Educ. 2011;2:53.

[88] Hajian-Tilaki K. Receiver operating characteristic (ROC) curve analysis for medical diagnostic test evaluation. Caspian J Intern Med. 2013;4(2):627.

[89] Henderson M. Predicting Performance on High Stakes Testing: Validity and Accuracy of Curriculum-based Measurement of Reading and Writing [Doctoral Thesis]. Baton Rouge: Louisiana State University; 2009.

[90] Fischer JE, Bachmann LM, Jaeschke R. A readers' guide to the interpretation of diagnostic test properties: Clinical example of sepsis. Intensive Care Med. 2003;29(7):1043–1051.

[91] Cassetta BD, Goghari VM. Ethical considerations of screening and early intervention for clinical high-risk psychosis. Ethics & Behavior. 2015;25 (1):1–20.

[92] O'Connor EA, Whitlock EP, Gaynes B, Beil TL. Screening for depression in adults and older adults in primary care. Evidence Syntheses, . 2009(75).

[93] Boyd RC, Mogul M, Newman D, Coyne JC. Screening and referral for postpartum depression among low-income women: A qualitative perspective from community health workers. Depress Res Treat. 2011;2011.

[94] Cook CR, Volpe RJ, Livanis A, Chafouleas SM, Kilgus SP, Wallach N. Ethical Dilemmas in School-based Behavioral Screening. Los Angeles: Sage Publications; 2010.

[95] Reynolds TM. The Ethics of Antenatal Screening: Lessons from Canute. The Clinical Biochemist Reviews. 2009;30(4):187.

[96] Maurer DM. Screening for depression. Depression. 2012;100:23.

[97] Trikalinos TA, Balion CM, Coleman CI, Griffith L, Santaguida PL, Vandermeer B, et al. Meta-analysis of test performance when there is a "gold standard". J Gen Intern Med. 2012;27(1): 56–66.

[98] Williams CC. Insight, stigma, and post–diagnosis identities in schizophrenia. Psychiatry: Interpersonal and Biological Processes. 2008;71(3): 246–256.

[99] Benedetti F, Lanotte M, Lopiano L, Colloca L. When words are painful: Unraveling the mechanisms of the nocebo effect. Neuroscience. 2007;147 (2):260–271.

[100] Ko JY, Farr SL, Dietz PM, Robbins CL. Depression and treatment among US pregnant and nonpregnant women of reproductive age, 2005–2009. Journal of Women's Health. 2012;21(8): 830–836.

[101] Leigh B, Milgrom J. Acceptability of antenatal screening for depression in routine antenatal care. Australian Journal of Advanced Nursing. 2007;24 (3):14.

[102] Wilkinson M, Mbuluma EL, Masache TG, Robins A. Mental Health Handbook for Malawi. Limbe: Assemblies of God Literature Centre Press; 1991.

[103] Steinforth AS. Troubled Minds: On the Cultural Construction of Mental Disorder and Normality in Southern Malawi. Frankfurt: Perter Lang; 2009.

[104] Sefasi A, Crumlish N, Samalani P, Kinsella A, O'Callaghan E, Chilale H. A little knowledge: caregiver burden in schizophrenia in Malawi. Social Psychiatry and Psychiatric Epidemiology. 2008;43(2):160–164.

[105] Stewart RC, Umar E, Gleadow-Ware S, Creed F, Bristow K. Perinatal distress and depression in Malawi: an exploratory qualitative study of stressors, supports and symptoms. Archives of Women's Mental Health. 2015;18(2):177–185.

[106] Crabb J, Stewart RC, Kokota D, Masson N, Chabunya S, Krishnadas R. Attitudes towards mental illness in Malawi: a cross-sectional survey. BMC Public Health. 2012;12(1):541.

[107] Kauye F, Udedi M, Mafuta C. Pathway to care for psychiatric patients in a developing country: Malawi. International Journal of Social Psychiatry. 2014;61(2):121–128.

[108] Udedi M, Swartz L, Stewart RC, Kauye F. Health service utilization by patients with common mental disorder identified by the Self-Reporting Questionnaire in a primary care setting in Zomba, Malawi: A descriptive study. The International Journal of Social Psychiatry. 2014;60(5):454–461.

[109] Kakuma R, Minas H, van Ginneken N, Dal Poz MR, Desiraju K, Morris JE, et al. Human resources for mental health care: current situation and strategies for action. The Lancet. 2011; 378(9803):1654–1663.

[110] Dambisya YM, Matinhure S. Policy and programmatic implications of task shifting in Uganda: a case study. BMC Health Services Research. 2012;12(1):61.

[111] Fulton BD, Scheffler RM, Sparkes SP, Auh EY, Vujicic M, Soucat A. Health workforce skill mix and task shifting in low income countries: A review of recent evidence. Human Resources for Health. 2011;9(1):1.

[112] Spedding M, Stein D, Sorsdahl K. Task-shifting psychosocial interventions in public mental health: A review of the evidence in the South African context. South African Health Review. 2014;15: 73–87.

[113] Petersen I, Lund C, Bhana A, Flisher AJ, Health M, Consortium PRP. A task shifting approach to primary mental health care for adults in South Africa: human resource requirements and costs for rural settings. Health policy and planning. 2011;27(1):42–51.

[114] Wright J, Chiwandira C. Building capacity for community mental health care in rural Malawi: findings from a district-wide task-sharing intervention with village-based health workers.

International Journal of Social Psychiatry. 2016;62(6):589–596.

[115] Kazdin AE, Rabbitt SM. Novel models for delivering mental health services and reducing the burdens of mental illness. Clinical Psychological Science. 2013;1(2):170–191.

[116] Chorwe-Sungani G. Development of a screening protocol for depresion in antenatal clinics in Malawi [Doctoral]. Bellville: University of the Western Cape; 2017.

[117] Kumbhar UT, Dhumale GB, Kumbhar UP. Self Reporting Questionnaire as a tool to diagnose psychiatric morbidity. Natl J Med Res, 2012;2:51-54.

Chapter 10

Associated Factors and Use of Health Services by Elderly Men in Northeast Brazil

Gisele Mariel de Sousa Vasconcelos, Alana Maiara Brito Bibiano, Lucas Fernando Rodrigues dos Santos and Rafael da Silveira Moreira

Abstract

The objective of the research was to analyze the factors associated with the use of health services by elderly men in the Northeast region of Brazil. Cross-sectional analytical study with a secondary database of elderly men (n = 3238). The dependent variable was composed of the profiles of the use of health services and the independent variables were factors of predisposition, capacity, and health need. The statistical association and effect were performed using the Rao-Scott test with $p < 0.05$ and multinomial logistic regression. Elderly men with worse social indicators had a risk effect for using medium/high complexity services and those who had better health indicators were associated with sporadic medical appointment, revealing that healthcare for elderly men is centered on curative and rehabilitative care and that the use of health services is associated with the worst social indicators.

Keywords: Health Services, Health of the Elderly, Men's Health, Cross-Sectional Studies

1. Introduction

The demographic transition is marked by a reduction in fertility and mortality and results, along with the epidemiological transition, in population aging. According to United Nations projections, the elderly population in Brazil will increase from 3.1% in 1970 to 19% in 2050. The increase in the elderly population generates the need for a new social, economic and health organization [1].

In this sense, it is observed that the elderly are major users of health services [2] and that this use has increased in recent years [3, 4]. Although in Brazil the National Health Policy for the Elderly and the National Policy for Comprehensive Care to Men's Health (PNAISH, in Portuguese) have been instituted which aim to organize, implement, qualify and humanize comprehensive healthcare for the elderly and the men, respectively, the demand for health services by this public are still low.

The use of health services represents the center of the health systems functioning and comprises all direct or indirect contact with health services. This process results from the interaction of the individual's behavior who seeks for care and the professional who leads him within the health system [5].

Andersen [6], in his classic model for the use of health services [7], points out the influence of access in the use of health services as mediated by individual factors, defined as predisposing factors (those that exist before the emergence of the health problem and affect the predisposition of people to use the services), enabling factors (the means available to obtain healthcare) and health needs (the health conditions perceived by people or diagnosed by health professionals).

Several studies show that men, in general, have more severe and chronic diseases than women [8–10]. Despite male rates responding significantly in the morbidity and mortality data, the presence of men in primary health care services is lower than that of women [11, 12] and although there is a wide discussion about masculinity in the health area, with research that refers to the need to reflect on this topic addressing to understand the risks to men's health [8, 13–16], there are few studies that explore the use of health services by elderly men and the associated epidemiological and socioeconomic factors.

Such data scarcity occurs especially in the Northeast of Brazil, a socioeconomically unequal region comparing to other regions of the country [17], making it necessary to analyze the theme. Thus, the present study analyzed the factors associated with the use of health services by elderly men in the Northeast region of Brazil.

2. Method

This is a cross-sectional, population-based study in the Northeast of Brazil, which used secondary data from the National Health Survey (PNS, in Portuguese), conducted by the Brazilian Institute of Geography and Statistics (IBGE, in Portuguese) in 2013. PNS is a household survey with national coverage, which was designed to represent the adult population, based on cluster sampling. Details of the design and sample selection process can be found in the PNS reports [18–24].

Altogether, 60.202 households in Brazil were visited and interviews conducted with individuals aged 18 years or older. A total of 205.546 individuals responded to the survey, among which 23.815 were elderly, and of these, 10.541 were male, 3238 from the Northeast [20]. This study included elderly male individuals (60 years of age or older) living in the Northeast region selected by the PNS-IBGE sampling process. Elderly men with missing information in the database were excluded.

The dependent variable of this study corresponded to the health service profile used by elderly men and was composed of ten questions from the PNS referring to the set of the use of health services. These questions were grouped and categorized through Latent Class Analysis (LCA) and were presented, after analysis, in a single health service use variable that represents a variety of phenomena to explain the outcome.

The LCA is a statistical approach that identifies distinct mutually exclusive groups (latent classes) based on the response patterns of categorical variables [25]. LCA works with heterogeneous data in which individuals are classified in the group by similar characteristics, that is, it is considered that individuals come from the same population and that the trajectory can be extrapolated to an entire population as well as the covariables that affect the trajectory will influence individuals in the same way [26]. Latent classes or trajectories aim to estimate the size and number of latent classes, the probability of the response of each individual and to assign latent class association to individuals in the population [27].

The independent variables were the PNS questions related to predisposing factors, capacity, and health needs of elderly men, organized according to the classic theoretical model for the Use of Health Services [7].

Predisposing factors were: North-eastern states; Condition of responsible or not for the domicile; Age; Color or race; Marital status; and Able to read and write. The capacity factors were: Possession of health insurance; and Participation in organized social activities (clubs, community or religious groups, elderly living centers). The necessity factors were: Diagnosis of any chronic, physical, or mental illness; Degree of difficulty in eating, bathing, use the bathroom, dressing, walking at home, lying, or getting out of bed, sitting or getting up from the chair, shopping, managing finances, taking medicine, go the doctor, and go out alone by transport; Occurrence of a fall in the last 12 months; and Perceived health status.

Regarding the variables referring to Basic and Instrumental Activities of Daily Living (ADLs and IADLs, respectively) there are some validated instruments [28–30] that evaluate these activities, however, not all the questions used in these scales were used in the PNS, such as urinary and fecal continence and the difficulty to use the phone. Thus, the set of questions that assessed ADLs and IADLs could not be grouped according to the instruments. As a result, the twelve variables referring to the degrees of difficulty to perform the ADLs and IADLs were also studied using the LCA method to form a single variable of the difficulty level to perform ADLs and IADLs.

To assess the latent class model and identify the number of classes that better define the object of study, some statistical criteria were considered. The first is entropy, the probability that the individual is perfectly classified in a particular latent class, whose measures can vary between 0 and 1, and the closer to 1 the value is, the more appropriate the model will be, indicating a good classification of the individual in the class [31].

Other criteria were considered such as the Akaike Information Criterion (AIC), Bayesian Information Criterion (BIC) and adjusted BIC, used for assessing the model's adjustments. In the analysis, the lower the value of AIC, BIC and adjusted BIC, the more suitable the model will be [32]. To assess the evolution of the testing model, the likelihood tests were used considering $p < 0.05$ as statistically significant values.

In this article, five models were tested, with two, three, four, five and six latent classes, to identify the number of classes that best represents the object of study according to the aforementioned statistical criteria. Weights and strata from the database for the LCA were considered.

In the descriptive statistical analysis, the quantitative variable corresponding to age was presented as a measure of central tendency and dispersion, with a 95% Confidence Interval (CI) being calculated. Qualitative variables were presented in the form of a frequency table and 95% CI.

In analytical statistics, the presence of an association between independent variables and the dependent variable (categorized through Latent Class Analysis) was investigated using the Rao-Scott test used in complex samples [33]. The significance level was 5%. The effect measures of the factors on the dependent variable were expressed by Odds Ratio (OR) and calculated by simple and multiple models of multinomial logistic regression, following the theoretical model of Health Services Utilization [7] from the assumption of the hierarchical approach.

Initially, a simple analysis was carried out on the blocks of predisposing factors, capacity factors and health needs. Within each block, variables with $p < 0.25$ were tested in multiple models [34]. In the end, the variables with $p < 0.05$ remained in the model for each block and were considered adjustment factors for the subsequent blocks.

The PNS-IBGE database is in the public domain and is available on the IBGE website (http://www.ibge.gov.br). The statistical programs used were IBM SPSS Statistics version 20 for data analysis, and Mplus 7.31 to establish latent classes in Latent Class Analysis (LCA).

The National Health Research (PNS) project was approved by the National Commission for Ethics in Research for Human Beings, of the National Health Council, under commission's opinion number 328159, on June 26, 2013. The Informed Consent Forms of the research participants were signed on the interviewers' handheld computers. The research project in this article did not require submission to the Ethics and Research Committee since it was subsidized by secondary data in the public domain.

3. Results

From the five models tested, the one that instituted four latent classes was the one with the best entropy, adjustment criteria and evolution of the testing model, in addition to greater parsimony in the regression model (**Table 1**). The four latent classes were identified and titled according to the observed response patterns: 1 - "Use of health services in the last two weeks" (3.2%; 95% CI 2.5–4.1%); 2 - "Use of health services for appointment in primary care" (12.6%; 95% CI 11.2–14.3%); 3 - "Use of health services for sporadic medical appointment" (77.0%; 95% CI 75.0–78.9%); and 4 - "Use of health services only for hospitalization in the last year" (7.1%; 95% CI 5.8–8.7%).

In the analysis of ADLs and IADLs, the model with three classes was selected, as it had a p-value < 0.05, the highest entropy value and the lowest values of AIC, BIC and adjusted BIC. The three latent classes entitled were: 1 - "Without difficulty to perform ADLs and IADLs"; 2 - "Intermediate degree of difficulty to perform ADLs and IADLs"; 3 - "High degree of difficulty to perform ADLs and IADLs".

In this study, 3238 elderly men were included. Most were from the state of Bahia (24.7%) followed by Ceará (18.0%) and were responsible for the household in which they lived (72.2%). The median age was 68 years old (1st quartile 63 years and 3rd quartile 74 years), and 51.2% of elderly men were above the median age. The most frequent color/race was "non-white" (71.8%); 64.2% were married and 57.5% could read and write.

	Number of Classes				
Statistical Criteria	**2**	**3**	**4**	**5**	**6**
AIC	103678.091	92431.330	**89423.056**	88908.037	88625.293
BIC	104092.083	93055.950	**90258.304**	89953.913	89881.797
Adjusted BIC	103910.945	92782.654	**89892.850**	89496.301	89332.026
Entropy	1.000	1.000	**1.000**	0.936	0.941
Vuong-Lo–Mendell–Rubin - LRT	p = 0.0000	p = 0.0000	**p = 0.0000**	p = 0.0000	p = 0.2148
Lo–Mendell–Rubin - LRT	p = 0.0000	p = 0.0000	**p = 0.0000**	p = 0.0000	p = 0.2164

AIC Akaike Information Criterion; BIC Bayesian Information Criterion; LRT Likelihood Test.
Source: The authors.
Bold font indicates the selected model.

Table 1.
Results of adequacy and adjustment of each of the tested models of the latent classes of use of health services, 2021.

Variable	Use of health services in the last two weeks % (IC95%)	Use of health services for appointment in primary care % (IC95%)	Use of health services for sporadic medical appointment % (IC95%)	Use of health services only for hospitalization in the last year % (IC95%)	p-value
			Block 1 - Predisposing Factors		
State of the Northeast Region					0.672
Maranhão	1.9 (0.6–5.3)	14.4 (9.9–20.4)	74.8 (67.9–80.7)	8.9 (5.1–15.2)	
Piauí	2.3 (1.0–5.2)	12.9 (9.6–17.2)	78.3 (73.6–82.4)	6.5 (4.2–10.0)	
Ceará	4.0 (2.5–6.3)	10.1 (7.3–13.9)	78.6 (74.4–82.4)	7.3 (5.0–10.5)	
Rio Grande do Norte	4.8 (2.3–9.5)	14.5 (10.6–19.6)	76.6 (70.7–81.7)	4.1 (2.5–6.6)	
Paraíba	4.6 (2.2–9.3)	12.4 (8.6–17.6)	73.7 (67.2–79.3)	9.3 (5.9–14.3)	
Pernambuco	3.0 (1.7–5.2)	12.9 (9.6–17.2)	78.2 (73.4–82.4)	5.8 (3.7–9.1)	
Alagoas	2.2 (0.9–4.9)	14.3 (10.2–19.7)	79.6 (73.5–84.6)	3.9 (2.2–6.8)	
Sergipe	1.3 (0.5–3.1)	16.2 (11.8–21.7)	75.2 (68.8–80.7)	7.3 (4.6–11.5)	
Bahia	3.4 (1.7–6.7)	12.2 (8.6–17.1)	75.7 (69.5–81.0)	8.6 (5.2–14.0)	
Condition of the elderly person at home					**0.006***
Responsible for the household	3.1 (2.2–4.3)	13.4 (11.7–15.4)	77.6 (75.1–79.9)	5.8 (4.6–7.3)	
Not responsible for the household	3.5 (2.3–5.3)	10.6 (7.9–14.1)	75.0 (70.3–79.1)	**10.9 (7.8–15.2) †**	
Age					0.484
Below the median	3.6 (2.5–5.0)	12.3 (10.2–14.8)	76.1 (72.9–79.0)	8.1 (6.4–10.2)	
Above the median	2.9 (1.9–4.3)	13.0 (11.0–15.4)	77.6 (74.7–80.4)	6.4 (4.8–8.6)	
Color/Race					0.698
White	4.0 (2.5–6.4)	12.8 (10.2–15.9)	76.3 (72.5–79.7)	6.9 (5.2–9.2)	
Not white	2.9 (2.1–4.0)	12.6 (10.9–14.6)	77.1 (74.6–79.4)	7.4 (5.7–9.4)	
Marital status					0.095
Married	**3.7 (2.7–5.1) †**	12.0 (10.3–14.0)	78.2 (75.7–80.5)	6.1 (4.8–7.6)	
Separately / Judicially Disqualified	4.2 (1.5–11.3)	22.2 (9.6–43.6)	70.7 (51.5–84.6)	2.8 (0.8–9.9)	
Divorced	2.3 (0.7–7.7)	10.5 (5.2–20.1)	79.7 (67.8–88.0)	7.4 (2.7–19.0)	
Widower	2.1 (1.0–4.6)	11.9 (8.0–17.4)	76.4 (69.8–82.0)	9.5 (6.1–14.6)	
Not married	2.2 (1.2–4.0)	14.5 (10.7–19.3)	73.0 (67.4–78.0)	10.3 (6.8–15.3)	

Variable	Use of health services in the last two weeks % (IC95%)	Use of health services for appointment in primary care % (IC95%)	Use of health services for sporadic medical appointment % (IC95%)	Use of health services only for hospitalization in the last year % (IC95%)	p-value
Can read and write					**0.002***
Yes	**4.2 (3.1–5.7)†**	13.5 (11.4–15.8)	76.7 (73.8–79.4)	5.6 (4.3–7.3)	
No	1.9 (1.2–3.1)	11.6 (9.4–14.2)	77.1 (73.6–80.1)	**9.4 (7.1–12.5) †**	
			Block 2 - Capacity Factors		
Health insurance					**0.005***
Yes	**6.9 (4.4–10.6)†**	14.0 (10.3–18.8)	71.2 (64.2–77.3)	8.0 (5.1–12.2)	
No	2.6 (1.9–3.6)	12.4 (10.8–14.3)	77.9 (75.7–79.9)	7.1 (5.7–8.9)	
Participation in organized social activities					0.898
Yes	2.6 (1.3–5.0)	13.1 (9.5–17.7)	76.4 (70.5–81.4)	7.9 (4.8–12.7)	
No	3.3 (2.5–4.4)	12.6 (10.9–14.5)	76.9 (74.6–79.1)	7.1 (5.8–8.8)	
			Block 3 - Necessity Factors		
Diagnosis of chronic, physical, or mental illness					**0.00***
Yes	**5.8 (4.1–8.1)†**	**17.9 (15.0–21.3)†**	66.9 (62.5–70.9)	**9.5 (7.1–12.4) †**	
No	2.0 (1.4–3.0)	10.2 (8.5–12.2)	**81.6 (79.1–83.9) †**	6.2 (4.7–8.2)	
Difficulty level to perform ADLs and IADLs					**0.00***
No difficulty	2.1 (1.5–3.1)	12.1 (10.5–14.0)	**80.1 (77.8–82.2) †**	5.6 (4.4–7.2)	
Intermediate degree of difficulty	**6.5 (4.2–9.9) †**	14.4 (10.4–19.7)	67.5 (61.6–72.8)	**11.6 (8.3–15.8)†**	
High degree of difficulty	**12.9 (6.7–23.2) †**	16.4 (9.2–27.4)	46.3 (34.4–58.6)	**24.5 (15.4–36.7)†**	
Fall in the last 12 months					**0.00***
Yes	**11.6 (6.0–21.4) †**	19.0 (12.3–28.2)	58.6 (48.0–68.4)	10.8 (6.6–17.2)	
No	2.7 (2.0–3.5)	12.2 (10.7–13.9)	**78.1 (75.9–80.1) †**	7.0 (5.7–8.6)	
Perceived health status					0.278
Very good	8.0 (2.1–26.5)	12.3 (6.7–21.5)	70.7 (57.4–81.1)	9.0 (4.6–16.9)	
Good	3.4 (2.3–4.9)	13.5 (10.7–16.9)	75.0 (71.0–78.6)	8.1 (5.9–11.0)	

Variable	Use of health services in the last two weeks % (IC95%)	Use of health services for appointment in primary care % (IC95%)	Use of health services for sporadic medical appointment % (IC95%)	Use of health services only for hospitalization in the last year % (IC95%)	p-value
Regular	2.8 (1.9–4.2)	12.0 (10.1–14.4)	78.5 (75.4–81.2)	6.6 (4.9–8.9)	
Bad	1.6 (0.7–3.4)	14.0 (9.7–19.7)	78.2 (72.1–83.3)	6.2 (4.0–9.7)	
Too bad-do not know how to answer	8.0 (3.3–18.1)	7.9 (4.0–15.1)	75.6 (62.8–85.0)	8.5 (2.8–22.9)	

95% CI - 95% confidence interval.
ADLs: Basic Activities of Daily Living; IADLs: Instrumental Activities of Daily Living.
$^{*}p < 0.05$ (Rao and Scott test).
†Standardized residual >1.96.
Source: The authors.
Bold font indicates statistical significance (p-value column) and/or dependency between categories (% columns).

Table 2.
Descriptive and analytical analysis of the use of health services by elderly men according to blocks of variables analyzed. Northeast, Brazil, 2021.

Regarding the possession of health insurance, 85.1% did not have it. Most elderly men did not participate in organized social activities (85.1%), had no diagnosis of chronic, physical, or mental illness (67.8%), had no difficulty in performing ADLs and IADLs (80.0%) and it did report a fall in the last year (93.7%). The perceptions of regular (46.4%) and good (34.6%) health status were the most frequent.

After the description of the dependent variable generated by the LCA, composed of four classes, a descriptive and analytical analysis of the independent variables was performed according to the dependent variable (**Table 2**).

The results of the simple and multiple multinomial logistic regression analysis according to each block of associated factors studied are shown in **Tables 3** and **4**, respectively. The use of services in primary care was considered as a reference category for the dependent variable.

In the simple logistic regression analysis, from the 12 variables analyzed, 7 had p-values <0.25 (**Table 3**) and were tested in the multiple model. By the end, six variables remained statistically significant, $p < 0.05$ (**Table 4**). In the multiple logistic regression to Block 1, elderly men not responsible for the home were approximately 2 times more likely to use the services for sporadic medical appointment compared to the appointment in primary care. Regarding being able to read and write, those who were not were approximately 1.8 times more likely to use the services only for hospitalization compared to the appointment in primary care.

In the analysis of Block 2, after adjusting the variables for Block 1, elderly men who did not have health insurance had about 54% less chance of using health services in the last two weeks compared to use in primary care.

In the last block, after adjusting the variables for Blocks 1 and 2, those who were not diagnosed with a chronic, physical, or mental illness had about 2 times more chance of using the services for a sporadic medical appointment. Those who did not have difficulty in performing ADLs and IADLs had approximately 79% less chance of using the services in the last two weeks and of being admitted in the last year compared to the appointment in primary care. Elderly men who did not report a fall in the last year were 1.9 times more likely to have a sporadic medical appointment compared to the primary care appointment.

Variable	Use of health services in the last two weeks OR (IC95%)	Use of health services for sporadic medical appointment OR (IC95%)	Use of health services only for hospitalization in the last year OR (IC95%)	p-value
		Block 1 - Predisposing Factors		
Condition of the elderly person at home				**0.020***
Responsible for the household	1.00	1.00	1.00	
Not responsible for the household	1.56 (0.83–2.96)	1.25 (0.86–1.82)	**2.25 (1.31–3.87)†**	
Marital status				0.459
Married	1.00	1.00	1.00	
Separately / Judicially Disqualified	0.57 (0.14–2.38)	0.49 (0.18–1.34)	0.26 (0.05–1.25)	
Divorced	0.63 (0.15–2.73)	1.19 (0.54–2.61)	1.53 (0.42–5.64)	
Widower	0.61 (0.24–1.57)	0.95 (0.59–1.53)	1.40 (0.70–2.77)	
Not married	0.51 (0.23–1.13)	0.73 (0.48–1.10)	1.12 (0.63–2.00)	
Can read and write				**0.011***
Yes	1.00	1.00	1.00	
No	0.57 (0.29–1.09)	1.19 (0.87–1.64)	**1.78 (1.09–2.90)†**	
		Block 2 - Capacity Factors		
Health insurance				**0.004***
Yes	1.00	1.00	1.00	
No	**0.42 (0.22–0.81) †**	1.23 (0.82–1.86)	1.00 (0.58–1.73)	
		Block 3 - Necessity Factors		
Diagnosis of chronic, physical, or mental illness				**0.00***
Yes	1.00	1.00	1.00	
No	0.72 (0.38–1.36)	**2.06 (1.49–2.85) †**	1.33 (0.79–2.24)	
Difficulty level to perform ADLs and IADLs				**0.00***
No difficulty	**0.28 (0.10–0.77) †**	1.77 (0.84–3.73)	**0.28 (0.12–0.65) †**	
Intermediate degree of difficulty	0.61 (0.21–1.76)	1.51 (0.68–3.35)	0.53 (0.21–1.38)	
High degree of difficulty	1.00	1.00	1.00	
Fall in the last 12 months				**0.026***

Variable	Use of health services in the last two weeks OR (IC95%)	Use of health services for sporadic medical appointment OR (IC95%)	Use of health services only for hospitalization in the last year OR (IC95%)	p-value
Yes	1.00	1.00	1.00	
No	0.47 (0.18–1.20)	**1.92 (1.04–3.54) †**	1.24 (0.62–2.48)	

OR - odds ratio; 95% CI - 95% confidence interval.
ADLs: Basic Activities of Daily Living; IADLs: Instrumental Activities of Daily Living.
**p < 0.05.*
†Category of the variable with p < 0.05.
Source: The authors.
Bold font indicates statistical significance.

Table 3.
Values of gross odds ratio and confidence interval obtained by simple analysis for the association between the variables presented in the hierarchical model and the use of the health service for appointment in primary care, 2021.

Variable	Use of health services in the last two weeks OR (IC95%)	Use of health services for sporadic medical appointment OR (IC95%)	Use of health services only for hospitalization in the last year OR (IC95%)	p-value
		Block 1 - Predisposing Factors[a]		
Condition of the elderly person at home				0.119
Responsible for the household	1.00	1.00	1.00	
Not responsible for the household	1.02 (0.52–2.01)	1.40 (0.94–2.08)	**1.97 (1.07–3.65)†**	
Can read and write				**0.009***
Yes	1.00	1.00	1.00	
No	0.52 (0.26–1.06)	1.10 (0.80–1.50)	**1.79 (1.07–3.00)†**	
		Block 2 - Capacity Factors[b]		
Health insurance				**0.048***
Yes	1.00	1.00	1.00	
No	**0.46 (0.23–0.93)†**	1.07 (0.68–1.68)	0.71 (0.39–1.28)	
		Block 3 - Necessity Factors[c]		
Diagnosis of chronic, physical, or mental illness				**0.000***
Yes	1.00	1.00	1.00	
No	0.86 (0.44–1.68)	**2.04 (1.48–2.82)†**	1.30 (0.76–2.20)	
Difficulty level to perform ADLs and IADLs				**0.000***
No difficulty	**0.21 (0.07–0.65)†**	**2.17 (1.02–4.64)†**	0.44 (0.18–1.10)	

Variable	Use of health services in the last two weeks OR (IC95%)	Use of health services for sporadic medical appointment OR (IC95%)	Use of health services only for hospitalization in the last year OR (IC95%)	p-value
Intermediate degree of difficulty	0.53 (0.18–1.54)	1.73 (0.76–3.95)	0.68 (0.25–1.86)	
High degree of difficulty	1.00	1.00	1.00	
Fall in the last 12 months				**0.020***
Yes	1.00	1.00	1.00	
No	0.46 (0.16–1.28)	**1.93 (1.06–3.52)†**	1.32 (0.65–2.72)	

OR - odds ratio; 95% CI - 95% confidence interval.
ADLs: Basic Activities of Daily Living; IADLs: Instrumental Activities of Daily Living.
$^{*}p < 0.05$.
†Category of the variable with $p < 0.05$.
[a]Adjusted by the variables in Block 1 – Predisposing Factors.
[b]Adjusted by the variables in Block 1 - Predisposing Factors and Block 2 - Capacity Factors.
[c]Adjusted for the variables in Block 1 - Predisposing Factors, Block 2 - Capacity Factors and Block 3 - Necessity Factors.
Source: The authors.
Bold font indicates statistical significance.

Table 4.
Values of adjusted odds ratio and confidence intervals obtained by multinominal logistic regression analysis for the association between the use of health services and the appointment in primary care and the three blocks of variables analyzed, 2021.

4. Discussion

According to the World Report on Aging and Health, the aging of the population demands a comprehensive public health action; however, the debate on the topic has been insufficient, even though there is sufficient evidence to act urgently at present [35]. When it comes to the aging of the male population, the situation becomes more worrying, as research is even scarcer.

In this study, the profile of the use of health services for elderly men in the Northeast of Brazil was analyzed through the LCA, which instituted four distinct classes of use profile based on the response patterns of the categorical variables of the PNS and allowed to study the phenomenon comprising the various aspects that involve the theme, with an innovative and safe statistical methodology, infrequently applied in epidemiological studies. Previous studies [36–39] defined the dependent variable by a single question about the use of health services that did not address the phenomenon in its entirety and complexity.

Regarding the latent classes, it was identified that most elderly men used the health service for sporadic medical appointments in the last year (77%), that is, they are not frequent users of the services. Only 12.6% used the services for appointment in Primary Care, and a minority was admitted in the last year or used the services of medium and high complexity in the last two weeks.

According to the National Primary Care Policy (PNAB, in Portuguese), primary care should be the user's main gateway to the Brazilian public health system and the communication center of the Health Care Network [40]. This fact was not found among elderly men in the Northeast of Brazil, and it is noteworthy that the search for healthcare by this population usually occurs much less than the female population [41]. Several studies have proven the fact that, compared to women, men are more vulnerable to diseases, especially to serious and chronic illnesses, in addition to dying earlier [8, 10, 38, 42].

In the hierarchical analysis of Block 1, elderly men who cannot read and write were about 1.8 times more likely to be hospitalized than to carry out appointments in primary care. According to studies of inequalities from the database of the Health, Well-Being, and Aging survey in Latin America [43, 44], elderly people with less education have worse health status due to worse habits, greater exclusion and lower level of information and socioeconomic conditions to access the health network early, which implies the use of services in more serious health conditions, such as hospitalization.

It was also analyzed the fact of being responsible or not for the home, identifying that those who were not responsible were approximately 2 times more likely to use the services for hospitalization compared to the appointment in primary care. This finding is lined with what PNAISH [45] presents: an issue pointed out by men for not looking for health services is linked to their position as the provider, claiming that the hours of services functioning coincide with their working time. In this sense, being responsible for the home keeps men away from preventive health services, which can result in the use of medium and high complexity services. However, in this research, the use of these services was related to men not responsible for the home.

In the analysis of Block 2, elderly men in the Northeast who had no health insurance had 54% less chance of using health services in the last two weeks compared to use in primary care. One study showed that having a referral doctor for routine care was strongly associated with having health insurance: 69.8% of individuals with health insurance declared that they had a referral doctor in contrast to 31.6% without insurance [38]. This may be because individuals with more serious health problems are more likely to buy health insurance (a phenomenon known in economic theory as adverse selection) [46]. Another possibility is that having health insurance increases the use of health services, especially for preventive or routine appointments [46].

Regarding the last block, elderly men who were not diagnosed with chronic, physical, or mental illness were approximately 2 times more likely to use the services for sporadic medical appointment. This demonstrates that the absence of clinical diagnosis is a conditioning factor for not using health services frequently. In a study carried out with sample data from the National Household Sample Survey, it was concluded that the probability of having had at least one medical appointment in the last 12 months was about 3 times higher among people with chronic diseases [47]. According to PNAISH, male entry into the health system occurs mainly through ambulatory and hospital care, which sets up a profile that favors morbidity aggravation due to the late search for care [45].

The prevalence of functional limitation varies between countries and according to the criterion adopted for its definition [48, 49]. A widely used definition is the reporting of difficulties in performing ADLs and IADLs. In this study, elderly men in the Northeast who had no difficulty in performing ADLs and IADLs were about 79% less likely to use the services in the past two weeks and 2.1 times more likely to check sporadically compared to the use in primary care.

These data corroborate with a study that identified the factors associated with the use of health services by elderly people with chronic diseases, which concluded that medical appointment among elderly people who are functionally incapable was 30% more prevalent when compared to those without functional limitations [50].

Regarding the occurrence of falls, those who did not suffer any type of fall in the last year were 1.9 times more likely to have a sporadic medical appointment compared to the appointment in primary care. A study carried out in four Brazilian states concluded that men, even in different social contexts, prefer to delay the search for assistance as much as possible and only do so when they are no longer able to deal with their symptoms alone [41]. This fact reinforces that, if elderly men do not have clinical complications, they do not use health services frequently, mainly in a preventive way.

As a methodological limitation, this study presented common restrictions to research using secondary databases, namely: the variables and objectives studied in the PNS database have already been established, which prevented new variables from being included; and long questionnaires, such as those applied in the PNS, can generate memory bias, in which the participant forgets or loses the desire to report past events.

However, despite the intrinsic limitations to the methodological design, this article is an essential contribution to the study of the aging of the male population in Northeast Brazil, with the possibility of a new look at the theme and can serve as an instrument for planning and institution of actions and public policies for this population.

Finally, it reinforces the importance of research on human aging aimed at the male population, as this study identified that healthcare and the use of health services by elderly men in Northeast Brazil are focused to medium and high complexity and in the presence of diseases or functional disabilities. Thus, intra-sectoral and inter-sectoral policies and actions should encourage the contact of the elderly male population with health services at an early stage, especially in Primary Care, addressing to reduce gender disparities in healthcare.

5. Conclusion

This study identified that healthcare and the use of health services by elderly men in Northeast Brazil are focused to medium and high complexity and in the presence of diseases or functional disabilities. Thus, intra-sectoral and inter-sectoral policies and actions should encourage the contact of the elderly male population with health services at an early stage, especially in Primary Care, addressing to reduce gender disparities in healthcare, and further studies should be carried out to analyze and reinforce the importance of research on human aging aimed at the male population.

Acknowledgements

For the scientific initiation scholarship granted by the Oswaldo Cruz Foundation.

Author details

Gisele Mariel de Sousa Vasconcelos[1,2]*, Alana Maiara Brito Bibiano[1], Lucas Fernando Rodrigues dos Santos[1] and Rafael da Silveira Moreira[1,2]

1 Instituto Aggeu Magalhães/Fiocruz, Recife, Pernambuco, Brazil

2 Universidade Federal de Pernambuco (UFPE), Recife, Pernambuco, Brazil

*Address all correspondence to: giselemsvasconcelos@gmail.com

References

[1] Nasri F. O envelhecimento populacional no Brasil. einstein, 2008; 6 (supl 1): S4-S6. , jan. 2008.

[2] Lima-Costa MF, Barreto SM, Giatti L. Condições de saúde, capacidade funcional, uso de serviços de saúde e gastos com medicamentos da população idosa brasileira: um estudo descritivo baseado na Pesquisa Nacional por Amostra de Domicílios. Cad. Saúde Pública 2003; 19(3): 735-743. https://doi.org/10.1590/S0102-311X2003000300006

[3] Mendoza-Sassi R, Béria JU. Utilización de los servicios de salud: una revisión sistemática sobre los factores relacionados. Cad. Saúde Pública 2001; 17(4): 819-832. https://doi.org/10.1590/S0102-311X2001000400016

[4] Veras R, Parahyba MI. O anacronismo dos modelos assistenciais para os idosos na área da saúde: desafios para o setor privado. Cad. Saúde Pública 2007; 23(10): 2479-2489. https://doi.org/10.1590/S0102-311X2007001000022

[5] Travassos C, Martins *M. uma* revisão sobre os conceitos de acesso e utilização de serviços de saúde. Cad. Saúde Pública 2004; 20(suppl.2): 190-198. https://doi.org/10.1590/S0102-311X2004000800014

[6] Andersen RM. Revisiting the behavioral model and access to medical care: does it matter?. J Health Soc Behav 1995; 36(1): 1-10.

[7] Andersen RM, Newman JF. Societal and Individual Determinants of Medical Care Utilization in the United States. The Milbank Quarterly 2005; 83(4): 95-124.

[8] Courtenay WH. Constructions of masculinity and their influence on men's well-being: a theory of gender and health. Soc Sci Med 2000; 50(10): 1385-1401. doi: 10.1016/s0277-9536(99)00390-1

[9] Laurenti R, Jorge MHPM, Gotlieb SLD. Perfil epidemiológico da morbi-mortalidade masculina. Ciênc. Saúde Coletiva 2005; 10(1). http://dx.doi.org/10.1590/S1413-81232005000100010

[10] Luck M, Bamford M, Williamson P. Men's Health: Perspectives, Diversity and Paradox. London: [s.n.], 2000. 288 p.

[11] Figueiredo W. Assistência à saúde dos homens: um desafio para os serviços de atenção primária. Ciênc. Saúde Coletiva 2005; 10(1): 105-109. https://doi.org/10.1590/S1413-81232005000100017

[12] Pinheiro RS, Viacava F, Travassos C, Brito AS. Gênero, morbidade, acesso e utilização de serviços de saúde no Brasil. Ciênc. Saúde Coletiva 2002; 7(4): 687-707. https://doi.org/10.1590/S1413-81232002000400007

[13] Gomes R. Sexualidade masculina e saúde do homem: proposta para uma discussão. Ciênc. Saúde Coletiva 2003; 8 (3): 825-829. https://doi.org/10.1590/S1413-81232003000300017

[14] Keijzer B. Hasta donde el cuerpo aguante: Género, Cuerpo y Salud Masculina. In: Cáceres CF, Cueto M, Ramos M, Vallas S, editors. La salud como derecho ciudadano: perspectivas y propuestas desde América Latina, Lima: Universidad Peruana Cayetano Heredia, p. 137-152, 2003.

[15] Schraiber LB, Gomes R, Couto MT. Homens e saúde na pauta da Saúde Coletiva. Ciênc. Saúde Coletiva 2005; 10 (1): 7-17. https://doi.org/10.1590/S1413-81232005000100002

[16] World Health Organization. What about boys?. Geneva: [s.n.], 2000. 58 p.

[17] Neto LG. Ciclos econômicos e desigualdades regionais no Brasil. Cad. Est. Soc. 2011; 14(2): 315-342.

[18] Souza-Junior PRB, Freitas MPS, Antonaci GA, Szwarcwald CL. Desenho da amostra da Pesquisa Nacional de Saúde 2013. Epidemiol. Serv. Saúde 2015; 24(2): 207-216. https://doi.org/10.5123/S1679-49742015000200003

[19] Silva AMM et al. Uso de serviços de saúde por idosos brasileiros com e sem limitação funcional. Rev. Saúde Pública 2017; 51(supl 1). https://doi.org/10.1590/s1518-8787.2017051000243

[20] Bibiano AMB. Fatores associados à utilização dos serviços de saúde pelos homens idosos no Brasil [dissertação de mestrado]. Recife: Universidade Federal de Pernambuco (UFPE); 2017.

[21] Freitas MPS, Lila MF, Azevedo RV, Antonaci GA. Amostra Mestra para o Sistema Integrado de Pesquisas Domiciliares. Ministério do Planejamento, Orçamento e Gestão. Instituto Brasileiro de Geografia e Estatística (IBGE), (Textos para discussão. Diretoria de Pesquisas, 23), Rio de Janeiro, 2007.

[22] Brasil. Ministério da Saúde, Ministério do Planejamento, Orçamento e Gestão, Instituto Brasileiro de Geografia e Estatística. Fundação Oswaldo Cruz – Fiocruz. Pesquisa Nacional de Saúde 2013 - Percepção do estado de saúde, estilos de vida e doenças crônicas. Rio de Janeiro: 2014, (1) p. 7-11.

[23] Brasil. Ministério da Saúde, Ministério do Planejamento, Orçamento e Gestão, Instituto Brasileiro de Geografia e Estatística. Fundação Oswaldo Cruz – Fiocruz. Pesquisa Nacional de Saúde 2013 – Acesso e utilização dos serviços de saúde, acidentes e violência. Rio de Janeiro: 2015a, (2) p. 7-11.

[24] Brasil. Ministério da Saúde, Ministério do Planejamento, Orçamento e Gestão, Instituto Brasileiro de Geografia e Estatística. Fundação Oswaldo Cruz – Fiocruz. Pesquisa Nacional de Saúde 2013 – Ciclos de vida. Rio de Janeiro: 2015b, (3) p. 7-11.

[25] Mastella JO. Análise de Classes Latentes: da Teoria à Prática. Porto Alegre: UFRGS, 2015.

[26] Jung T, Wickrama KAS. An Introduction to Latent Class Growth Analysis and Growth Mixture Modeling. Social and Personality Psychology Compass 2008; 21(10): 302–317. https://doi.org/10.1111/j.1751-9004.2007.00054.x

[27] Ducan TE, Ducan SC, Strycker LA. An Introduction to Latent Variable Growth Curve Modeling. 2ª ed. Mahwah: Lawrence Eribaum Associates, 2011.

[28] Araújo F, Pais-Ribeiro J, Oliveira A, Pinto C. Validação do Índice de Barthel numa amostra de idosos não institucionalizados. Rev. Portuguesa Saúde Pública 2007; 25(2): 59-66.

[29] Araújo F, Pais-Ribeiro J, Oliveira A, Pinto C, Martins T. Validação da escala de Lawton e Brody numa amostra de idosos não institucionalizados. In I. Leal, J. Pais-Ribeiro, I. Silva & S. Marques (Eds.), Actas do 7° Congresso Nacional de Psicologia da Saúde, 2008, Lisboa: ISPA, p. 217-220.

[30] Duarte YAO, Andrade CL, Lebrão ML. O Índex de Katz na avaliação da funcionalidade dos idosos. Revista da Escola Enfermagem da USP 2007; 41(2): 317-325.

[31] Cover TM, Thomas JA. Elements of Information Theory. 2ª ed. Hoboken: John Wiley & Sons, 2006.

[32] Dziak JJ, et al. Sensitivity and Specificity of Information Criteria. Peer J preprints 2015; p. 1–20.

[33] Snijders TAB, Bosker RJ. Multilevel analysis. An introduction to basic and advanced multilevel modelling. 2ª ed. London - SAGE Publication: 1999.

[34] Hosmer DW, Lemeshow S. Model-Building strategies and methods for logistic regression. In: HOSMER, D. W.; LEMESHOW, S. Applied logistic regression. 2ª.ed. Hoboken: John Wiley & Sons, 2000. p. 91-142.

[35] World Health Organization - WHO. World Report on Aging and Health. Luxembourg: 2015.

[36] Arruda GO, Marcon SS. Inquérito sobre a utilização dos serviços de saúde por homens adultos: prevalências e fatores associados. Rev. Latino Americana de Enfermagem 2016; 24: 2685. DOI: 10.1590/1518-8345.0296.2685

[37] Arruda GO, Mathias TAF, Marcon SS. Prevalência e fatores associados à utilização de serviços públicos de saúde por homens adultos. Ciênc. Saúde Coletiva 2017; 22(1): 279-290. https://doi.org/10.1590/1413-81232017221.20532015

[38] Chiavegatto Filho ADP, Wang YP, Malik AM, Takaoka J, Viana MC, Andrade LH. Determinantes do uso de serviços de saúde: análise multinível da Região Metropolitana de São Paulo. Rev. Saúde Pública 2015; 49(1): 1-12. https://doi.org/10.1590/S0034-8910.2015049005246

[39] Kim JL, Cho J, Park S, Park EC. Depression symptom and Professional mental health service use. BioMed Central Psychiatry 2015; 15: 261.

[40] Brasil. Ministério da Saúde. Política Nacional de Atenção Básica. Brasília: Ministério da Saúde, 2012. (Série E. Legislação em Saúde).

[41] Gomes R et al. O atendimento à saúde de homens: estudo qualitativo em quatro estados Brasileiros. Physis: Revista de Saúde Coletiva 2011; 21(1): 1-10. https://doi.org/10.1590/S0103-73312011000100007

[42] Nardi AC, Glina S, Favorito LA. Estudo epidemiológico sobre câncer de pênis no Brasil. Int Braz J Urol. 2007; 33 (Suppl 1): 1-7.

[43] Noronha KVMS, Andrade MV. Desigualdades sociais em saúde e na utilização dos serviços de saúde entre os idosos na América Latina. Rev. Panamericana de Salud Publica 2005; 17 (5/6): 410-8.

[44] Wallace SP, Gutiérrez VF. La equidad del acceso de adultos mayores a la atención de salud en cuatro grandes ciudades latinoamericanas. Rev. Panamericana de Salud Publica 2005; 17 (5/6): 394-409.

[45] Brasil. Ministério da Saúde. Departamento de Ações Programáticas Estratégicas. Política Nacional de Atenção Integral à Saúde do Homem (PNAISH). Brasília (DF): Ministério da Saúde; 2008.

[46] Zhang L, Wang H. Dynamic process of adverse selection: evidence from a subsidized community-based health insurance in rural China. Soc Sci Med. 2008; 67(7): 1173-1182. DOI: 10.1016/j.socscimed.2008.06.024

[47] Almeida MF, Barata RB, Montero CV, Silva ZP. Prevalência de doenças crônicas auto-referidas e utilização de serviços de saúde, PNAD/1998, Brasil. Ciênc. Saúde Coletiva 2002; 7(4): 743-756. https://doi.org/10.1590/S1413-81232002000400011

[48] Organização Mundial de Saúde. Mental Health: New Understanding, New Hope. 1ª ed, Lisboa; 2002.

[49] Alves LC, Leite IC, Machado CJ. Conceituando e mensurando a

incapacidade funcional da população idosa: uma revisão de literatura. Ciênc. Saúde Coletiva 2008; 13(4): 1199-207. https://doi.org/10.1590/S1413-81232008000400016

[50] Rodrigues MAP, et al. Uso de serviços básicos de saúde por idosos portadores de condições crônicas, Brasil. Rev.Saúde Pública 2009; 43(4): 604-612. https://doi.org/10.1590/S0034-89102009005000037

Chapter 11

Access to Emergency Healthcare

Abdulnasir F.H. Al Jazairi and Guillaume Alinier

Abstract

Access to emergency services is essential for the health and well-being of people. The World Health Organization (WHO) made it a human right for everybody to have access to emergency care and it is an ethical obligation for governments to provide this service for the whole population. In recent years, the overcrowding in emergency departments has become a prominent issue that needs proper solutions. There have been several attempts resolving this ongoing issue. One of those is the patients' distribution according to the severity level of their chief complaint, since more than half of the urgent cases are of low acuity and can be managed in less equipped facilities. Primary healthcare centers are perfectly suited to look after a significant proportion of cases for many reasons such as their scope of service, their wider geographical distribution, and are a more cost-effective resource for such cases than the use of higher acuity facilities. In Qatar, we have been implementing such model of patient distribution to release the burden on emergency departments since 1999. In this chapter we are proposing a full protocol to distribute emergency patients involving the ambulance service, primary healthcare centers, and emergency departments. Cooperation of all these services with the help of higher authorities and media is expected to show great improvements in patient care and better crowd control in emergency departments.

Keywords: healthcare access, emergency care, urgent care, ambulance service, triage

1. Introduction

The World Health Organization (WHO) made it a human right for everybody to have access to emergency care and it is an ethical obligation for governments to provide this service for the whole population [1]. It is an instinct for human beings to search better living place for themselves and family. There are several criteria to consider regarding the suitability of a place or city to live in. One important indicator is quality of life in general and an essential part of it is accessibility to high quality healthcare services. Part of quality assessment of healthcare in modern medicine is the time factor and easy access to healthcare services especially in emergency situations, such as serious traumatic injuries, myocardial infarction, stroke, infection ...etc. Putting such system in place relies on an infrastructure which encompasses the provision to the general public of an emergency services contact number managed by a call center. The emergency medical dispatchers answering the calls should ideally have oversight of the status and location of the response vehicles around the caller so they can send the required help in the shortest amount of time as possible [2]. The expectation of the caller is to then be attended to by a team of well-trained professionals

IntechOpen

coming in a vehicle equipped to deal with a wide range of medical emergencies. If transportation of the patient is needed, the next requirement is to have local and appropriately resourced facilities that can provide emergency and potentially definitive care. There are many factors to account for, a multitude of potential stakeholders, and several health delivery system models to consider for the provision of emergency care. This chapter will discuss access to emergency care and relate to our experience of working in the State of Qatar, a country which has been developing very fast since the beginning of the 21st century across several sectors, including healthcare [3].

2. Background

Early in the history of medicine, "healers", who we would now call physicians, had a general scope of practice and were looking at every all types of complaints from patients [4]. Before the widespread of telecommunication technology, patients were often expected to report to the physician as opposed to the physician receiving an emergency call to then travel to meet their patient. Then there was specialization into medicine and surgery. Those main branches were gradually divided into many others increasing number of subspecialties [5] and lead to the advancement of medical care in general. This has played a role into increasing our life expectancy, especially in the most developed countries. On the other hand, it has also led to the fragmentation of health services. There is a tendency for each service to concentrate on their narrow scope of practice, generally limiting patient access to other services. Some patients' health issues may not be diagnosed and the complaints they might raise may not be carefully considered and addressed. There was a need for a specialty to look at patients as a whole entity so they can be appropriately referred and benefit from the best line of management from other more specialized physicians or other healthcare professionals. Acting as a patient advocate is often the role of the modern family physician or general practitioner, but it can also be perceived as a gatekeeping activity which raises concerns [6, 7].

Furthermore, there was difficulty in accessing health services in emergency situations. This elicited the need for out of hospital emergency services, primarily started as a transport service, eventually with first aid capability, to pick up patients wherever they were and take them to a hospital where they could be seen by a medical professional [8]. This was followed by the development of the emergency medicine specialty. The role of the emergency medicine specialist is not to provide long-term care and follow up patients until they recover from their illness or injury, but simply to provide immediate urgent care and act as one of the possible entry points into the healthcare system. That healthcare system can then provide longer terms support with follow up appointments organized with the appropriately specialized department(s) and clinicians, or if necessary, the patient may be admitted as an in-patient into the hospital for longer-term care. The issue is that many patients are either playing with the system to their personal advantage to gain quicker treatment to the detriment of others or that they do not understand the real function of an ambulance service and the emergency department (ED). Many people call an ambulance or use emergency departments to obtain quicker service and avoid long delays in obtaining appointments in outpatient clinics. The crowding of EDs has become a growing global problem [9, 10]. There is a need for a new way of dealing with the varying degrees of emergency cases to decongest emergency departments so patients in a real emergency condition can be seen in a timely matter. It could play a significant role in decreasing mortality and morbidity, and making more cost-effective use of healthcare resources.

3. Qatar experience in emergency health access

Qatar is a small country and has a special population distribution. Around 80% of the population is concentrated in the capital city Doha and its immediately neighboring district of Al Rayyan [11]. For a long time, before the rapid expansion of the country in the last 15 years, there was only one ED, in Hamad Medical Corporation (HMC) Hamad General Hospital (HGH), situated in Doha. Patients needed to come from distant places for any medical emergency. This was challenging for many people, especially during nighttime and weekends, as the road network was limited. The Chairman of the HGH Emergency Department, at that time, lead a project to have an emergency room in selected primary healthcare centers. The basis for this decision was to bring emergency services closer to people and decrease unnecessary visits to the main ED in Doha, especially as more than 50% of emergency cases were of low acuity and did not need clinical investigations or admission. The project started during early October 1999 in one center. The services provided were considered a success and these minor emergency rooms were developed in nine primary healthcare centers in the following few years according to the population distribution as illustrated in **Figure 1**. They were called Adult Urgent Care Centers (AUCC).

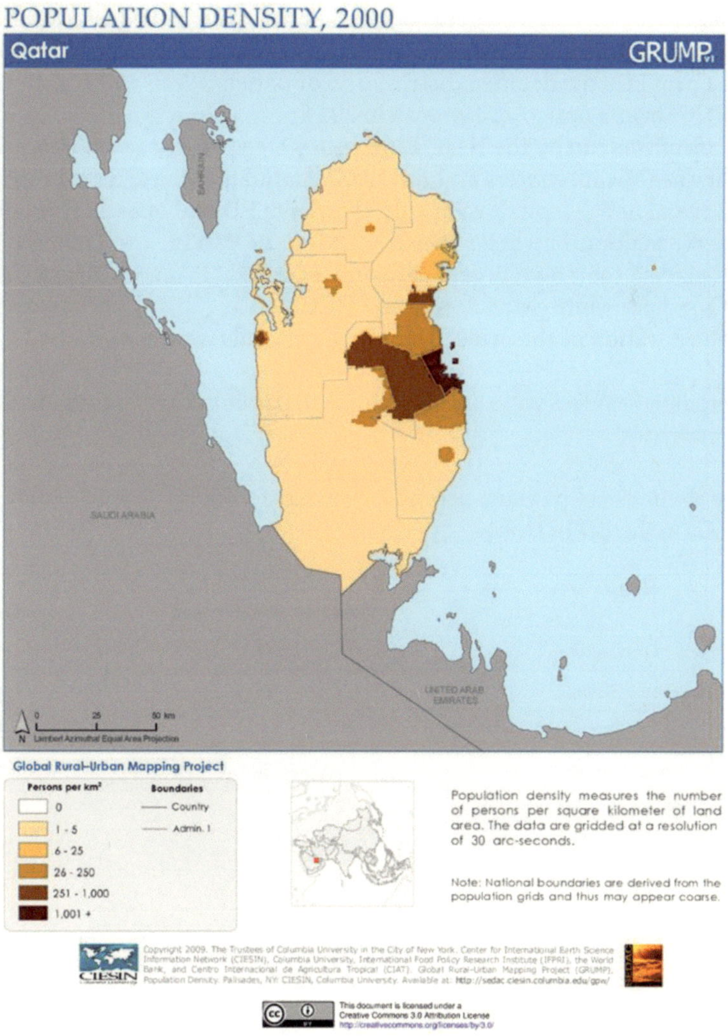

Figure 1.
Population distribution in Qatar in the year 2000.

The AUCC emergency room in each of the Primary Healthcare Centers included the following:

1. Space: An area near the entrance for easy access and evacuation of critical patients. Doctors were regularly rotated between the AUCC and the main HGH ED in order to maintain their skills. Moreover, the doctors needed to have experience in working alone to make clinical decisions and undertake simple investigations.

2. Staffing: Doctors and nurses were from the ED. The ancillary services (e.g. laboratory, radiology, and pharmacy) were supported by the primary healthcare center.

3. Patient transfer: Arrangements were made with the Ambulance Service to have an ambulance on standby in the vicinity for rapid transfer of patients.

4. Working hours: The AUCC emergency rooms was opened the whole week continuously, day and night.

The AUCCs distributed around Qatar collectively received around 6,000 patients per month. About 97% were treated directly by the AUCC staff and discharged home with the possibility of a referral to the outpatient clinics according to the patients' complaint and needs. Only 3.% were referred and transported to the ED by ambulance.

Table 1 provides the detailed distribution of patients seen and transferred across all the AUCCs over a period of 1 month in 2014.

The project was run by the HMC Emergency Department in collaboration with the primary healthcare centers and the HMC Ambulance Service from 1999 to 2016. By 2016, several new hospitals each with their own ED had opened throughout Qatar to serve major urban areas such as Al Khor, Al Wakra, and Dukhan. Moreover the PHCC started their own urgent care project called "Primary Urgent Care", and the AUCCs' responsibility transferred to PHCC.

Over the duration of the project, a number of goals were achieved:

1. Emergency services were brought closer to patients hence saving travel time and expenses.

2. Only about 3% of patients needed to be transferred by ambulance from the AUCCs to the ED in Doha.

AUCC	Patients transferred to ED	Patients encounters
Primary Healthcare Center 1	49	486
Primary Healthcare Center 2	18	407
Primary Healthcare Center 3	8	323
Primary Healthcare Center 4	5	181
Primary Healthcare Center 5	15	712
Primary Healthcare Center 6	30	888
Primary Healthcare Center 7	53	1714
Primary Healthcare Center 8	22	1363
Primary Healthcare Center 9	0	29
Total:	200	6103

Table 1.
Sample of AUCC patient encounters corresponding to October 2014.

3. Treatment in AUCCs is less expensive than in the main emergency department, so it facilitated a more cost-effective use of resources.

4. This project served as a training opportunity for doctors to practice medicine with limited resources.

Patient transfers to the emergency department from primary healthcare centers after 2016 was 10% (personal contact).

4. New project proposal

According to the above-mentioned data, we are proposing a new project for distributing patients with urgent complaints according to the level of severity of their medical complaint. This project depends on a common triage system used by the Ambulance Service, the Primary Healthcare system, and the Emergency Department to dispose of patients appropriately.

5. The triad of emergency healthcare

In most countries, there are three health services that deal with patients regardless of their chief health complaint, age, or gender. Those are the prehospital emergency medical services (EMS), commonly managed by one more ambulance services, the hospital emergency departments, and the primary healthcare centers or clinics (PHC).

Traditionally, patients, who require emergency care seek treatment in an emergency department. They may either directly report there using their own means of transportation or may have been brought in by ambulance. Each approach has its own advantages and disadvantages depending on how the system operates and what resources are available. Ambulance services and hospital EDs around the world are often overwhelmed [12, 13] and this is where the primary healthcare system can play an important role in sharing the burden as described above where we presented the Qatar experience. In turn, this relies on facilities being appropriately resourced and the general public being educated to make the correct use of the services available based on the urgency of their apparent or suspected health related complaint.

We propose that the ideal solution to providing patients with effective access to emergency care relies on a collaborative triad composed of a clinically focused ambulance service, a network of primary healthcare centers with a minor illnesses and injury unit, and geographically distributed hospital-based emergency departments, also based on patient density. Their respective scope could be defined as follows:

1. Ambulance service: Mobile team of well-trained clinicians able to deal with all urgent and critical cases in the community setting, supported by appropriate medical equipment, therapeutic drugs, and various means of transportation. Ambulance resources are centrally managed and crews are dispatched from a call center after receiving an emergency call [14]. Upon careful consideration, thorough physical patient assessment, and remote clinical advice from a more senior clinician, ambulance crews may determine if a patient requires or not transportation to hospital or a primary healthcare centre for emergency treatment.

2. Primary healthcare centers: Facilities traditionally focusing on providing non-critical patient care, generally dealing with acute and chronic illnesses, but also delivering preventive care and patient health education. They usually

have limited diagnostic equipment capability (e.g. X-ray, ultrasound) because of their holistic approach to patient assessment and care. They cannot admit patients, but can refer to other specialties. They are generally staffed by nurses and family physicians who may also have additional subspecialties such as women's health and dermatology to cite a few examples.

3. Emergency departments: Hospital department that can be accessed by any patient without prior appointment and that is staffed by a multi-professional team of clinicians able to deal with all emergency conditions. It reacts faster than other specialties in the hospital and provides rapid access to radiology and other urgent services such as cardiology and trauma surgery. They can facilitate admission of patients into the relevant department for definitive care.

6. How to make the primary healthcare centers suitable to manage urgent medical cases

The primary healthcare centers are ideally located in residential areas to be easily accessible to patients for routine checkups and to receive treatment for minor ailments, but others may seek consultations for more urgent medical conditions. To offer this service, primary healthcare centers need to meet a number of criteria with the way they operate, especially in the domains of:

1. Patient screening: As a starting point, a triage nurse should be able to perform some basic assessment to determine if the patient's condition can be dealt with through a normal clinic appointment, as an emergency suitable for the primary healthcare center to deal with, or if an emergency transfer by ambulance should be arranged to a hospital ED.

2. Space management: There needs to be an area near the entrance of each primary healthcare centre set up to receive patients seeking emergency care. It should be equipped to deal with a few patients with minor injuries or other medical complaint at a time. Ideally, the primary healthcare center could also serve as an ambulance service standby location with dedicated parking and welfare facilities for the crew, so if an emergency transfer to hospital is required, there is a chance for an ambulance to be already available within the premises and ready to take a critically ill or injured patient to the nearest ED.

3. Staffing: Staff (doctors, nurses, and ancillary staff) assigned to treat patients in such urgent care clinic should be trained to deal with a wide range of complaints. Following the initial screening, duties will be either to immediately treat patients and discharging them home, or noticing red flags and transferring them to ED for more advanced treatment and possible hospitalization. Ideally, a qualified emergency physician from the nearby ED should have short rotations (maximum of 1 month) in the urgent care clinic of a primary healthcare center so they do not lose their skills in dealing with more critical patients.

4. Administrative issues: There are several administrative requirements for primary healthcare centers to be able to deal with urgent cases and help relieve the pressure on hospital emergency services. For examples:

   a. Agreement with an ambulance service to transfer patients to and from the primary healthcare center if and as required.

b. Agreement with a local hospital to accept critically ill patients referred by a primary healthcare center urgent care clinic.

c. Agreement on a common patient triage system across all the three services to ensure patients are appropriately managed.

d. Staff duty roaster of primary healthcare centers needs to accommodate for extended working hours in order to accept urgent cases as per the local population's needs. The required operational hours could be continuous day and night and including weekends, or less depending on needs.

7. Providing access to effective emergency care

"Access" is a multifaceted term. From the patient's perspective it may start by picking up the phone to either call an emergency number, a healthcare advice number, or a clinic to book a primary care appointment. Each country, state, or community operates slightly differently but some of the possible decision pathways from call takers in the case of a potential medical emergency are illustrated in **Figure 2**. It may range from the call taker simply providing advice to a patient over the phone regarding a minor ailment, to dispatching an ambulance crew, sometimes with a rapid response vehicle if a higher level of response is required. Call takers may also advise the caller to either call another healthcare assistance number or to call their primary healthcare clinic [15]. Call takers may either be clinicians (nurse, physician…), Emergency Medical Dispatchers (EMDs) with or without clinical training, or even clerical staff [16, 17]. Advice they provide and decisions they make are often based on a scripted series of questions aimed at getting information from the caller to eventually select the most appropriate protocol to follow and potentially dispatch an ambulance or determine that no face to face help was needed [18].

Once an ambulance crew reaches the patient and the assessment is performed. The paramedics can decide of the most appropriate patient disposition which may be one of four possibilities as illustrated in **Figure 3**. Such practice varies vastly between ambulance service providers and from country to country [15, 19]. Many factors may impact on the patient transport decisions made by ambulance crews, such as

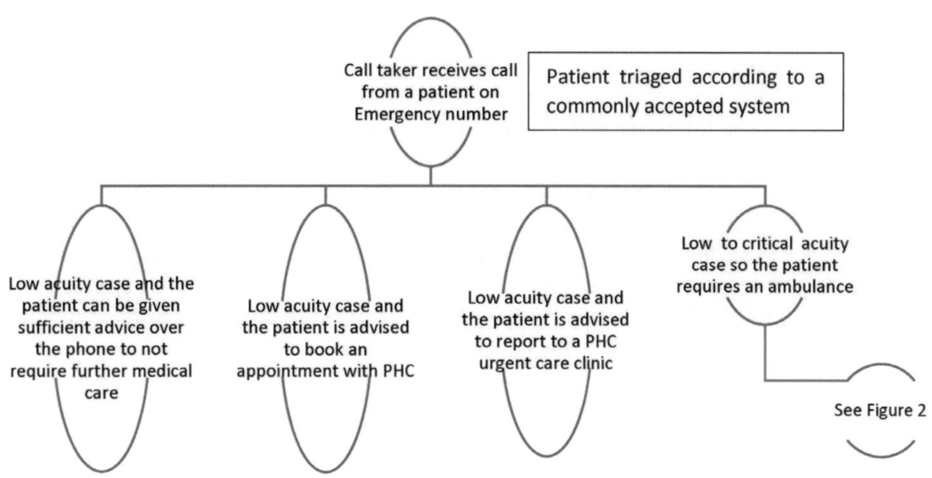

Figure 2.
Proposed call taker decision tree when communicating with a patient or caller.

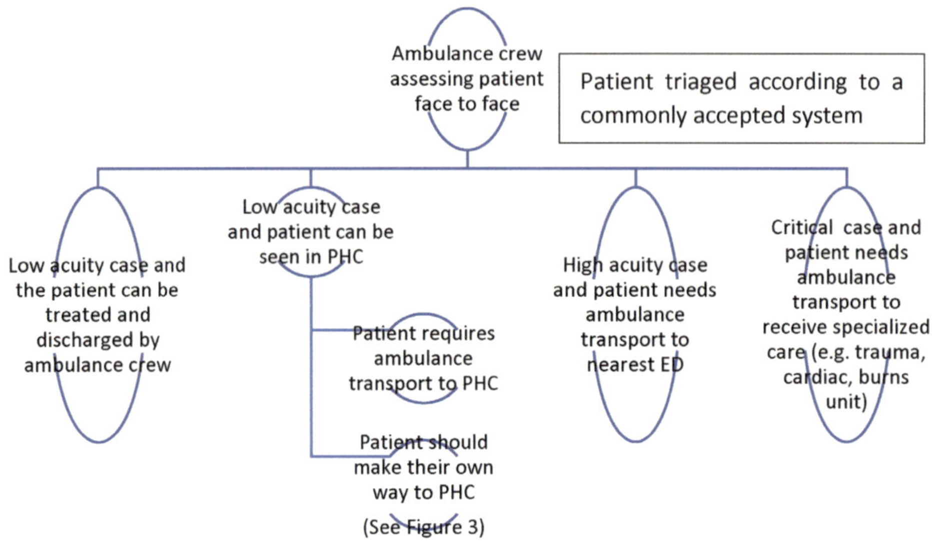

Figure 3.
Possible ambulance crew decisions after assessing a patient face to face.

operating procedures, patient triage algorithms, healthcare policies, relationships with other healthcare entities, staff training, but also the pressure of the call volume the ambulance service is experiencing at the time. In some cases the patient may be provided with reassurance, treated on scene, and discharged by the ambulance crew [10]. The paramedics may advise the patient to seek further medical help if needed, but there are potential negative implications such as subsequent emergency call, delayed care, or even mortality [20]. Another possibility is that the ambulance crew might not be the best suited clinical team to address the patient's needs so they may be offered transportation to their local PHC or advised to report there by their own means of transportation so the crew can instead deal with more critical cases. Then comes what should be the most common scenario, corresponding to a real emergency call, whereby the ambulance crew needs to provide immediate care and transport the patient to an ED. There are also highly critical cases which require the prehospital intervention of additional clinicians with a wider scope of practice before the patient can be safely transported to an ED or other highly specialized facility. Some specific triage or scoring system based on physiological, motor, and mental status parameters if often used to identify the level of severity of the patient condition [21]. For such cases and depending on the country's prehospital response model adopted, the call taker may dispatch a prehospital emergency physician with a nurse anesthetist or a critical care paramedic who will help stabilize the patient or perform other lifesaving procedures before urgent transportation to a more specialized facility such as a high level trauma centre, cardiac centre, or severe burns unit.

PHC services in general can play a big role in reducing the number of ED visits [10, 22]. Whether a patient has been referred over the phone to report to a PHC Urgent Care Clinic (UCC) by a call taker (**Figure 2**) or by an ambulance crew advising them to self-transport there (**Figure 3**), or a patient is directly self-reporting there, the triage nurse will first assess them. The possible outcomes of a visit to the PHC UCC are illustrated in **Figure 4**. The patient may be immediately treated (depending on how busy the UCC is) and discharged. If the case is a more complex, treatment may be initiated and the patient will be reassessed after a short period of time (e.g. 2 hours). Depending on the evolution of the patient's condition, they may either be discharged or an ambulance transfer may be arranged to the nearest ED. If from the

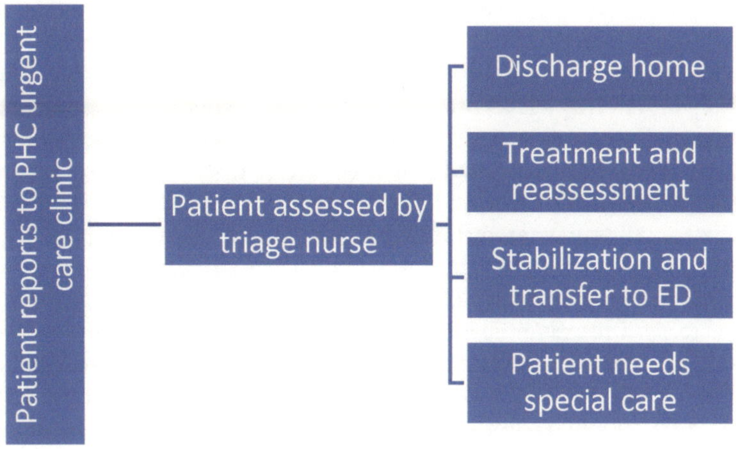

Figure 4.
Disposition of patients reporting to a primary healthcare center urgent care clinic.

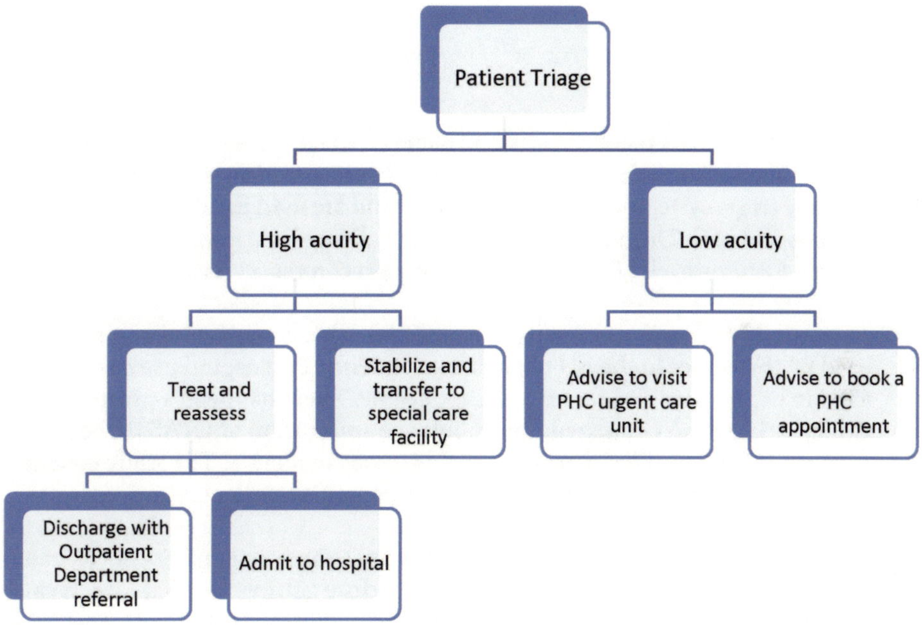

Figure 5.
Emergency Department triage algorithm incorporating the recommendation for low acuity patients to report to a Primary Healthcare Center Urgent Care Clinic.

initial assessment, the patient is determined to have deteriorated from the previous interaction with the call taker or ambulance crew, only stabilization measures will be performed and arrangements will be made to transfer the patient to ED without delay. Lastly, if the patient requires special emergency care (e.g. myocardial infarction), an emergency call will be made so they will be transported by ambulance to a specialized facility as a high priority case, possibly with a more medically advanced team (e.g. accompanied by a critical care paramedic). The presence of an ambulance on standby near the PHC is an important element for the rapid transfer of such cases.

Lastly, the case when a patient reports directly to an ED needs to be considered. Again some form of triage needs to be implemented to determine if the patient is trying to make use of the most appropriate service. There are several triage systems, for example the Canadian Triage and Acuity Scale (CTAS) and many other validated triage systems are commonly used in emergency departments worldwide [23, 24]. Most systems result in EDs seeing all patients, even those with a very low acuity level, but their non-urgent triage level often results in them experiencing a potentially very long wait time before being seen after their initial assessment. This is usually not a pleasant experience for patients and will affect their satisfaction level with the overall care experience eventually received [25]. **Figure 5** proposes an ED triage algorithm incorporating a pathway whereby low acuity patients are asked to report to a Primary Healthcare Center Urgent Care Clinic or to book a primary care appointment. Probably not the desired outcome of a patient's visit to the ED, this approach would be expected to significantly relieve the pressure on EDs and contribute to a better use of the ED resources and expertise. Higher acuity patients will however be treated more rapidly, according to the severity of their health condition, and reassessed to determine if they should be discharged with or without a referral for a follow up out-patient consultation, or be admitted into hospital for definitive care. In some particular cases, if the patient walked-in, was wrongly transported to hospital by ambulance, or their condition changed, they may need to be urgently transferred to a specialized emergency facility (e.g. trauma, cardiac, burns unit) after having been stabilized.

8. Triage systems

The baseline for this process depends on having a triage system accepted by all services. Until now there is no single internationally accepted triage system [26] and instead many triage systems have been developed and are used in different countries all over the world [24]. The most widely used and validated triage systems divide patients into 5 acuity levels [27, 28]. Some of the most commonly used systems include:

1. The Canadian Triage and Acuity Scale (CTAS): this is a 5-level acuity system used by the nurses in the ED to prioritize patients. Prehospital use has been tired in paper cases and found to be applicable. There has been a prospective clinical trial which compared the ambulance application of CTAS to the ED nurses application. The interrater reliability was moderate. The study concluded that CTAS can be used reliably in the prehospital setting [29].

2. The Australian triage system: It is also a 5-level triage system that concentrates on the maximum time the patient can wait before getting hospital care. It can be used by paramedics in prehospital cases for prioritization of patients [30].

3. The Manchester triage system (MTS): It depends on flow charts which the nurse choose according to the patient's complaint. Following those charts helps the nurse to determine to which of the five categories the patient belongs to [31].

4. The emergency severity index (ESI): This is an easy to implement 5-level triaging system used mainly in the United States. It uses one algorithm for all patients to determine the patient's triage severity level [32].

There are many other triage systems used by emergency departments and pre-hospital care services, some are validated while others are not [33]. Until now there is no single internationally accepted triage system [26]. This is probably because not all countries are equally equipped and prepared to implement a common triage system and act according to the findings of the triage levels, however they simply try to deliver the best possible care to all patients.

The use of the primary healthcare centers and family physicians in providing emergency care has been practiced in several countries, especially in small cities and rural areas [10, 34]. The American Association of family physicians published a position paper highlights the many benefits of using "family medicine centers" (i.e. primary healthcare centers) and family physicians for the delivery of emergency and urgent care [35]. They also mention that the provision of emergency care "require a cooperative relationship between among a variety of health professional". Some of the benefits include:

1. Delivering urgent care is part of the comprehensive patient care model adopted by the family physician.

2. The geographical distribution of primary healthcare centers nearby people facilitates their easy and rapid access to their healthcare needs.

3. More than 50% of urgent cases are simple and can be managed efficiently by family physicians.

4. PHC are more cost-effective facilities to treat minor emergency cases as it has been determined that, in the United Kingdom, treating one patient costs 124 Great Britain Pounds (GBP) in the ED while it costs only 32 GBP in a primary care clinic setting [36].

9. The key pieces to effective emergency service provision

To implement the proposed solution the following needed:

A. Ambulance service and call center: The key factor in this system is the presence of a good ambulance service with an optimal distribution of its resources at standby locations situated around the state or country (**Figure 6**) and skilled staff, coordinated by EMDs responding to the emergency calls gathering information form patients, providing them with advice, and dispatching ambulance crews as required (**Figure 7**) [14, 37]. Whether it is through a emergency or medical advice phone number, healthcare call center staff can play a key role in addressing a large number of simple medical cases by providing telephone advice and consultations [17, 38]. When an ambulance is dispatched, upon reaching the patient(s), paramedics can assess their health condition using a validated triage system, and

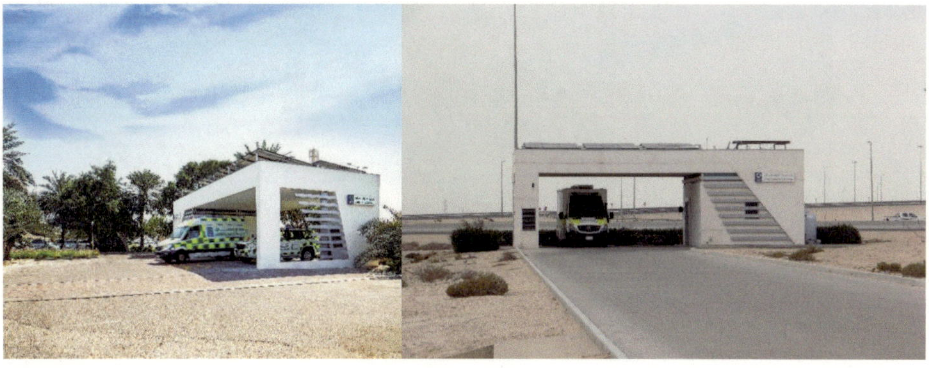

Figure 6.
Standalone ambulance standby locations geographically distributed based on call volumes in urban and rural areas to reach patients rapidly.

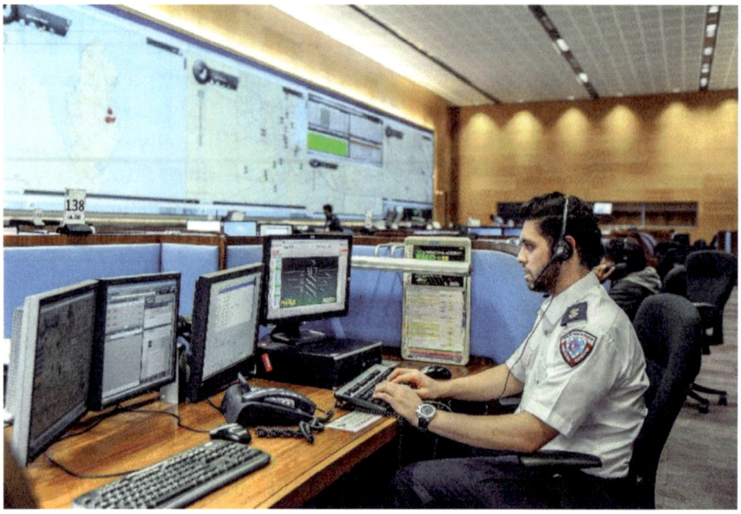

Figure 7.
Emergency medical dispatcher in the Ambulance Service control room.

initiate treatment before deciding of the most appropriate patient disposition (**Figure 3**). We recommend the use of the emergency severity score (ESI) because it is easy, fast, and requires little training on the part of the clinicians [28, 32].

B. Primary Healthcare Centers: an urgent care room should be available 24/7 in primary healthcare centers to receive minor emergency cases (**Figure 8**). The source of these cases may be walk- in patients or low acuity patients transported by ambulance. An ambulance standby location should ideally be located near the PHC to facilitate the rapid transfer of patients who require a higher level of care to the nearest hospital ED or other specialized medical facility.

C. Emergency Department: The ED should be available and have the capacity to receive high acuity emergency patients coming by road or air ambulance, but

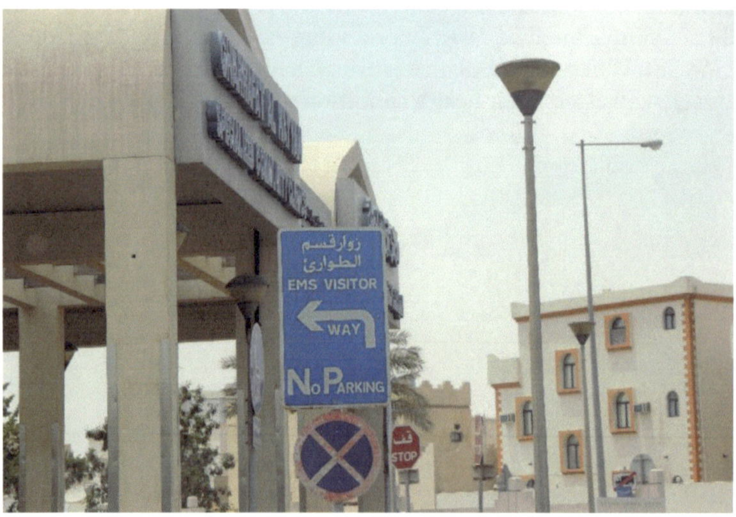

Figure 8.
Emergency room in primary healthcare center. It is near an entrance for easy dropping and transfer of patient by ambulance.

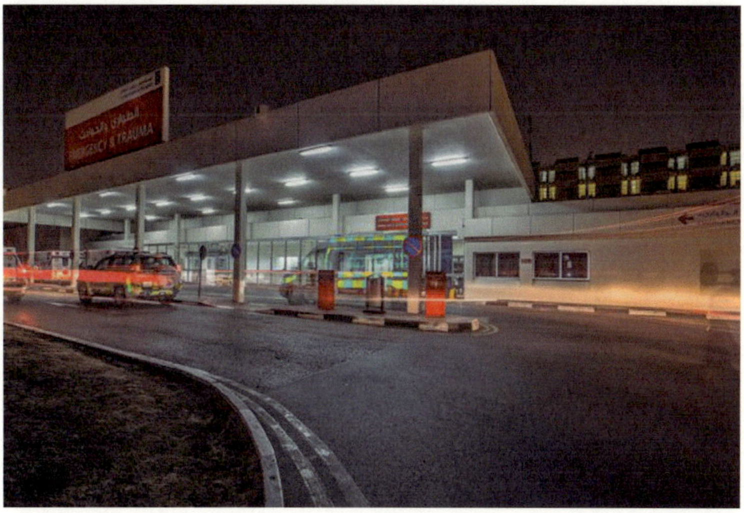

Figure 9.
Emergency department available 24/7 with the capacity to receive patients coming by ambulance or by their own means of transportation.

also by their own means of transportation (**Figure 9**). At the point of entry it is now common good practice to have a triage area for walk-in patients. The lowest acuity patients should be advised to visit their local PHC urgent care clinic (**Figure 5**). This will keep space and resources available for the patients with more severe conditions and need to be managed in the ED.

D. Support: The successful implementation of such initiativerequires the support from higher authorities that can promote the collaboration between the various institutions involved. There is also a need for public education to explain how emergency services provided by the various institutions should be used effectively.

10. Conclusion

The World Health Organization (WHO) made access to emergency care services a part of human rights that should be available for everybody regardless of gender, nationality, or condition [1]. This proposal is a method to decongest the emergency departments and make it easy for people to get emergency care or advice in timely manner. This would enable EDs to have a surge capacity in case it is needed. There are difficulties in the implementation of such processes due to general public behaviours and expectations, and operational changes required of PHC, call centers, and clinical staff from a training perpective.. These difficulties can be managed by political will, staff training, and educating the general public.

Acknowledgements

We would like to thank Dr. Loua Al Shaikh, Medical Director in the Hamad Medical Corporation Ambulance Service for encouraging to collaborate on this chapter and to Dr. Azza Awadh Mujally Manager of Gharrafat Al Rayyan Primary Health Care Center for his input in this chapter.

Author details

Abdulnasir F.H. Al Jazairi[1,2,3,4]* and Guillaume Alinier[5,6,7,8]

1 Emergency Department, Hamad General Hospital Doha, Qatar

2 Hamad Medical Corporation Doha, Qatar

3 Head of ED Major Incident Planning Committee, Qatar

4 Member of the Expert Panel member, Ministry of Public Health, Doha, Qatar

5 Director of Research, Hamad Medical Corporation Ambulance Service, Doha, Qatar

6 Professor of Simulation in Healthcare Education and National Teaching Fellow (2006), School Health and Social Work, University of Hertfordshire, Hatfield, UK

7 Adjunct Professor of Education in Medicine, Weill Cornell Medicine - Qatar, Doha, Qatar

8 Visiting Fellow, Faculty of Health and Life Sciences, Northumbria University, Newcastle Upon Tyne, UK

*Address all correspondence to: drhowaidi@gmail.com

References

[1] Burkholder TW, Hill K, Hynes EJC. Developing emergency care systems: a human rights-based approach. Bulletin of the World Health Organization. 2019;97(9):612-9.

[2] Hutton D, Alinier G. Ambulance service operational improvement. International Paramedic Practice. 2013;3(3):61-3.

[3] Goodman A. The development of the Qatar Healthcare System: A review of the literature. International Journal of Clinical Medicine. 2015;6(03):177-85.

[4] Weisz G. Divide and conquer: a comparative history of medical specialization: Oxford University Press, USA; 2006.

[5] Rosser W. The decline of family medicine as a career choice. CMAJ: Canadian Medical Association Journal. 2002;166(11):1419-20.

[6] Greenfield G, Foley K, Majeed A. Rethinking primary care's gatekeeper role. BMJ. 2016;354:i4803.

[7] Foster NE, Hartvigsen J, Croft PR. Taking responsibility for the early assessment and treatment of patients with musculoskeletal pain: a review and critical analysis. Arthritis research & therapy. 2012;14(1):1-9.

[8] Pollock A. Ambulance services in London and Great Britain from 1860 until today: a glimpse of history gleaned mainly from the pages of contemporary journals. Emergency Medicine Journal. 2013;30(3):218-22.

[9] Yarmohammadian MH, Rezaei F, Haghshenas A, Tavakoli N. Overcrowding in emergency departments: A review of strategies to decrease future challenges. J Res Med Sci. 2017;22:23-.

[10] Van den Heede K, Van de Voorde C. Interventions to reduce emergency department utilisation: a review of reviews. Health Policy. 2016;120(12): 1337-49.

[11] Hashem N, Balakrishnan P. Change analysis of land use/land cover and modelling urban growth in Greater Doha, Qatar. Annals of GIS. 2015;21(3):233-47.

[12] Mahmood MA, Thornes JE, Pope FD, Fisher PA, Vardoulakis S. Impact of air temperature on London ambulance call-out incidents and response times. Climate. 2017;5(3):61.

[13] Salway R, Valenzuela R, Shoenberger J, Mallon W, Viccellio A. Emergency department (ED) overcrowding: evidence-based answers to frequently asked questions. Revista Médica Clínica Las Condes. 2017;28(2): 213-9.

[14] Wilson P, Alinier G, Reimann T, Morris B. Influential Factors on Urban and Rural Response Times for Emergency Ambulances in Qatar. Mediterranean Journal of Emergency Medicine. 2017; 26:4-9.

[15] Knowles E, Bishop-Edwards L, O'Cathain A. Exploring variation in how ambulance services address non-conveyance: a qualitative interview study. BMJ Open. 2018;8(11):e024228.

[16] Wheeler SQ, Greenberg ME, Mahlmeister L, Wolfe N. Safety of Clinical and Non-Clinical Decision Makers in Telephone Triage: A Narrative Review. Journal of Telemedicine and Telecare. 2015;21(6):305-22.

[17] Anderson A, Roland M. Potential for advice from doctors to reduce the number of patients referred to emergency departments by NHS 111 call handlers: observational study. BMJ Open. 2015;5(11):e009444.

[18] Lindfors R, Bolton M, Gardett I. Comparison of EMD selections of Sick

Person Chief Complaint Protocol with on-scene responder findings. Ann Emerg Dispatch & Response. 2018;6(3):15-20.

[19] Coster J, O'Cathain A, Jacques R, Crum A, Siriwardena AN, Turner J. Outcomes for patients who contact the emergency ambulance service and are not transported to the emergency department: a data linkage study. Prehospital Emergency Care. 2019; 23(4):566-77.

[20] O'Cathain A, Jacques R, Stone T, Turner J. Why do ambulance services have different non-transport rates? A national cross sectional study. PloS one. 2018;13(9):e0204508.

[21] Campbell C, Al Shaikh L, Saifeldeen K, Bowen J, Pap R, Alinier G, et al. Validation of the pre-hospital Qatar Early Warning Score (QEWS) to determine transport priority. Journal of Emergency Medicine, Trauma and Acute Care. 2016;2016(2-International Conference in Emergency Medicine and Public Health-Qatar Proceedings):104.

[22] Kellermann AL, Hsia RY, Yeh C, Morganti KG. Emergency care: then, now, and next. Health affairs. 2013;32(12):2069-74.

[23] Ding Y, Park E, Nagarajan M, Grafstein E. Patient prioritization in emergency department triage systems: An empirical study of the Canadian triage and acuity scale (CTAS). Manufacturing & Service Operations Management. 2019;21(4):723-41.

[24] Hinson JS, Martinez DA, Cabral S, George K, Whalen M, Hansoti B, et al. Triage performance in emergency medicine: a systematic review. Annals of emergency medicine. 2019;74(1):140-52.

[25] Abolfotouh MA, Al-Assiri MH, Alshahrani RT, Almutairi ZM, Hijazi RA, Alaskar AS. Predictors of patient satisfaction in an emergency care centre in central Saudi Arabia: a prospective study. Emergency Medicine Journal. 2017;34(1):27-33.

[26] Lidal IB, Holte HH, Vist GE. Triage systems for pre-hospital emergency medical services-a systematic review. Scandinavian journal of trauma, resuscitation and emergency medicine. 2013;21(1):1-6.

[27] Kuriyama A, Urushidani S, Nakayama T. Five-level emergency triage systems: variation in assessment of validity. Emergency Medicine Journal. 2017;34(11):703-10.

[28] Storm-Versloot MN, Ubbink DT, Kappelhof J, Luitse JS. Comparison of an informally structured triage system, the emergency severity index, and the manchester triage system to distinguish patient priority in the emergency department. Academic Emergency Medicine. 2011;18(8):822-9.

[29] Leeies M, Strome T, Weldon E, Bullard M, Grierson R. Prehospital application of the Canadian triage and acuity scale by emergency medical services. Canadian Journal of Emergency Medicine. 2017;19(1):26-31.

[30] Sprivulis PC. Evaluation of the prehospital utilisation of the Australasian Triage Scale. PhD. Diss.: University of Western Australia; 2003.

[31] Grouse A, Bishop R, Bannon A. The Manchester Triage System provides good reliability in an Australian emergency department. Emergency Medicine Journal. 2009;26(7):484-6.

[32] Eitel DR, Travers DA, Rosenau AM, Gilboy N, Wuerz RC. The emergency severity index triage algorithm version 2 is reliable and valid. Academic Emergency Medicine. 2003;10(10):1070-80.

[33] Gottschalk S, Wood D, DeVries S, Wallis LA, Bruijns S. The cape triage score: a new triage system South Africa. Proposal from the cape triage group.

Emergency Medicine Journal. 2006; 23(2):149-53.

[34] Banks GC, Gerard AW, Yu K, Bullock KA. From the American Academy of Family Physicians: FAMILY PHYSICIANS PLAY INTEGRAL ROLE IN EMERGENCY MEDICINE. Annals of Family Medicine. 2017;15(1):84.

[35] American Association of Family Physicians. Family Physicians Delivering Emergency Medical Care - Critical Challenges and Opportunities (Position Paper). AAFP; 2018 https://www.aafp.org/about/policies/all/family-physicians-emergency-care.html Accessed on 19/05/2021.

[36] Pinchbeck EW. Convenient primary care and emergency hospital utilisation. Journal of Health Economics. 2019;68: 102242.

[37] Gangaram P, Menacho AM, Alinier G. Crisis resource management in relation to empowering people to speak up in emergency medical service clinical practice settings. Journal of Paramedic Practice. 2017;9(2):60-5.

[38] Hicks LL, Boles KE, Hudson ST, Madsen RW, Kling B, Tracy J, et al. Using telemedicine to avoid transfer of rural emergency department patients. The Journal of Rural Health. 2001;17(3):220-8.

Chapter 12

A New Approach to Surgical Gowns

Yüksel Atay, Oktay Pamuk, Bekir Boyaci, Esra Zeynep Yildiz, Tuncay Göksel, Dilek Yeşim Metin, Servet Gül, Gökberk Devrim and Özlem Topbaş

Abstract

Emerging diseases such as Ebola hemorrhagic fever, hepatitis B, hepatitis C, SARS, and most recently the Covid 19 epidemic have increased the importance of hygiene in the world, bringing the need for personal protective equipment (PPE) to the forefront. An important part of PPE in healthcare is surgical gowns, which are worn by doctors and nurses in the operating room to serve a dual function of preventing the transmission of microorganisms and body fluids from surgical staff to patients and from patients to staff. This chapter presents the history and importance of surgical gowns. The factors to be considered in the selection of surgical gowns are discussed. The model characteristics and fabric properties of surgical gowns currently on the market and the environmental impact of reusable and disposable gowns are outlined. Finally, shortcomings in available gowns are discussed, a new knitted surgical gown design is introduced, and recommendations are given in the final section. The chapter provides broad coverage of surgical gowns for both experienced readers and those new to the field.

Keywords: Surgical gown, reusable, disposable, design analysis, performance characteristics, environmental effect

1. Introduction

As a result of the Covid-19 epidemic, the importance given to hygiene has increased in the world, thus the necessity of personal protective equipment (PPE) has come to the fore. The type of PPE that should be used in the health field varies depending on three factors:

- the body part at risk (e.g. face, legs, hands) and type of exposure (e.g. pressure, liquids, droplets, aerosols),
- the amount of exposure to blood or body fluid (i.e., large volumes of fluid with a few drops)
- possible duration of exposure (i.e. short exposure such as initiation of an intravenous route or long exposure such as cardiothoracic surgery) [1].

An important part of PPE in the field of health; it forms surgical gowns that are worn by healthcare professionals to prevent the transfer of blood, body fluids and other potentially infectious materials and to help maintain the integrity of the sterile field. These gowns are the second most frequently used PPE item after gloves in this area [2–4].

Surgical gowns are defined by the United States (USA) Food and Drug Administration (FDA) as: "Equipment intended to be worn by operating room staff during surgical procedures to protect both the surgical patient and operating room staff from the transfer of microorganisms and bodily fluids" [5]. Surgical gowns are the most important part of the surgical clothing system that covers a large part of the body, and besides protection, they also affect the comfort condition of the healthcare personnel and thus the operational success [6].

Surgical gowns have been used by healthcare professionals for more than a century. Although these gowns are considered the leading item of protective equipment today, surgical gowns and clothing were not used regularly in the surgical profession until the 1800s. At that time, surgeons performed their operations in an auditorium or amphitheater-style rooms, in rooms where the operation would be performed in the center and where the audience would sit in the surrounding seats. Surgeons typically wore street clothes and sometimes wore something similar to a butcher's apron to protect their clothes from stains. In fact, surgeons in those years typically performed surgeries with bare hands and non-sterile surgical instruments and supplies. In the late 1800s, after Joseph Lister's pioneering research, the carbolic acid solution was used to sterilize surgical instruments, surgical cuts and dressings to prevent gangrene and other infections. In 1867 he published numerous articles on "Antiseptic Surgery Practice" describing these procedures and also encouraged surgeons to wear clean gloves and wash their hands before and after surgery. However; surgical gowns and other protective equipment did not see wide use until much later. Advances in the knowledge of antisepsis and infection until the 1940s led to the use of antiseptic dressings and surgical gowns. In 1952, when William C. Beck warned the surgical circles that these gowns lost their bacterial barrier property while wet, researches on developing materials in this area increased.

Surgical gowns used from the late 19th century until the 1970s; It is made from a loosely woven, readily permeable, reusable fabric known as cotton muslin fabric. Three types of fabric were commonly used at that time. All-cotton muslin (140 thread muslin); it is a soft, absorbent, draped and highly porous, loosely woven fabric. Because it is easily permeable, this material does not have any liquid resistance properties. It also tends to wear easily and create lint. It is a blended layered (180 thread) polyester and cotton blend fabric that has a permanent print quality but otherwise performs similar to muslin. Finally, it is the first reusable fabric with a water-repellent chemical coating, a tightly woven cotton or polyester/cotton blend fabric (with 175–280 threads). However, with repeated washing cycles, it has been shown that resistance to liquid penetration is reduced in this fabric [7].

While initially worn surgical garments were white to emphasize cleanliness; the combination of bright lights, white rooms, and white clothing caused eye strain on surgeons and staff. For this reason, the use of white surgical gowns and other clothing used in the early days has been abandoned and hospitals have started to use various shades of green and blue surgical clothing. As surgical procedures progressed during the twentieth century, surgical garments saw more use and improvement, but the biggest increase in surgical garment use did not occur until the 1980s. The Occupational Safety and Health Administration (OSHA) [8] introduced a rule in 1991 to minimize the risk of healthcare workers acquiring blood-borne pathogens. This rule required employers to provide appropriate personal protective equipment (PPE) to healthcare workers. It is stated that the AIDS epidemic has a lot to do with this [9].

2. Performance features required in surgical gowns

Surgical gowns are worn by doctors and nurses in the operating room to fulfill a dual function of preventing the transfer of microorganisms and body fluids from the surgical staff to the patient as well as from patient to staff [10]. These gowns, which are used to protect the surgical team, must have some protective properties. Most of the performance requirements for surgical gowns are clearly stated in the standards. Performance characteristics required from these aprons can be listed as follows:

- It must be resistant to the penetration of blood and other body fluids as required by its intended use (gown materials should contain protective barriers to minimize the passage of microorganisms, particles and fluids),
- It should be designed considering liquid repellency, liquid impermeability, air permeability and similar properties,
- It must be resistant to tears, punctures and abrasions,
- It must have an acceptable level of quality (i.e. no holes, tears, etc. in the garment),
- It must be made of materials suitable for the sterilization method/methods (e.g. radiation, steam and ethylene oxide),
- It must be resistant to fire (i.e. gowns chosen for use must be consistent with accepted flammability standards that will provide the safest environment for patients and healthcare professionals),
- It should contribute to maintaining the user's desired body temperature, that is, have the ability to maintain an isothermal environment for the user,
- It should not generate dust and fly or allow them to pass through,
- It should fit tightly but does not restrict movement.
- In general, it should be free from toxic ingredients and allergens,
- It should be soft and flexible, light, which does not cause discomfort during use,
- It must be large enough to allow full closure at the back,
- It should be of sufficient arm length to prevent exposure of the sleeve outside of the sterile glove,
- It should have an appropriate cost–benefit ratio, that is, it should not be a priority in the cost selection process,
- It should also meet some ergonomic requirements. It should be comfortable and functional, have sufficient freedom of movement and adapts to changes in heat and sweat when necessary,

- Surgical gowns should be ankle-long, the design of the collars and straps should not disturb the person wearing the garment and should not restrict the person's movements,
- It should provide high wearing comfort, should not lose its protection performance as a result of repeated washing and sterilization processes,
- As hospitals only stock in limited quantities, they should be designed to fit a variety of body shapes and sizes with a limited size range,
- It should help to protect the sterile area required in the operating room,
- It should be easy to donning and doffing without contamination,
- Whether single or reusable, the garment must be durable enough to maintain its intended useful life,
- The integrity of the garment must be preserved [9, 11–16].

Each of these characteristics can be measured in one or more "standardized" tests. These standardized tests have been developed by various organizations such as the American Society for Testing and Materials (ASTM; e.g. ASTM F-1670, ASTM F-1671), the American Textile Colorists and Chemists Association, the Health Industry Manufacturers Association, and the National Fire Prevention Association.

For the structural requirements of surgical gowns, structural analysis is performed first to evaluate the design features of existing products and to characterize the market. Comfort issues with product design are particularly alarming, as comfort is a critical product requirement for surgical gowns. While comfort is somewhat dependent on the permeability and flexibility of the fabric, it has a design effect. Researches done; emphasizes the sustainability of reusable gowns as they are more cost-effective throughout their life cycle in terms of production costs, waste and carbon footprints [17–19].

3. Design analysis of surgical gowns

Today, different gowns are designed to handle different surgeries. **Figure 1** shows the front and the back of a simple disposable surgical gown. The model and cost of aprons vary depending on the amount of protection provided.

The successful production of functional apparel products is a matter of a disciplined, structured approach to design and development. An effective, integrated approach proceeds through researching the design problem, defining design requirements and critical analysis of those requirements before arriving at a design solution [14].

Plumlee and Pittman [14] carried out a design analysis of 13 disposable and 2 reusable surgical gowns. They devised an analysis strategy to evaluate whether surgical gowns were of appropriate size. With this analysis, the model features of the surgical garments were examined and measurement analyzes were made. Kilic et al. conducted a study to determine the model characteristics of functional surgical suits to be worn in the surgical setting. For this purpose, samples were taken from surgical clothes used in hospitals in Izmir and design analysis was applied to these clothes. As a result of this analysis, suggestions were made about the model features and dimensions of surgical suits [20].

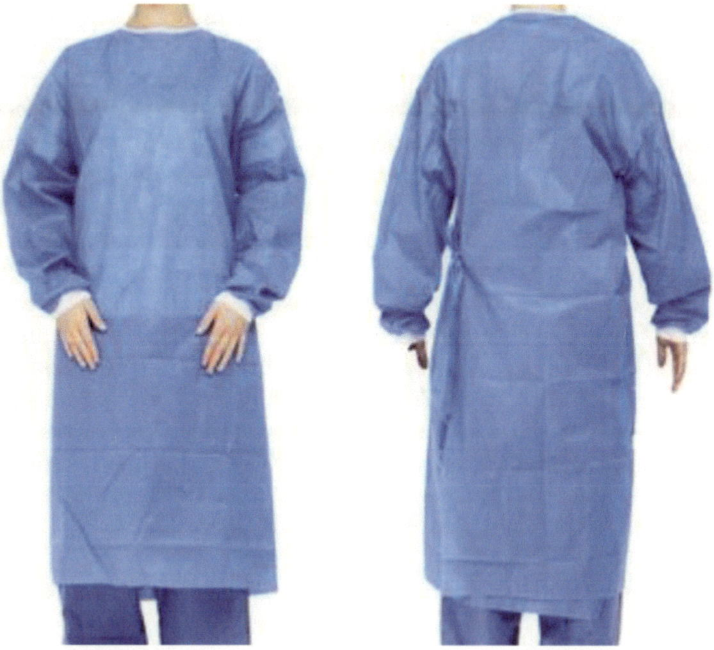

Figure 1.
Front and back of a surgical gown.

The model characteristics (size-sleeve length, closure properties, etc.) and fabric properties of surgical gowns worn in surgical settings vary according to the characteristics specified in the technical specifications of the Ministry of Health. **Figure 2** includes various surgical gowns.

3.1 Sleeves and cuffs

In general, there are two different kinds of sleeves in the gowns sold in the market at present: Raglan sleeves and set-in sleeves. A raglan sleeve, which can be identified by the diagonal seam line from the neckline to the armpit, is the most common type of sleeve used in surgical gowns [21]. Another type of sleeve construction found in many garments is commonly referred to as a set-in sleeve. The set-in sleeve is more difficult to construct and offers less freedom of movement

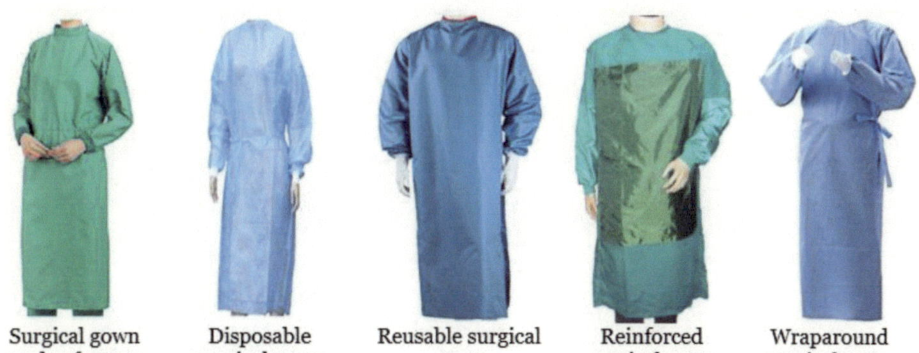

Figure 2.
Various surgical gowns.

for the wearer. The set-in sleeve is tight and results in high garment pressure in the armpit.

Since surgical gowns are worn over the scrubs, it is extremely important that they provide freedom of movement. The necessary comfort and freedom of movement are achieved by raglan sleeves as they create a large area in the armpit and provide more fit for the shoulder and arm [21–23]. In addition, raglan sleeves make donning and doffing easier compared to set-in sleeves because the deep armholes of raglan sleeves make it easier to reach into the sleeves when donning [21].

The sleeve edges were trimmed with a wrist cuff. Generally, three different types of cuffs are used, elastic cuffs around the wrist (disposable), knit cuffs made of cotton or cotton-polyester blend (disposable and reusable), and thumb loops (disposable and reusable) [3]. **Figure 3** contains different cuff designs.

According to the ANSI/AAMI PB70 classification, cuffs are not considered a critical area, so the material used on the cuff does not necessarily have barrier protection. In order to eliminate the strike-through through the cuffs, surgical gloves are worn pulled up over the cuffs so that the cuffs must fit snugly. One of the latest solutions to keep the gown wrist in place are thumb loops [3, 14].

3.2 Neck closures

The necklines of the gowns are closed in various ways: Tie, snaps, and hook and loop neck closures, all of which provide some adjustability for fit. The different types of closures are shown in **Figure 4**.

The most commonly used method is the tie back closure. The back contains a tie band at the neckline edge and another inside the neckline near the shoulder. The corresponding ties are located outside the left back piece, near the shoulder or at the edge [14]. The reusable surgical gowns made of slippery materials tend to slide down when worn. The back tie(s) can sometimes become loose, which would cause the surgical gown to slide down slightly and make the medical staff feel

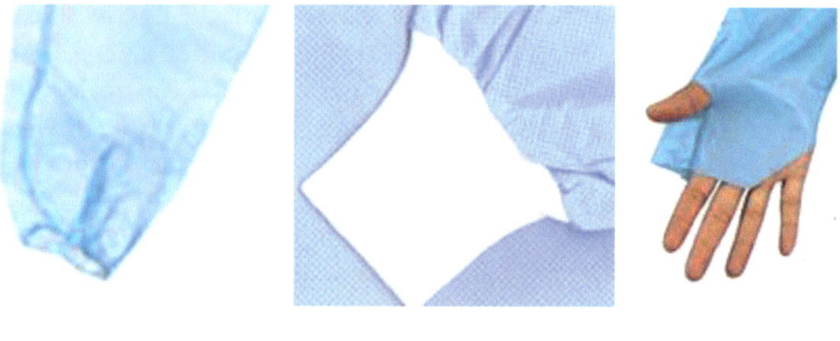

Figure 3.
Different cuff designs.

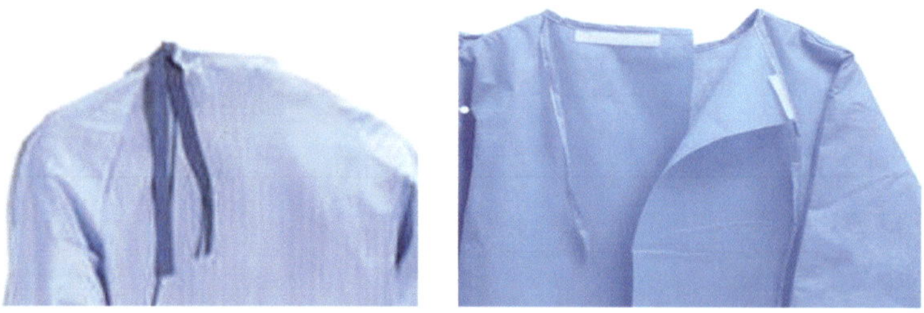

Figure 4.
Different closure types.

uncomfortable [24]. For this reason, Chang et al. [24] proposed a new combined tie fastening method for the reusable surgical gowns with two tie straps to prevent the tendency of the surgical gowns to loosen and slide down.

Snap fasteners provide closure of the gown neckline. The right back includes two male snap components, while the female components are located near the neckline of the left back. The snap components are spaced 1–1.5 inches apart to provide four adjustment options and flexibility in fit. Closer spacing of the snaps allows for more precise adjustment of the neckline area [14].

Some gowns with hook and loop neck closures are made for easy adjustability. This type of neck closure allows for easy adjustment of the neckline to fit a variety of sizes. The look components of the tape are located at the neckline of the left back. The corresponding hook component is located on the right back piece. Hook and loop closures offer great ease, flexibility, and accuracy in neckline fit, but often cause discomfort to surgical staff as hair is easily caught in the closure [3, 14].

It has been observed that reusable surgical gowns are subjected to heavy washing and sterilization steps after each use and various difficulties are encountered in models with hook and loop and snap fasteners. Due to the rough surface of the hook and loop fastener, it is difficult to clean its surface, it can be deformed quickly, and its outer surface can cause linting. In addition, the hook and loop can get caught in the garment during the washing process, which can cause damage. On the other hand, snaps can damage both the garment and the machine during wash and sterilization cycles. If the snap is damaged, it is unlikely that it can be repaired. There is also the possibility that the snap will not provide the desired degree of closure. So there is a risk that the gown will be tight/loose for the user. Since the tie is made from the fabric structure of the gown or a more durable fabric, there are no problems during washing and sterilization. It also ensures a complete closure for people of different sizes and avoids the problem of loose/tight fit.

3.3 Sizing/fit

Sizing/fit is also one of the features that is critical to surgeon protection and comfort. Gowns must allow the surgeon adequate freedom of movement, fit a variety of body shapes and sizes, and be easy to put on and take off without contaminating the worker or the workplace. Poorly fitting gowns can cause blood to easily get on the skin or other clothing [3].

Nowadays, surgical gowns are made with different size options (medium, large, extra-large, etc.) in addition to the universal fit (one size fits all). One-size-fits-all gowns are designed to fit a range of people with different sizes. However, they are usually not efficient for surgeons and are too large. The CDC recommends that multiple gown types and sizes be available in a healthcare facility to ensure adequate coverage for staff.

3.4 Stitches-seam

The characteristics of the seams of surgical gowns determine the overall performance of the product as a barrier to the spread of microorganisms. The seam provides a barrier against particulate, liquid, and gas/vapor, as well as potential chemical resistance and a biological barrier [22].

Traditional sewing with needles and threads is the most widely used method to join textiles together. Most of the reusable gowns are partially joined using traditional stitches and seams, usually a 401 double-thread chain stitch with a simple superimposed seam. Exceptions to this generalization include a reusable gown assembled with a lapped seam structure and two parallel rows of 401 stitches [14].

A low stitch density is used to minimize puncturing of the fabric and needle holes to avoid loss of barrier effect. Traditional sewing is not preferable in the manufacture of reinforced surgical gowns or some critical zones, such as sleeve seams, as needles can leave holes and cause seam leakage, leading to loss of barrier effect of the gowns [22, 25].

Eryuruk et al. [26] found that in traditionally sewn garments with membrane reinforcement, water can penetrate through the seams due to the needle holes in the fabric, which poses a risk to medical personnel in real-life use of the garment. To prevent this, the seams need to be sealed or a new joining technique based on welding such as ultrasonic welding can be used to create a fully sealed seam. Ultrasonic sewing is even more preferred than other conventional sewing methods in the manufacture of nonwoven based products. By using ultrasonic welding, seams with high waterproof properties can be obtained [25, 27, 28].

Mistik et al. compared the tensile properties of ultrasonic, lock and chain sewing methods. In their study, woven fabric was used, and the result of their study shows that the tensile properties of ultrasonic sewing were lower than traditional sewing methods [27]. Eryuruk et al. [29] compared bond strength and permeability properties of ultrasonically welded nonwoven fabrics with traditional sewing techniques. They found that ultrasonic welding technique is a suitable method for joining layers in the manufacture of surgical gowns, with acceptable bonding strength. Moreover, no water penetration was observed in the ultrasonically welded joints of the membrane-reinforced fabrics [26].

As a result, it can be said that while traditional sewing methods are preferred for reusable gowns, ultrasonic welding gives better results for disposable gowns. Although the seam strength values obtained in traditional sewing are high, the ultrasonic welded seams show higher performance in terms of liquid impermeability.

4. Fabrics used in surgical gowns

The surgical gowns on the market are made of different fabrics and a variety of fibers to reduce microbial contamination of the incision and protect the surgical staff from infection. These gowns are classified as "disposable/single-use" or "reusable/multi-use/multiple". These two basic types of each product have advantages and disadvantages in terms of protection, maintenance, comfort, cost and environmental impact. Within each of these categories, there are significant differences in design and performance characteristics [3, 30–32].

Reusable gowns, typically made of 100% cotton, 100% polyester, or polyester/cotton blends, are tightly woven plain weave fabrics; after each use, they are laundered, sterilized, and packaged for reuse. They can generally be used for 50 or more washing and sterilization cycles. Reusable gowns meet several requirements, such as comfort, drapability, good tensile strength, steam permeability, and steam sterilizability. While reusable surgical gowns are desirable for their comfort, their protectiveness is a critical factor. The pore size is large enough to allow fluid or viruses to pass through, thus providing no barrier effect until or unless a specific measure is taken [3, 30, 33–36].

Disposable surgical gowns and drapes are usually made from nonwovens alone or in combination with materials that provide greater protection against fluid penetration (e.g., plastic films). Nonwoven fabrics are made from various forms of natural fibers (wood pulp, cotton) and synthetic fibers (polyester, polyolefin) that can be adjusted to desired properties through specific fiber types, bonding processes, and fabric finishing. There are a variety of nonwoven fabrics of all types, including hydroentangled, bonded, stitched, and laminated nonwovens, which vary in quality depending on the manufacturer's intended use. The three most commonly used nonwovens for surgical gowns and drapes are: Spunlace, a hydroentangled material often composed of wood pulp and polyester fibers; Spunbond/Meltblown/ Spunbond, a fabric composed of three layers thermally or adhesively bonded together; and Wet-laid, a nonwoven fabric composed of wood pulp or a blend of polyester and wood pulp fibers [1, 30, 37].

Additional materials in the form of coatings, reinforcements, laminates or plastic films are often added to reusable and disposable products to improve their performance in terms of barrier resistance, absorbency and slip resistance. For some surgical gowns and drapes, the barrier properties of one layer of a material may not be sufficient for the application; in these cases, additional materials are often added in the form of additional layers of material, coatings, reinforcements, or laminates. Rutala and Weber [1] provide the following categorization of reinforcement approaches: reinforced fabric (second fabric layer to reinforce base materials); impermeable fabric with liquid repellent finish; layered fabric with a highly resistant membrane between two layers; and fabric reinforced with liquid-proof protection membrane. These approaches improve the protective performance of gown materials, but whether they address the thermal comfort of wearers is questionable. Membranes and coatings tend to compromise wearer comfort [1].

These two basic types of products each have advantages and disadvantages. Criteria for the selection of gowns and drapes include protection of medical personnel and patients from surgical site infections or nosocomial infections, barrier efficacy, clothing comfort, cost effectiveness, and environmental life cycle analysis. Moreover, the appropriate gown should be selected according to the duration of surgery and surgical status [1, 7, 18, 34].

The reusable gowns are mostly preferred by the clinicians due to their comfort, color etc. Disposable gowns are generally perceived by them as "paper-like" gowns and they do not want to wear them. Reusable gowns are also preferable in terms of tear resistance and liquid absorption. Independent studies have found that the use of disposable gowns can be 4–10 times more expensive than reusable materials on a per benefit cost basis. The potential problems with reusable surgical items can be listed as: perception of lower barrier protection, actual loss of barrier properties due to wear, abrasion and degradation of the fabric during laundering and sterilization, uneven consistency of the product when reprocessed multiple times [34, 38, 39].

The disposable gowns are used only once so there is no concern of damage to the barrier due to reprocessing and the product quality is very uniform. These gowns offer the advantage that hospitals can quickly dispose of the contaminated textiles, they reduce the cost of laundering, and they can be donned and doffed quickly in a place like the emergency room. In addition, nonwoven fabrics can prevent almost all possible strike-through of blood and body fluids. While disposable textiles are often perceived as having protective advantages over reusable textiles, there are some problems that arise with disposable textiles. For one, they tend to tear and break. Also, due to their barrier properties to liquids, the textiles are not permeable to air and moisture, making them uncomfortable to wear, especially during prolonged surgeries. Disposable gowns and drapes often receive negative feedback from surgeons and OR technicians due to thermal comfort and size issues. Finally, inexpensive disposables also tend to shed more particles than reusable ones, which in turn increases cleaning and maintenance costs [34, 38–40].

So, in conclusion, the gown type should be selected according to the different expectations of the users, the different operating environment conditions and the duration of operation. In the study where Behera and Arora made a general assessment, they stated that high density reusable synthetic fibers which are beneficial in terms of comfort and have adequate barrier performance should be preferred for high-risk surgical procedures with bleeding and disposable gowns with low barrier performance and lower comfort performance should be used for less risky procedures.

5. Environmental effects of reusable and disposable surgical gowns

The environmental impact of surgical gowns has had an increasing influence on the decision-making process in recent years. As environmental issues have become increasingly important, the environmental impacts of surgical gowns are discussed in this section.

Climate change and other environmental threats have become more prominent in recent years. As a result, environmental sustainability has gained much importance in many sectors. As one of the most polluting industries in the world, sustainability issues have received much attention in the textile and apparel industry. Textile and apparel products impact the environment at every point of the product life cycle, from fiber extraction to disposal (which is referred to as cradle to grave) and threaten our planet and its resources through the consumption of energy, chemicals, and water [41–44]. The textile industry causes significant environmental impacts throughout the life cycle of textile products.

Environmental sustainability, which considers the trade-off between economic productivity and environmental impact, should be an important perspective in business decisions. It refers to the ability of something to continue to exist without disturbing the ecological balance of the earth. Environmental sustainability in business refers to longevity, but in terms of what natural resources the production process relies on, how the resources are used and replenished, the overall impact of the final product on the environment, and where the product ends up after it is disposed of. Many tools and indicators have been developed to assess and benchmark the environmental impact of different systems. Life cycle assessment (LCA) is an environmental management tool that is increasingly used to understand and compare how a product or service is provided "from cradle to grave". The technique quantifies the environmental impact of a product, service or commodity at each stage of the Life Cycle, from raw material sourcing through manufacturing, distribution, use, potential reuse/recycling and then final disposal [29, 43, 45–47].

Furthermore, each operation or process unit within a stage is included. For each process within a stage, inputs (raw materials, resources, and energy) and outputs (emissions to air, water, and solid waste) are calculated. These inputs and outputs are then aggregated across the Life Cycle [47].

From a material life cycle perspective, reusable textiles have the advantage of a longer life span, they can withstand more than 50 commercial laundering cycles and therefore offer an additional saving to the user and the environment. In the case of reusable gowns, the final products are biodegradable when cotton or biodegradable polyester fibers such as polylactic acid (PLA) are the main components. The reusable textiles are used more frequently and therefore offer significant environmental advantages over disposable materials in terms of waste. However, these processes require more labor and facilities for washing and sterilizing and may contribute to water pollution. They also generate more volatile organic compounds as air emissions [1, 35, 39].

On the other hand, disposable products consume more raw materials and energy and generate more solid waste than reusable products. Moreover, disposable materials release more toxic compounds such as dioxins and mercury into the environment during the disposal process. In addition, disposable gowns require a larger inventory. Most of the air emissions (nitrogen oxides, sulfur oxides, and particulate matter) from the manufacturing and transportation of both types of products result from energy production; therefore, the disposable products generate more energy-related air emissions. These types of air emissions are associated with air pollution that leads to acid rain [1, 35, 39].

Both disposable and reusable gowns have an impact on the environment that has been evaluated by researchers. Vozzola et al. analyzed all activities from the extraction of fossil materials from the earth to the end-of-life disposal of reusable and disposable surgical gowns. The results of the study showed that choosing reusable gowns instead of disposable gowns reduced the energy consumption of natural resources (64%), greenhouse gas emissions (66%), blue water consumption (83%) and solid waste generation (84%). In addition, the reusable surgical gown system was found to consume approximately 83% less water (blue water) than the disposable surgical gown system. This result differs from some published information indicating that reusable garments are more water intensive [48].

Comparative life cycle studies by McDowell, Carre, Van den Berghe and Zimmer, and Overcash compared the manufacturing, sterilization, and transportation of reusable and disposable surgical gowns. All of these studies found that reusable textile systems had a significantly better environmental profile than disposable systems. Reusable gowns were found to produce lower environmental impacts in terms of global warming, photochemical oxidation, eutrophication, carcinogens, land use, water consumption, solid waste and fossil fuels. In general, disposable gowns had higher impacts in most categories because of the environmental impacts associated with gown production for each gown use. In a study also found that when these disposable products were replaced with reusable products, there was an average 64.5% reduction in surgical waste generated [40].

The European Textile Services Association (ETSA) reviewed the environmental impact of reusable and disposable surgical gowns in a LCA study considering a number of environmental impact categories. In the overall comparison, reusable products were found to have a lower negative environmental impact [49].

Another study conducted by American Reusable Textile Association (ARTA) and International Association for Healthcare Textile Management (IAHTM) found that reusable surgical gowns were significantly better for the environment than disposable gowns in areas such as energy consumption, water use, greenhouse gas emissions, and waste management. The study found that choosing reusable isolation gowns instead of disposable alternatives reduces the environmental footprint by; 28% lower energy consumption of natural resources, 30% lower greenhouse gas emissions (measured as CO2 emissions), 41% lower total water consumption (blue water), 93–99% lower waste generation in the healthcare facility [50, 51].

In summary, both disposable and reusable gowns and drapes have an impact on the environment. However, the existing literature on comparative studies for surgical gowns and drapes generally concludes that reusable textiles result in a lower environmental impact than disposable textiles. Comparing the two systems above, reusable gowns have advantages over disposable gowns in terms of natural resource consumption, waste generation, emissions and sustainability.

6. Shortcomings in available gowns, the design of knitted surgical gowns and recommendations

Garments used in the surgical environment are available in the market as single-use and multi-use. As mentioned before, reusable surgical garments are more preferable in terms of tensile strength, liquid absorption and bacterial protection performance. At the same time, they provide more comfort to the user because they are breathable. However, although the procurement processes of single and reusable products are simultaneous, the reusability of reusable products makes these products more advantageous due to the increasing needs in the field of health in today's conditions.

Sun Tekstil San. ve Tic. A.S. and Ekoten Tekstil San. ve Tic. A.S. in the study carried out by the companies within the scope of cooperation; the development of knitted fabric structures with different constructions produced from functional fiber structures, which will replace the woven fabrics used in the production of reusable surgical gowns according to the state of the art, that provide high wearing comfort in accordance with different types of surgical operations, do not lose their protection performance as a result of repeated washing and sterilization processes, and this reusable surgical gowns have been produced using functional fabric structures. Surgical garments have been developed by using knitted fabric structures in order to increase wearing comfort, breathability and comfort features. Thanks to the knitted fabric of the fabric used in clothing, it has an advantage over woven fabrics in terms of lightness and flexibility. The use of knitted fabric structures in the production of surgical clothing and the use of knitted fabric structures developed in different constructions from functional fibers in different parts of the garment have created the innovative aspect of the study.

With this study, knitted fabrics of different constructions were developed by using different fiber structures, thus the production of surgical garments with improved protection and comfort properties was achieved. In the production of fabrics; cotton, polyester, cotton-polyester, cotton-polyester-carbon fiber blends and nilite, coolmax, tencel, etc. fibers are used to increase the comfort feature. Antistatic thread is used to prevent static electricity of the fabrics. With these yarn raw materials, fabrics with a single jersey knit structure were obtained and the characteristics of these fabric structures regarding performance and comfort were compared with each other. As a result of the tests, it has been observed that 100% cotton fabric gives worse results than other fabrics in relation to moisture transmission, thermal resistance and size stability in washing. The rubbing fastness and pilling values of the tencel/cotton blend fabric are very low in terms of usage. When the results were examined, it was seen that 100% Coolmax and 100% Nilit fabrics are advantageous in terms of comfort properties such as moisture transmission and thermal resistance. In addition, the results of moisture transmission, bursting strength and size stability in washing of 100% polyester and 99% -1% polyester-carbon fabrics were better than other fabrics. It is seen that it has the best results after 100% Coolmax and 100% Nilit fabrics in terms of thermal resistance. Although the test results of the micro-polyester fabric seem good, due to its fast moisture absorbing structure, its moisture transmission properties are quite low. Dimension change properties of 65–34–1% polyester-cotton-carbon blended fabric in washing gave worse results than Nilit, Coolmax, polyester and polyester-carbon fabrics. Comfort features are very important in surgical garments. In the literature, the expected value for comfort from fabrics in terms of moisture management performance properties is above 0.4. For this reason, it has been observed that 100% Coolmax, 100% Nilit, 100% Polyester and 99–1% polyester-carbon fabrics provide these values, while other fabrics are poor in terms of moisture management in terms of comfort. For this reason, fabric structures with these 4 different raw materials have been selected for lamination.

Multiple film structures (PTFE, microporous PU film, hydrophilic PU film and ether-based polyester film) were used to use the surgical gowns obtained with the study for multiple purposes. The advantages provided by each film structure in terms of its technical properties also vary. In order to make the barrier properties of the film structures more effective, dot lamination studies were carried out with reactive polyurethane adhesive as 2-layer (Fabric + Film) and 3-layer (Fabric + Film + Fabric) together with the fabric structures of the films. Due to the insufficient test and sterilization resistance of the 2-layer structures, the lamination studies of the 3-layer structures were continued. However, different performance criteria were met with the different film structures used in the studies. Adhesives with high resistance to sterilization were preferred in studies on film structures with different performance properties.

After lamination processes, antibacterial finishing process to give antibacterial properties to the fabrics, water repellent finishing that is resistant to washing at high temperatures to give water repellency and membrane coating to increase the protection feature.

In order to determine the physical-mechanical, protection and comfort properties of the fabrics produced; thickness, liquid repellency, liquid impermeability, bursting strength, linting, porosity and microorganism permeability were investigated. At the same time, bending strength, air permeability, thermal resistance and water vapor resistance tests were applied to determine the clothing comfort properties of the fabrics. The sterilization strength of the products obtained was also examined. These tests to be applied to fabric structures also shed light on the tests applied in EN 13795 and PB70 standards, which are a requirement for surgical gowns.

Along with these; the designs of the existing surgical gowns were examined, and in line with the interviews with surgeons, new designs were created for different types of operations (intense fluid, low fluid, etc.), that can be easily put on and taken off and provide body movement comfort.

It has been observed that the 3-layer laminated fabric structure obtained with the knitted fabric design and film lamination within the scope of the study has fulfilled both the comfort and protection parameters with the test studies. In the light of this information, it was decided to use a film laminated knitted fabric structure in the entire surgical gown. In this way, the protection and barrier feature of the user is not only specific to the body and arms of the user, but a protection that covers the whole body will be provided. The fact that the fabric structure is extremely light in weight will not create a weight on the user in terms of comfort.

Surgical garments developed; It will be used as personal protection equipment to minimize the transmission of viruses to patients and the exposure of healthcare personnel to pathogens, especially blood-borne pathogens. Within this scope, there is no product in which knitted fabric structures are used in the production of surgical garments in the international market. In this respect and according to the advantages it provides compared to reusable woven fabrics, surgical garments have been obtained from knitted fabric that stands out in the market.

Author details

Yüksel Atay[1], Oktay Pamuk[2], Bekir Boyaci[3], Esra Zeynep Yildiz[4*], Tuncay Göksel[1], Dilek Yeşim Metin[1], Servet Gül[3], Gökberk Devrim[3] and Özlem Topbaş[3]

1 Faculty of Medicine, Ege University, Izmir, Turkey

2 Textile Engineering Department, Ege University, Izmir, Turkey

3 Sun Tekstil, R&D Center, Izmir, Turkey

4 Emel Akın Vocational Training School, Ege University, Izmir, Turkey

*Address all correspondence to: esra.zeynep.yildiz@ege.edu.tr

References

[1] Rutala WA, Weber DJ. Mint: A review of single-use and reusable gowns and drapes in health care. Infection Control and Hospital Epidemiology. 2001;4:248-257.

[2] Leonas KK. Microorganism protection. In: Scott RA, editor. Textiles for Protection. BocaRaton, FL: Woodhead Publishing-CRC Press; 2005. p. 441-464.

[3] Kilinc FS. Mint: A review of isolation gowns in healthcare: Fabric and gown properties. Journal of Engineered Fibers and Fabrics. 2015;10:180-190.

[4] Gruendemann B. Single-use vs. Reusable Gowns and Drape [Internet]. 2020. Available from: https://www.infectioncontroltoday.com/general-hais/taking-cover [Accessed:2020-01-12]

[5] U.S. Food and Drug Administration. Code of Federal Regulations Title 21 Subchapter H-Medical Devices [Internet]. 2020. Available from: https://www.fda.gov/health-professionals [Accessed: 2020-01-04]

[6] Aslan S. An investigation about comfort and protective performances of medical protective structures [thesis]. Suleyman Demirel University; 2011.

[7] Association for the Advancement of Medical Instrumentation. Selection of Surgical Gowns and Drapes in Health Care Facilities. Arlington, VA: Association for the Advancement of Medical Instrumentation; 1994. Technical Information Report No 11-1994.

[8] Occupational Safety and Health Administration. Occupational Exposure to Bloodborne Pathogens: Final Rule. Federal Register. 1991;56:235,64175-64182.

[9] Chinta SK, Veena KV. Mint: Significance of textiles in surgical gowns. International Journal of Engineering Research & Technology. 2012;7:1-8.

[10] Schoenberger LCH. Liquid barrier and thermal comfort properties of selected surgical gowns [thesis]. Kansas, USA: Kansas State University; 1990.

[11] Medical/Surgical Technical Committee. Guide to Nonwoven Medical Products. Association of the Nonwoven Fabrics Industry; 1984. New York.

[12] Ondogan Z. Mint: Cerrahi giysilerde özellikler. Tekstil & Teknik Dergisi. 1999;175:76-79.

[13] Kavusturan Y. Mint: Hastanelerde kullanılan kumaş yapıları. Tekstil Maraton. 2002;63:71-80.

[14] May-Plumlee T, Pittman A. Mint: Surgical gown requirements capture: A Design Analysis case study. Journal of Textile and Apparel, Technology and Management. 2002;2:1-10.

[15] Cireli A, Kılıç B, Sarıışık M, Okur A. Tıbbi tekstiller ve test yöntemleri, paketleme malzemelerinde TSE standartları. In: 5. Ulusal Sterilizasyon Dezenfeksiyon Kongresi; 2007; Izmir.

[16] Kishwar F, Kalsoom S, Khan FZ, Alam S, Sohail MT. Mint: Surgical apparels comparison of some physical parameters. The Professional Medical Journal. 2011;3:390-395.

[17] Baykasoglu A, Dereli T, Yilankirkan N. Mint: Application of cost/benefit analysis for surgical gown and drape selection: A case study. American Journal of Infection Control. 2009;37:215-226.

[18] Overcash M. Mint: A comparison of reusable and disposable perioperative textiles. Anesthesia & Analgesia. 2012;114:1055-1066.

[19] Vozzola E, Overcash M, Griffing E. Mint: Environmental considerations in the selection of ısolation gowns: A life cycle assessment of reusable and disposable alternatives, American Journal of Infection Control. 2018;46:881-886.

[20] Sen Kılıc A, Ondogan Z, Dirgar E. Mint: Design Analysis of Reusable Surgical Clothes and New Product Development. Tekstil. 2019;1-3:22-28.

[21] Cho K. Mint: Redesigning hospital gowns to enhance end users' satisfaction. Family and Consumer Sciences Research Journal. 2006;4: 332-349.

[22] Rogina-Car B, Budimir A, Katovic D. Mint: Microbial barrier properties of healthcare professional uniforms. Textile Research Journal. 2017;15:1-9.

[23] Liu K, Kamalha E, Wang J, Agrawal TK. Mint: Optimization design of cycling clothes' patterns based on digital clothing pressures. Fibers and Polymers. 2016;9:1522-1529.

[24] Chang KH, Chen YL, Dai SY. Mint: A combined tie-fastening method for the reusable surgical gown with two neck tie belts to improve wearing comfort. 2020:1-7.

[25] Ashour S, Gabr B, Abdel Megeid ZM. Mint: Investigating the effect of joining techniques on waterproof and comfort properties. International Journal of Scientific & Engineering Research. 2017;11: 1319-1327.

[26] Eryuruk SH, Karaguzel Kayaoglu B, Kalaoglu F. Mint: A study on ultrasonic welding of nonwovens used for surgical gowns. International Journal of Clothing Science and Technology. 2017;4:539-552.

[27] Kayar M. Mint: Analysis of ultrasonic seam tensile properties of thermal bonded nonwoven fabrics. Journal of Engineered Fibers and Fabrics. 2014;3:8-18.

[28] Sevkan Macit A, Tiber B. Mint: Investigation of water permeability of ultrasonic seaming on PU coated fabrics. Int. Per. of Recent Tech. in App. Eng. 2019;1:25-29.

[29] Daystar J, Chapman L, Moore M, Pires S, Golden J. Mint: Quantifying apparel consumer use behavior in six countries: Addressing a data need in life cycle assessment modeling. JTATM Journal of Textile and Apparel, Technology and Management. 2019;1:1-25.

[30] Abreu MJ, Silva ME, Schacher L, Adolphe D. Mint: Designing surgical clothing and drapes according to the new technical standards. International Journal of Clothing Science and Technology. 2003;1:69-74.

[31] Pamuk O, Ondogan Z, Abreu MJ. Mint: The thermal comfort properties of surgical gown fabrics. Tekstilec. 2009;1-3:24-30.

[32] Kilinc Balci FS. Mint: Isolation gowns in health care settings: Laboratory studies, regulations and standards, and potential barriers of gown selection and use. American Journal of Infection Control. 2016;1:104-111.

[33] Song, MK. Liquid barrier and thermal comfort properties of reusable and disposable surgical gowns [thesis]. Kansas State University; 1992.

[34] Behera BK, Arora H. Mint: Surgical gown: A critical review. Journal of Industrial Textiles. 2009;38:205-231.

[35] Song MK, McCullough EA. Mint: The liquid and viral barrier properties of reusable and disposable surgical gowns. Journal of the Korean Society of Clothing and Textiles. 1993;1:37-47.

[36] Leonas KK. Mint: Effect of laundering on the barrier properties of reusable surgical gown fabrics. American Journal of Infection Control. 1998;5:495-501.

[37] Pamuk O. The development of functional medical products for using of surgical team and patients [thesis]. Ege University; 2006.

[38] Eiff. How do the costs of disposable and reusable surgical drapes and gowns compare? [Internet]. 2009. Available from: https://www.textile-services.eu/_common/file.cfm?id=5B31BC1AE3C4A6F289A91E8E356A3FC4 [Accessed: 2021-02-21]

[39] Sun G. Mint: Disposable and reusable medical textiles. Textiles for Hygiene and Infection Control. 2011:125-135.

[40] Moving (Back) to Reusables in the OR [Internet]. 2019. Available from: https://practicegreenhealth.org/sites/default/files/2019-03/gorimpmod-reusablegowns_r5_web.pdf [Accessed: 2021-03-10].

[41] Shen B, Li Q, Dong C, Perry P. Mint: Sustainability issues in textile and apparel supply chains. Sustainability. 2017;9:1-6.

[42] Ozek HZ. Mint: Sustainability: Increasing impact on textile and apparel industry. Journal of Textile Engineering&Fashion Technology. 2017;5:506-509.

[43] Khan MR, Islam, M. Mint: Materials and manufacturing environmental sustainability evaluation of apparel product: Knitted t-shirt case study. Textiles and Clothing Sustainability. 2015;1:1-12.

[44] Jung S, Jin B. Mint: A theoretical investigation of slow fashion: Sustainable future of the apparel industry. International Journal of Consumer Studies. 2014;38:510-519.

[45] Luo Y, Song K, Ding X, Wu X. Mint: Environmental sustainability of textiles and apparel: review of evaluation methods. Environmental Impact Assessment Review. 2021; 86.

[46] Finnveden G, Hauschild M, Ekvall T, Guinee J, Heijungs R, Hellweg S, Koehler A, Pennington D, Suh S. Mint: Recent developments in life cycle assessment. Journal of Environmental Management. 2009;1:1-21.

[47] McDougall FR, White PR, Franke M, Hindle P. Integrated Solid Waste Management: A Life Cycle Inventory. 2nd ed. Blackwell Publishing Company; 2001. 544 p.

[48] Vozzola E, Overcash M, Griffing E. Mint: An environmental analysis of reusable and disposable surgical gowns. AORN Journal. 2020;3:315-325.

[49] Zins HM, Howard M. Reusable medical textiles. In: Bartels VT, editor. Handbook of Medical Textiles. Woodhead Publishing Series in Textiles; 2011. p. 80-105.

[50] Study Finds Reusable Surgical Gowns are Better for the Environment than Disposable Gowns [Internet]. 2018. Available from: https://www.medicleanse.com/blog/reusable-surgical-gowns-study/#:~:text=An%20investigative%20study%20by%20the,consumption%2C%20water%20use%2C%20greenhouse%20gas [Accessed: 2021-02-21]

[51] Life Cycle Analysis of Isolation Gowns Gives the Advantage to Reusables [Internet]. 2018. Available from: https://www.infectioncontroltoday.com/view/life-cycle-analysis-isolation-gowns-gives-advantage-reusables [Accessed: 2021-02-21]

Chapter 13

Occupational Health and Safety in Operating Rooms

Hülya Gül

Abstract

Nurses are one of the most endeavored members of healthcare services. Operating rooms, on the other hand, require special caution and contain various hazards for healthcare professionals. Operating rooms contain various risk factors related to applications, infrastructure and humans. It is one of the areas that need nursing care the most since patients are dependent on their nurses to meet their personal needs. Nurses are exposed to various risk and health problems in operating rooms. Healthcare service provided by nurses working in a healthy environment directly affects the health and quality of life of those who receive the service. In order to prevent these problems, intensive up-to-date educations on occupational risks and employee safety should be provided for the nurses working in operating rooms. In addition to the general occupational hygiene measures, different precautions should be taken for the operating rooms. Working in a healthy and safe environment is a human right that every individual must have. Managers of the medical institutions should be attentive to follow the laws and sanctions on occupational health and safety, institutions should be inspected frequently and monitored carefully. In this section, this subject will be studied in line with actual data and resources.

Keywords: Nurses, hospitals, operating room, occupational health, occupational safety

1. Introduction

It is a legal requirement that employers must provide a safe and healthy working environment their employees. In terms of public health, it is important to control occupational and environmental factors in all workplaces [1]. Health sector is one of the dangerous lines of work in which occupational health and safety (OHS) are becoming increasingly important. Healthcare professionals are faced with many occupational risks while performing their duties. There are also many risk factors for those who work in operating rooms. These include inconvenient physical environment, heavy physical work, working in shifts and working in non-ergonomic positions [2–5]. Employee health is also threatened by stress, mobbing, violence, malnutrition etc. For example, being in close contact with the patient in the operating room increases the risk of infection. Nurses who are likely to come into contact with blood and bodily fluids of the patients during their daily activities at the hospital are in the high risk group for blood-borne diseases. Thus, researches indicate that nurses are mostly faced with biological and psychological risk factors [6].

Operating room employees may experience occupational accidents due to sharp object injuries, contamination with blood and bodily fluids, heavy lifting, falling, hitting, tripping, slipping, being injured etc. [7, 8]. Moreover, traffic accidents during commute and all kinds of accidents that happen at work such as musculoskeletal system wounds, violence, allergic reactions, burnt, poisoning, fire, explosion and electric shock can also be listed among these [9].

However, the duties of healthcare professionals are mostly considered as providing service to patients who need healthcare. Therefore, it is mostly neglected that healthcare professionals can have occupational problems. In this respect, institutions that provide healthcare service are generally organized to achieve patient care, treatment and satisfaction instead of prioritizing the health and safety needs of healthcare personnel. Work environment, occupational health and safety of the healthcare professionals, who provide service for patients, are mostly overlooked.

The risks of the operating rooms may cause a decrease in productivity, economic loss of the institution, increase in occupational accidents, and putting the people who receive care from healthcare professionals directly at risk. Therefore, hospitals need to be suitable for health and safety measures, environmental precautions should be taken, risk factors should be eliminated or controlled and personal protective equipment should be paid attention to by performing risk assessment and management.

2. Occupational and environmental risk factors

2.1 Physical risk factors

Physical factors take an important place in healthcare institutions. Primary physical factors affecting work in operating rooms can be listed as temperature, noise, lighting, humidity, air-conditioning, air pollutants, ionizing radiation, non-ergonomic work conditions etc. [10].

Work environment should be adequately lighted in order for the healthcare personnel to do their jobs properly and comfortably. Especially in working areas critical for human health such as operating rooms, inadequate lighting negatively affects the personnel's vision and excessive lighting can cause personnel to get exhausted. Researches show that light and electromagnetic fields affect the function of pineal gland. In the long term, this may lead to problems in reproductive functions, depression and especially breast cancer in women. Exposure to light at night or electromagnetic fields decreases the melatonin production of pineal gland which increases the production of estrogen from the ovaries and may cause malignant transformation in breast epithelial cells. Therefore, lighting in healthcare institutions is important especially for those who work in shifts, have night shifts and work at intensive care units.

Operating rooms are desired to be quiet environments. Sound level should not exceed 35–40 decibels in the units where patients are lying. However, it can be noisy during patient visit hours, crowded polyclinic hours and some operations. It is observed that sound level in the operating rooms reaches maximum especially during the preparation to the operation and using the surgical tools during the operation [11]. A study by Juang et al. states that physiological states of the nurses working at intensive care units for over five years are severely affected [12]. It is also stated that these nurses, especially the ones working in different shifts, are extremely sensitive to noise and cannot tolerate it. Varicose vein, the main risk factor of which is to stand still, is seen very often especially in nurses working in operating rooms.

Sharp object injuries, which are generally preventable risk factors for nurses, are mainly caused by tools that disrupt skin integrity. Inadequate number of nurses in operating rooms, shifts, high work circulation, and long working hours also increase the risk of sharp object injuries. Because more risky surgical tools are used in these units besides the tools used by other healthcare personnel. Operating rooms have a risk of fire due to factors such as use of lasers and oxygen. Heating flammable preparation materials pose a serious risk for fire. These agents can easily catch fire with increased temperature. If a flammable preparation material is being used, additional precautions should be taken to avoid surgical fires and burns in patients. Operating room staff should have sufficient knowledge on laser and oxygen use, factors causing fire and how to use fire extinguishers.

Surgical site infections are one of the most difficult postoperative complications which threaten millions of lives every year. Current evidence presents a positive relationship between the infection rate and the concentration of the bacteria-carrying particles in air [13]. Ventilation of the operating room is important to decrease the concentration of bacterial pollutants in air and control the risk of infection. Advanced air conditioning systems are needed to minimize the risk of infection and keep the concentration of microorganisms at the minimum values specified by standards. To that end, ventilation systems of operating rooms should be designed and organized in a way to prevent occupational and healthcare institution originated infections by considering the biological and physical characteristics of the microorganisms.

Air conditioning installation should be performed in frequent intervals determined by laws and elaborately controlled in order to minimize the microorganisms, dust, narcotic gases and bad odors in the hospital, as well as providing comfort conditions in the operating rooms. Inadequate or improper ventilation may cause health problems and employees to breathe more air pollutants.

2.2 Chemical risk factors

Various chemical substances are used in operating rooms to provide healthcare service. These substances are especially used to take hygienic precautions as well as diagnosis and treatment. Healthcare professionals can get exposed to the chemical substances in various ways such as respiratory system, gastrointestinal tract, absorption (skin, eyes) and pinpricks. These chemical substances have acute or chronic effects on healthcare personnel [14, 15]. Effects of chemical substances on healthcare personnel may vary according to duration of contact, way of contact, physical and chemical characteristics of the substance. The effectiveness of the substance can especially vary by the presence of different chemical substances in the work environment, genetic and personal characteristics of the employee and addictions such as alcohol and smoking.

Disinfectants, anesthetic agents, cytotoxic agents, drugs, some heavy metals such as mercury and latex are primary chemicals used in operating rooms [16]. Glutaraldehyde, formaldehyde, ethylene oxide are commonly used in operating rooms for chemical sterilization. Some of them, for example alcohol, have a relatively low toxicity. On the other hand, glutaraldehyde and formaldehyde are extremely irritant for skin, eyes and airways even at very low concentrations and their increased concentrations may result in increased heart rate and pulmonary edema. Formaldehyde belongs to "Group-1 Carcinogenic to humans", which includes factors proven to cause cancer by International Agency for Research on Cancer [17]. Ethylene oxide, used for the sterilization of heat sensitive materials, shows mutagenic and carcinogenic characteristics as well as toxic and explosive effects. Ethylene oxide is a combustible gas which explodes when it reaches %3 concentration.

Its acute effects are respiratory problems and neurological symptoms. High level of exposure causes cataract. Moreover, the need for a relatively long time for sterilization causes the risk factors to extend over time. Nurses can be exposed to risk while they break the ampoule containing the medicine, dilute the medicine in powder form, spilling the medicine by accident etc. Allergic reactions in nurses working in operating rooms mostly develop as latex energy due to frequent use of gloves. Latex gloves are flexible, easy to wear and used for every process in the operating room. Latex can cause allergic reactions ranging from mild contact dermatitis to urticaria, conjunctivitis, bronchospasm and anaphylactic shock.

Anesthetic gases take an important place in chemical risks that healthcare professionals are exposed to [18]. Operating room is constantly contaminated by the leakage from the valves of anesthetic devices and even by the anesthetic gases of the expiratory air of the patients. Healthcare professionals are chronically exposed to these gases in operating rooms. Anesthetic gases are highly volatile compounds and especially small indoor places such as operating rooms can get highly contaminated with these gases in a short amount of time. Anesthetic gases can affect employees in the operating room and recovery room [19]. Anesthetic gases spread in a way that harms the environment by leakage from the anesthetic devices, accidental spilling and spreading of the gas, using an unsuitable mask on the patient, poorly inflating the intubation tube and the gas spread by the expiration of the patient. Epidemiological studies show that chronic exposure to anesthetic gases is an occupational risk which has consequences like spontaneous abortion, congenital malformations, premature birth, cancer, liver and kidney diseases, regression in mental functions, headache, fatigue and irritability [20]. Therefore, nurses working in operating rooms, surgical doctors and other personnel working in operating rooms are at high risk of anesthetic gases (nitrous oxide, halothane, isoflurane etc.)

On the other hand, healthcare personnel may be exposed to chemical substances in the hazardous medicine during the preparation, transfer, application, storage and disposal of the medicine. Cytotoxic drugs have the potential to cause serious health problems for people and personnel who come into contact with them. The risks include cancer, malformed, abnormal birth, recurring toxic effects, organ or tissue damage, chromosomal abnormalities. More women are employed in healthcare sector compared to other sectors and majority of the chemically risky actions are performed by nurses, the majority of whom are women. Therefore, another dimension of the danger of the chemical substances is that most of these substances have genotoxic effects (mutagenic, carcinogenic and/or teratogenic) and they may cause spontaneous abortions, low birth weight, babies with anomalies by affecting the reproductive health of the women working in operating rooms.

2.3 Biological risk factors

Healthcare employees are at risk of various infectious diseases at the daily work environment. Thousands of healthcare employees are caught in numerous serious infections such as Hepatitis B, Hepatitis C and AIDS. Respiratory transmitted diseases, which are among the occupational risks for employees in healthcare sector, are huge reasons of loss of work and power. There are two main ways for respiratory transmission which are droplet contact and airborne transmission. Droplet contact refers to contact of the droplets carrying microorganisms from an infected person to conjunctiva, nasal or oral mucosa (by coughing, sneezing, speaking, bronchoscopy or aspiration). Airborne transmission refers to the spread of the droplets carrying microorganisms through air by suspending in air for a long time or contacting dust particles.

A newly identified coronavirus, SARS-CoV-2, has caused a worldwide pandemic. Coronavirus was first identified in December 2019 in China. In February 2020, the World Health Organization (WHO) named it COVID-19. Covid-19 with high transmission level, it has become a serious public health issue. COVID-19 easily is transmitted by respiratory system which causes numerous deaths and it is a serious threat for healthcare professionals. Nurses should act carefully to protect both themselves and the patients from contamination in operating rooms. Personal Protective Equipment (PPE) should be used in accordance with the rules. Surgical nurses should carry out this challenging process with a multidisciplinary approach in issues such as restructuring in operating rooms and reviewing in-hospital triage [21–24]. Surgical smoke may be effective in the spread of coronavirus [25]. Surgical smoke is a potential risk factor for patients, personnel and environment. Mutagen gases, carcinogens, particles containing DNA components or HPV (Human Papilloma Virus) may spread in air via smoke when lasers or electrocauteries are used [26, 27].

Nosocomial infection occurs when pathogens are transmitted by nurses and healthcare personnel who came into contact with intubated patients in intensive care units and patients with intravascular catheters. Nosocomial infections emerge as direct or indirect microbial spread (cross infection) or spread from one's own infected tissue to another tissue (self-infection). Studies show that nosocomial infections are mostly caused by microorganisms in the environment outside of patient and healthcare employees are the primary source of infections. Both the bacteria found in these individuals and the ones that are transmitted to other patients are important sources of nosocomial infections.

Studies on infection prevalence and risk analysis are increasing and new information is obtained day by day. Another of these infections is blood-borne infections [28–30]. Blood-borne infections are of particular importance because of their frequency and long term negative effects. Serious precautions should be taken to protect healthcare professionals from blood-borne infections. Personnel at risk should be included in vaccination program. Hygiene is very important. The labels of bags and containers used to transport waste with risk of contamination should be colored in red and clearly indicate danger. Sharp and penetrating tools should be carried in labeled, special containers in conformity with the standard. There should be no risk of contamination or leakage in these containers. Contaminated laundry should be carries in special, marked bags which should be labeled as dangerous. The use of gloves is very important. Biological risk factors can be controlled as well as employee safety if risk factors are known by all employees and necessary precautions are taken.

2.4 Psychological risk factors

Nurses have a very active role in every field of healthcare service present in operating rooms. Nurses are under more pressure and experience more psychological reactions due to the occupational differences in working conditions [31–34]. Therefore, more satisfied, happier and more productive nurses are important to increase the quality of the service provided. However, job satisfaction of nurses can be negatively affected by hopeless thoughts on the future of occupation, the fact that nursing is considered as an auxiliary occupation and difficult work conditions, which is the foremost problem in nursing. Nurses need to work in shifts since healthcare institutions provide service for 24 hours. This may have negative effects on the biological, psychological and social lives of nurses. Working in shifts disrupts body's normal biological rhythm and may cause chronic fatigue and disruption in person's family and social lives. The fact that nurses have to work at nights and on the weekends besides the traditional working hours is a cause of stress on its own. Nurses may have problems in communication due to the way they work. Moreover, reversed biological clock may cause chronic fatigue, tiredness and depression. Overtime work causes a decrease in attention level in operating rooms where attention is very important and this causes an increase in the possibility of making mistakes and decrease in the quality of work. Therefore, operating room nurses experience stress and homeostatic deterioration comes with sleep disorders and have significant effects on the quantity of life and performance of people.

Surgical teams in the operating rooms generally differ by the type of operation. However, anesthetic team generally remains constant and works longer times in shifts. Thus, health problems are more common in this group.

Workplace violence is the most common situation that healthcare professionals encounter. Violence against doctors and healthcare personnel have been rapidly increasing in recent years. Healthcare employees are a specific group in terms of facing stress and exposure to violence is quite high in this group. There many different factors of violence such as patients, relatives, coworkers in healthcare institutions. Hospitals are becoming more dangerous for healthcare personnel day by day [35]. In that case doctors and healthcare personnel do not feel safe themselves in their workplaces. In a Turkish study by Ayranci et al., on healthcare professionals, it was identified that 50.8% of the healthcare professionals were subjected to one or more type of violence while they were working, practitioners were subjected to violence the most (67.6%) and 58.4% of the nurses were subjected to violence [36]. A research in Turkey by Gokce and Dundar on doctors and nurses stated that 71.4% of the doctors and 90% of the nurses were subjected to violence [37].

2.5 Ergonomic risk factors

Healthcare professionals try to do their best in their jobs, just like the employees in other sectors. In order for healthcare personnel to efficiently perform what is expected from them, work environment should be designed in a way that allows moving comfortably. Ergonomics refers to designing and organizing the workplace and equipment in the most physically suitable way for the users. No matter how perfect they are technically, if the tools and equipment, tables, chairs and methods used by healthcare personnel are not suitable for themselves, a high performance should not be expected. In other words, if they are designed without considering the characteristics, abilities and disabilities of the people, employees cannot perform with high performance. Ergonomic stress factors are very common in operating rooms. Especially the nurses who provide service to the complete dependent patients help them with all activities such as getting dressed, eating, going to bathroom etc. This may cause musculoskeletal injuries, especially due to overload, in healthcare personnel. Researches on nurses identified that bad back problems are more common in nurses compared to the people working in fields requiring heavy physical work. Hospital employees are in the risk group for backache; occupational activities such as lifting patients in improper positions, leaning forward, turning around and standing still for a long time may cause biomechanical stress in vertebra and backache [38–41].

2.6 Radiation risk factors

Another important risk factor in hospitals is radiation. Regulations on this subject must be followed carefully [42–45]. Radiation in operating rooms can be emitted from mobile rontgen devices, fluoroscopy devices and non-ionizing devices like lasers [46]. Radiation exposure is caused by working with fluoroscopy and radioactive substance application in operating rooms. Long term effects of low dose radiation use for a long time in operating rooms are not known. Biological effects of the ionizing radiation in the tissue differ by the total dose, dose rate, amount of body receiving radiation, radio sensitivity and the type of radiation and it may have stochastic and deterministic (non-stochastic) effects. Adverse effects of radiation exposure can occur within hours or years. Thyroids, eyes, hands and gonads are among the regions that are most affected by radiation. Radiation safety is important for employee safety as it is for patient safety. In studies conducted on operating room workers, it was determined that healthcare workers ignored protective measures regarding radiation safety [47–49]. The main reason for this was explained by the lack of knowledge of the employees on the physical characteristics and biological effects of radiation. Yet, setting and applying basic principles of radiation protection is important for employee and patient safety. Therefore, attention should be paid for in-service trainings for operating room personnel, inspection of the application and having informed and certified personnel to use fluoroscopy.

3. Conclusion

OHS aims to minimize occupational accidents and diseases and to keep the health of employees at the best level in all the world. With OHS studies, dangers and risk factors should be determined and controlled at their source. Operating rooms are complex places where the most advanced technology and systems are used and qualified employees work at. The most threatening factors for employee safety in operating rooms are contaminated, sharp object injuries and material splashes. The most common ones are pinprick injuries. Allergies to latex gloves and hand washing solutions in the operating rooms may cause serious problems. Ergonomics is an important yet ignored topic. If the actions such as positioning and lifting patients, transferring patients from the bed to the stretcher and carrying patients are performed without being careful, they may cause serious musculoskeletal problems for employees. Factors such as excessive amount of time spent in work environment, shifts and insufficient number of nurses may cause an increase in work intensity and a decrease in motivation for nurses.

Critical decisions on the lives of patients are taken and applied in operating rooms which have high level of psychological and physical stress. Therefore, they require concordant team work and moderate work environment. Use of too many technological devices, necessity to make fast decisions and risks caused by the nature of the operating rooms also pose some risks for the employees. Nurses working in operating rooms may encounter various risky conditions as explained above. Unsuitable physical environment, heavy physical work, frequent criminal activities, working late at night with fewer people, working in non-physiological positions, non-ergonomic conditions, stress, discomfort, workplace conditions which makes healthy diet difficult, commute problems are factors threatening employee safety. Since numerous factors might have negative effects on the safety and health in operating rooms, risk assessment should be performed and reformative-preventive actions should be taken in order to identify characteristics such as what these factors are, at what level they are present and who they affect. Occupational health problems caused by the risks in the workplace can be reduced and the rates of serious injuries and damages can be decreased with proper and efficient risk management.

Operating room nurses should be trained on subjects such as general environmental pathogens, ergonomics, blood-borne pathogens, protective equipment, radiation safety, fire safety, general safety, use of hazardous material (substances), emergency situation management, protection against airborne diseases, mobile liquefied oxygen, communication and enlightenment on dangers, medical equipment care and safety of tap water.

Primary precautions to reduce exposure to chemical substances include using materials with low danger potential, paying attention to the allowed concentrations, frequently ventilating the environment, hand washing, using personal protective equipment such as aprons and masks, updating old methods and equipment, measuring and monitoring samples taken regularly, biological monitoring. In addition to these, there are many precautions that are customized according to the characteristics and risks of the chemical substances.

Preoperative, intraoperative and postoperative management of the patients with suspected or diagnosed new coronavirus pneumonia should be known and defined in detail. All healthcare professionals, particularly surgeons and nurses, should be provided with advantages in protection from the disease. All patients should be managed as Covid-19 patients until the results are confirmed. Risk of Covid-19 should be considered for general surgery emergencies and personal protective equipment should be used accordingly. Patients should be transferred to the operating rooms by service nurses and nurses should wear N95 masks, goggles/face shields, waterproof aprons and overshoes. Patients should also wear a surgical mask and transferred to the operating room via the shortest way with least contact with others.

Hospital management should take precautions against the risk of infection, nurses should gain more awareness and pay attention to using protective equipment such as gloves and masks. Ventilation of the healthcare institutions is important to protect patients and healthcare personnel and to prevent the infections caused by the institution. For this purpose, various air conditioning systems are developed, each of which has its pros and cons. It is thought that improving environmental conditions of the operating rooms would increase the chance of preventing surgical infections, decrease complications, increase the quality of the operation, increase the quality of healthcare service by decreasing cost and reduce the stress of the operating room personnel.

Multidimensionality of the concept of health and the need for interdisciplinary cooperation and several approaches are some of the most important elements that form the basis of nursing education. Nurses who are educated on occupational risks and employee safety can have the ability to define and control the possible risk factors. Nurses undertake many duties besides patient care in operating rooms, which are not their essential duties. Excessive workload and transfer of the duties of other disciplines to nurses leads to the emergence of an unhappy occupational group which works hard yet does not have time to practice their own profession. This situation should be prevented and it should be ensured that nurses do the duties they have been trained for.

Concordance and productivity of the team depend on the position and role of each member of the team being defined and recognized. It also depends on each member having the capability and possibility to perform their own roles at their best. Therefore, nurses' roles should be defined and nurses should be capable of performing those, and roles of nurses should be known, recognized, accepted and respected by the other members of the team. In order to establish such an environment, besides following the law and legislation, employees and employers should accept their roles that prioritize health and safety, believe that safety would be maintained in the institution, adopt an appropriate attitude and display social responsibilities.

As described above safe working environment is important for all hospital workers, especially for those who work in operating rooms. Necessary precautions should be taken and controlled regularly in order for surgical nurses to perform their duties successfully. Employees should be informed about work safety precautions and most importantly push for these precautions. In addition to patient and employee safety in operating rooms, environmental safety also has an important place. Environmental risk analysis should be performed by experts in the operating rooms at regular intervals and risk management should be implemented by the occupational health and safety committees in the hospital.

Conflict of interest

The author declares no conflict of interest.

Author details

Hülya Gül
Public Health Department, Istanbul Medical Faculty, Istanbul University, Fatih Istanbul, Turkey

*Address all correspondence to: hulyagul@istanbul.edu.tr

References

[1] Gül H, Atlı ZC. A public health approach to environmental and occupational health problems in developing countries, In: Health of People, Places and Planet: Reflections based on Tony McMichael's four decades of contribution to epidemiological understanding, 2015, Chapter 5, p: 95-106, Editor: Colin D Butler, Jane Dixon, Anthony G Capon, ISBN: 9781925022407 (paperback) 9781925022414 (ebook), Canberra, Australia, ANU E Press.

[2] Gates MA, et al. Operating room nursing and lung cancer risk in a cohort of female registered nurses. Scand J Work Environ Health. 2007. PMID: 23357728

[3] Walts LF, Forsythe AB, Moore G. Critique: occupational disease among operating room personnel. Anesthesiology. 1975; 42(5):608-11.

[4] Azizoğlu F, Köse A, Gül, H. Self - Reported environmental health risks of nurses working in hospital surgical units, International Nursing Review, 2018; (2):10-18, 2018, https://doi.org/10.1111/inr.12467.

[5] Le Moual N, Varraso R, Zock JP, Henneberger P, Speizer FK, Camargo AC. Are operating room nurses at higher risk of severe persistent asthma? The Nurse s' Health Study. J Occup Environ Med. 2013. PMID: 3977115.

[6] Walton A and Rogers B. Workplace hazards faced by nursing assistants in the United States: a focused literature review. Int J Eenviron Res Pu; 2017; 14(5): 544.

[7] Lee JH, Cho J, Kim YJ, Im SH, Jang ES, Kim JW, Kim HB, Jeong SH. Occupational blood exposures in health care workers: incidence, characteristics, and transmission of blood borne pathogens in South Korea. BMC Public Health. 2017; 18; 17(1):827.

[8] Memon AG, Naeem Z, Zaman A, Zahid F. Occupational health related concerns among surgeons. Int J Health Sci (Qassim). 2016; 10(2):279-91.

[9] Patz JA, Jodrey D. Occupational health in surgery: risks extend beyond the operating room. Aust N Z J Surg. 1995; 65(9):627-9.

[10] Gül H. Sick Building Syndrome from Perspective of Occupational and Public Health İn: Sick Building Syndrome in Public Buildings and Workplaces Y Springer, USA, Chapter: 5, 2011, p: 89-104, Editor: Sabah A. Abdul-Wahab Al-Sulaiman, ISBN: 978-3-642-17918-1, DOI: 10.1007/978-3-642-17919-8,

[11] Keller, S., Tschan, F., Semmer, N.K. et al. Noise in the Operating Room Distracts Members of the Surgical Team. An Observational Study. World J Surg 42, 3880-3887 (2018). https://doi.org/10.1007/s00268-018-4730-7.

[12] Juang DF, Lee CH, Yang T. et al. Noise pollution and its effects on medical care workers and patients in hospitals. Int. J. Environ. Sci. Technol. 7, 705-716 (2010). https://doi.org/10.1007/BF03326180.

[13] Liu Z., Liu H, Yin H. et al. Prevention of surgical site infection under different ventilation systems in operating room environment. Front. Environ. Sci. Eng. 15, 36 (2021).

[14] Dehghani F, Kamalinia M, Omidi F, Fallahzadeh RA. Probabilistic health risk assessment of occupational exposure to isoflurane and sevoflurane in the operating room. Ecotoxicol Environ Saf. 2021 (1); 207:111270.

[15] Jafari A, Bargeshadi R, Jafari F, Mohebbi I, Hajaghazadeh M. Environmental and biological measurements of isoflurane and sevoflurane in operating room personnel. Int Arch Occup Environ Health 2018; 91(3):349-359. https://doi.org/10.1007/s00420-017-1287-y.

[16] Hoerauf, K., Koller, C., Taeger, K, Hobbhahn J. Occupational exposure to sevoflurane and nitrous oxide in operating room personnel. Int Arch Occup Environ Health, 1996 (69); 134-138. https://doi.org/10.1007/s004200050127

[17] IARC. IARC Monographs on the identification of carcinogenic hazards to humans, Available from https://monographs.iarc.who.int/cards_page/contact-us/ Accessed date: 22.02.2021.

[18] Buring JE, Hennekens CH, Mayrent SL, Rosner B, Greenberg ER, Colton T. Health experiences of operating room personnel. Anesthesiology. 1985;62(3):325-30.

[19] Herzog-Niescery J, Steffens T, Bellgardt M, Breuer-Kaiser A, Gude P, Vogelsang H, et al., HM. Photoacoustic gas monitoring for anesthetic gas pollution measurements and its cross-sensitivity to alcoholic disinfectants. BMC Anesthesiol. 2019 (9); 19(1):148.

[20] Nilsson R., Björdal C., Andersson M., Björdal J, Nyberg A, Welin B, Willman A. Health risks and occupational exposure to volatile anesthetics – a review with a systematic approach. Journal of Clinical Nursing, 2005 ;(14):173-186. https://doi.org/10.1111/j.1365-2702.2004.01032.x.

[21] Barrett ES, Horton DB, Roy J, Xia W, Greenberg P, Andrews T, et al., Risk Factors for Severe Acute Respiratory Syndrome Coronavirus 2 Infection in Hospital Workers: Results From a Screening Study in New Jersey, United States in Spring 2020. Open Forum Infect Dis. 2020 Oct 31; 7(12):ofaa534.

[22] Baker JM, Nelson KN, Overton E, Lopman BA, Lash TL, Photakis M, et al., Quantification of Occupational and Community Risk Factors for SARS-CoV-2 Seropositivity Among Health Care Workers in a Large U.S. Health Care System. Ann Intern Med. 2021 Jan 29. doi: 10.7326/M20-7145. Online ahead of print.

[23] Rubbi I, Pasquinelli G, Brighenti A, Fanelli M, Gualandi P, Nanni E, D'Antoni V, Fabbri C. Healthcare personnel exposure to COVID - 19: an observational study on quarantined positive workers. Acta Biomed. 2020 Nov 30; 91(12-S):e2020012.

[24] Sanghera J, Pattani N, Hashmi Y, Varley KF, Cheruvu MS, Bradley A, Burke JR The impact of SARS-CoV-2 on the mental health of healthcare workers in a hospital setting-A Systematic Review. J Occup Health. 2020; 62(1):e12175.

[25] Quaedackers JSLT, Stein R, Bhatt N, Dogan HS, Hoen L, Nijman RJM, et al. Clinical and surgical consequences of the COVID-19 pandemic for patients with pediatric urological problems. Statement of the EAU guidelines panel for pediatric urology, Journal of Pediatric Urology, 2020; 16(3):284-287. https://doi.org/10.1016/j.jpurol.2020.04.007.

[26] Swerdlow BN. Surgical smoke and the anesthesia provider, Journal of Anesthesia, 2020 (34):575-584 https://doi.org/10.1007/s00540-020-02775-x.

[27] Bree K, Barnhill S, Rundell W. The Dangers of Electrosurgical Smoke to Operating Room Personnel: A Review. Workplace Health & Safety. 2017; 65(11):517-526. doi:10.1177/2165079917691063.

[28] Panlilio AL, Foy DR, Edwards JR, Bell DM, Welch BA, Parrish CM, et al. Blood contacts during surgical procedures. JAMA. 1991; 27; 265(12):1533-7.

[29] Lin H, Wang X, Luo X, Qin ZA. Management program for preventing occupational blood-borne infectious exposure among operating room nurses: an application of the PRECEDE-PROCEED model. J Int Med Res. 2020; 48(1):300060519895670.

[30] Fry DE. Occupational risks of blood exposure in the operating room. Am Surg. 2007; 73(7):637-46.PMID: 17674933 Review.

[31] Gül H. Mobbing at Workplaces and the Mental Health Effects on Employees Essential Notes in Psychiatry chapter one, Editor: Victor Olisah, ISBN: 978-953-51-0574-9, 2012, p: 3-12, InTech - Open Access Publisher, Croatia.

[32] Xu D, Zhu S, Li, H, Gao J, Mou H, Wang K. Relationships among occupational stress, toileting behaviors, and overactive bladder in nurses: A multiple mediator model. J Adv Nurs. 2019; 75: 1263– 1271. https://doi.org/10.1111/jan.13940.

[33] Yang Y-M, Zhou L-J. Workplace bullying among operating room nurses in China: A cross-sectional survey. Perspect Psychiatr Care. 2021; 57: 27– 32. https://doi.org/10.1111/ppc.12519.

[34] Zheng R, Zhou Y, Fu Y, Xiang Q, Cheng F, Chen H, et al. Prevalence and associated factors of depression and anxiety among nurses during the outbreak of COVID-19 in China: A cross-sectional study. Int J Nurs Stud. 2021; 114:103809.

[35] Ozsaker E, Kaya A, Okgun Alcan A, Yavuz van Giersbergen M, Aktas. EO.J Forensic Cases in the Operating Room: Knowledge and Practices of Physicians and Nurses. Perianesth Nurs. 2020; 35(1):38-43.

[36] Ayrancı U, Yenilmez C, Balcı Y, Kaptanoğlu C. Identification of violence in Turkish health care settings. J Interpers Violence 2006; 21:276-96.

[37] Gökçe T, Dündar C. The frequency of exposing to violence and ıts effects on state and trait anxiety levels among the doctors and nurses working in Samsun Psychiatry Hospital. Journal of Turgut Ozal Medical Center 2008; 15:25-28.

[38] Clari M, Garzaro G., Di Maso M., Donato F., Godono A., Paleologo M. et al. Upper Limb Work-Related Musculoskeletal Disorders in Operating Room Nurses: A Multicenter Cross-Sectional Study. Int. J. Environ. Res. Public Health 2019, 16, 2844.

[39] Cavdar I, Karaman A, Ozhanli Y, Ozbas A. Low Back Pain in Operating Room Nurses and Its Associated Factors. Pak J Med Sci. 2020 Sep-Oct; 36(6):1291-1296.

[40] Rypicz, Ł, Karniej, P, Witczak, I, Kołcz, A. Evaluation of the occurrence of work-related musculoskeletal pain among anesthesiology, intensive care, and surgical nurses: An observational and descriptive study. Nurs Health Sci. 2020; 22: 1056– 1064. https://doi.org/10.1111/nhs.12767.

[41] Rypicz Ł, Karniej, P, Witczak I, Kołcz A. Evaluation of the occurrence of work-related musculoskeletal pain among anesthesiology, intensive care, and surgical nurses: An observational and descriptive study. Nurs Health Sci. 2020; 22: 1056– 1064. https://doi.org/10.1111/nhs.12767.

[42] Frane N, Bitterman A. Radiation Safety and Protection. In: Stat Pearls [Internet]. Treasure Island (FL): StatPearls Publishing; 2021 Jan-. Available from: https://www.ncbi.nlm.nih.gov/books/NBK557499/.

[43] EPA: Radiation Protection Available: https://www.epa.gov/radiation.

[44] US. NRC: Part 20—Standards for protection against radiation. Available: https://www.nrc.gov/reading-rm/doc collections/cfr/part020/full-text.html.

[45] American College of Radiology (ACR): Radiation Safety Available: https://www.acr.org/Clinical-Resources/Radiology-Safety/Radiation-Safety. https://www.acr.org/-/media/ACR/Files/Radiology-Safety/Radiation-Safety/Dose-Reference-Card.pdf

[46] Rajabi Pour M, Fardid R, Zare T, Kargar Shouroki F, Mosleh-Shirazi MA, Behzad Behbahani A. Assessment of Adaptive Response of Gamma Radiation in the Operating Room Personnel Exposed to Anesthetic Gases by Measuring the Relative Gene Expression Changes Ku80, Ligase1 and P53. J Biomed Phys Eng. 2020; 10(2):225-234. doi: 10.31661/jbpe.v0i0.1273.

[47] Kahkhaei FR, Sarani H. Surgical technologists' knowledge and performance about radiation protection in Zahedan educational hospitals. A descriptive-analytical study. J Educ Health Promot. 2020; 9:283. doi:10.4103/jehp.jehp_162_20.

[48] Jeong KW, Jung Jang HJ. Correlation between Knowledge and Performance of Radiation Protection among Operating Room International Journal of Bio-Science and Bio-Technology, 2016; (1):8:275-284 http://dx.doi.org/10.14257/ijbsbt.2016.8.1.24.

[49] Zindrou K, Kelesi M, Toulia G, Stoufis N, Babatsikou F, & Marvaki A. Knowledge of nursing stuff on radiation protection in a public hospital. Health & Research Journal, 2016; 2(3):244-258. doi:https://doi.org/10.12681/healthresj.19706.

Section 3

Healthcare Delivery

Chapter 14

Accessing Oral Healthcare within a Context of Economic Transition

Kasusu Nyamuryekung'e and Febronia Kahabuka

Abstract

In many low-mid income settings, accessibility of health services remains inadequate and inequitable. These observed disparities in accessibility are particularly evident for oral healthcare services. The access to oral healthcare is influenced by the responsiveness of the health system, including availability of human resources for health, oral health facilities' infrastructure, geographical distribution, equipment and materials as well as community's awareness and affordability of the provided services. The evolution of oral healthcare access in Tanzania; from the early post-colonial phases of independence to current transition that the country is undergoing from low to a low-mid income economy is presented. The major health policies' transition from "Free Healthcare" services to "Cost-sharing" and ultimately to "Health Insurance" are presented within the context of their influence towards oral healthcare access.

Keywords: Access, Oral Health Services, Economic, Utilization

1. Introduction

Being healthy is a prerequisite for enjoyable and productive life of any human being. It is an invaluable resource for all human activities and is considered one of the fundamental basic rights. Attaining and maintaining health is a complex endeavor. At its most basic level, it requires an individual to have access to health information which is necessary to prevent diseases and demand care when needed. A bit more complicated is the ability to obtain timely, responsive, adequate, appropriate, and accessible health services whenever in need. Despite the importance of oral health to general well-being, many countries have not managed to avail equitable healthcare services to all their citizens. The factors responsible for this regrettable situation vary greatly across and even within countries. Generally, the prevailing health situation of a specific setting is an outcome of the historical background, policies, and sociocultural issues. This brief chapter presents the various stages of provision of healthcare access in Tanzania within the context of major health policy implementations and unique historical perspectives underpinning the evolution of oral healthcare services within the country.

2. Accessibility of Oral health services in Tanzania

The United Republic of Tanzania was formed in 1964 following a union between Tanganyika and Zanzibar. It is one of the East Africa countries of the African Great

Lakes region. It borders to the north by Uganda; the northeast by Kenya; to the east by Comoro Islands and the Indian Ocean; to the south by Mozambique and Malawi; to the southwest by Zambia; and to the west by Rwanda, Burundi, and the Democratic Republic of the Congo. It is 945,087 km^2 in size inhabited by more than 60,000,000 people (2021 United Nations estimates). The country consists of about 125 ethnic groups with a wide range of traditions and customs.

From the year 2020, Tanzania started to be classified as a lower middle-income country. This highlights tremendous development strides that the country has made in its 59 years of existence as an independent state. Nevertheless, like many other countries found in sub-Saharan Africa, Tanzania experiences a high proportion of the global disease burden, but also have an insufficient number of human resources for health. Furthermore, the health system is burdened due to the high prevalence of communicable and rapidly increasing rates of non-communicable diseases. Despite the marked improvements in increasing access to healthcare services, they remain inadequate and inequitably distributed. These impediments become amplified several folds with respect to oral care services. Oral healthcare facilities are disproportionately distributed geographically, have exceedingly limited human resources and few facilities that provide the services.

Healthcare accessibility is a broad concept and does not simply imply ability to visit a health facility as need arises. Affordability of health services, Availability of health facilities and services, Appropriateness of provided health services according to need, Adequacy of the provided services as well as Accessibility in terms of reachability and geographical considerations are all pertinent factors which determine health service accessibility. Oral health service provision in many areas within the country is limited to predominantly emergency care. There is insufficient provision of restorative care, and lack of sustained preventive care which is the cornerstone of controlling all the major oral diseases.

Currently, Tanzania does not have a mandatory health insurance policy. Therefore, accessing oral health services and overall financing of the health system relies mostly on out-of-pocket payments (cash payments at the point of health service). It immediately becomes noticeable that in settings such as this, with high poverty levels, requiring cash at the point of health service provision prohibits many from accessing it. Overtly, where large proportions of the population are poor, a requirement of cash in lieu of access to healthcare may lead to considerable accessibility issues.

One can expect that poor people especially, may face financial difficulties because of required out-of-pocket payments for oral healthcare services. Many people in sub-Saharan countries only go to oral health facilities after a prolonged period of wait-and-see. Their first points when seeking oral healthcare may be folk remedies, traditional healers or over the counter drugs from drug stores. Reluctance in usage of formal oral healthcare services is usually due to several accessibility challenges including lack of, and uncertainty regarding the financial resources that would be required to obtain treatment for their health problem, low levels of knowledge regarding their ailment (and the corresponding care), as well as poor attitudes towards available oral healthcare.

Even in situations whereby the patients overcome these formidable financial and structural hurdles and manage to attend oral health facilities, they are not guaranteed of the best available care. Low-level oral health facilities within Tanzania, which are the first (and for some, the only) points of contact with the health system, may experience frequent medication and equipment stock-outs, are understaffed, and lack the necessary investigative tools. Generally, the most prevalent dental conditions (dental caries and periodontal diseases) are not associated with mortality. Thus, in many cases, and because of need of maximization of limited resources, policymakers frequently overlook oral health; despite its strong linkages to general health and significant contribution to an individuals' quality of life.

The latest statistics from the Ministry of Health (2021) reveal that there are less than 1,000 oral health personnel working at public health facilities in the country. This figure encompasses several cadres, including dental surgeons and specialists, assistant dental officers, dental therapists, and dental laboratory technicians. Furthermore, oral healthcare services are offered in only about 5% of all available public health facilities countrywide.

2.1 Chronology of oral health services formation in Tanzania

2.1.1 Traditional healthcare in Tanzania (1800s and beyond)

"Traditional medicine" is defined by WHO as sum of the knowledge, skills, and practices based on the theories, beliefs, and experiences indigenous to different cultures, whether explicable or not, used in the maintenance of health, as well as in the prevention, diagnosis, improvement, or treatment of illnesses (WHO Executive Board EB134/24).

In Tanzania, historically traditional medicines are provided by traditional healers who are usually trusted and respected by communities. These healers are purported to have gaine insight about the medicines from their parents or grandparents. Therefore, the practice usually runs within a clan.

The various ethnic groups employ diverse traditional medicines in managing oral ailments. They include a wide assortment of tree barks, leaves or roots. Depending on the nature of the ailment, fresh traditional products may be squeezed or boiled to make solutions for drinking, ground into poultices used for topical application or boiled for medicinal steam inhalation. The products are sun dried for preservation purpose; either in their original form or ground into a powder. Treatment of oral diseases is usually done by applying a freshly ground product or powder on the area of complaint or on the oral mucosa, tooth or in the tooth cavity. Occasionally it may be in form of liquid for drinking.

Indeed, traditional medicines and remedies have persisted and continue to be utilized in high rates even with the advent of modern oral healthcare services in Tanzania. It is common to have street vendors and self-appointed healers offering various wares purported to treat all manner of oral conditions. For many people in the Tanzanian community, these traditional remedies serve as their first foray towards their quest of addressing oral health complaints.

2.1.2 Modern healthcare services during colonial times (1884–1961)

Tanganyika was a colony of Germany (1884–1919) and later a British Protectorate (1919–1961). Modern healthcare was introduced in Tanganyika during colonial time. This healthcare arrangement was primarily envisioned to suit economic, social, and political requirements of colonial rulers rather than the health needs of the native Tanganyika population [1]. Auspiciously, in the 19th century Christian missionaries brought hospitals with them among other services. The missionaries desired to give services to native communities as well [2]. Moreover, only facets of indigenous people enjoyed these health services because the missionary hospitals were few, health professionals scarce and transportation infrastructures extremely poor.

However, as missionary health services increased within the country, and partly driven by the altruistic nature of the establishments, some facilities started to offer oral care services to the local population. Due to the very real limitations during that period, the only treatment that the local population could realistically receive was emergency care in the form of tooth extractions. Thus, for the very first time that the population is being introduced to institutionalized oral healthcare services, tooth extractions were the one and only service available. No concerted efforts were made to establish basic oral healthcare services with restorative or routine preventive components. Thus, it remains until this day to a large swathe of the Tanzanian population the belief and sentiment borne out of community-acquired historical experience that "the only cure for a tooth ache is extraction".

2.2 "Free" health for all

2.2.1 Health services post-independence (1961–1995)

When Tanganyika became independent in 1961, the government expanded accessibility to modern health services aiming to improve the health and wellbeing of all her citizens. The health system was intended to be more responsive to the needs of the people focusing on those most at risk. The general goal was to facilitate provision of equitable, quality, and affordable basic health services.

Over the years, since independence in 1961 and soon afterwards, the government of Tanganyika and later the United Republic of Tanzania placed emphasis on the health sector and especially the key targets of eliminating diseases, eradicating poverty and illiteracy with the objective of achieving a universal health to all Tanzanians. In 1967, the country adopted a party declaration "Arusha declaration of 1967" which marked the start of a series of health sector reforms with the intention of increasing universal access to social services to the poor and those living in marginalized rural areas.

The implementation of the Arusha declaration entailed countrywide banning of private-for-profit medical practice in 1977 upon which the government took on the ambitious task of providing health services to all citizens free of charge. Further deliberate restructuring of the health sector included making health services more effective, accessible, and affordable with specific attention to most underprivileged groups of population including women, children under five-year age group and those living in abject poverty. Naturally, this policy necessitated prioritization of healthcare services due to the reality of limited resources. Considerable, deliberate, and focused efforts were directed towards combating communicable diseases which were seen to have high mortality rates.

Additionally, the country established and adopted an extensive network of health facilities throughout the country, which follows a pyramidal structure, from village dispensaries and community-based activities at the base followed by health centers, district hospitals, regional level hospitals, zonal hospitals and referral and national hospitals at the summit. This pyramidal structure of health services persists up to this very day and forms the backbone of healthcare facilities' distribution countrywide.

2.2.2 Financing system for "Free health services"

Free health services were enjoyed by Tanzanians until early 1990s. At this time, it became apparent that provision of free healthcare for all was neither tenable nor possible. The main explanation to this situation was the rising healthcare costs along with low economic growth. This sobering situation led to the government's adoption of health sector reforms in early 1990s. The reforms changed the financing system from free services to cost sharing policies in the form of user fees which was introduced in four phases from July 1993 to January 1995. The cost sharing policy put in place exemption and waiver for special groups.

2.2.3 Intended and unintended effects of "free health policy"

Provision of free medical services in Tanzania recorded several achievements. Among the major successes of the free services and the policy implemented during that period was significant progress in reducing infant and child mortality through declines in morbidity and mortality from malaria and other childhood diseases. Other achievements include progress in aspects of child malnutrition, expansion of vaccine coverage, decline in HIV prevalence as well as Neonatal and Maternal Mortality [3, 4].

Despite the recorded accomplishments, there were unintended outcomes of the free health services regime. They include occurrence of healthcare service disparities due to intensification of social and economic inequalities, limited availability of equipment, medicines and supplies, equipment breakdown and lack of accountability in service provision or reduced performance [3].

2.2.4 Implications of "Health for all" on accessibility to oral healthcare services

All Tanzanians enjoyed free oral healthcare services at all government facilities under free healthcare regime. Nevertheless, the bulk of care being offered was emergency care in form of tooth extractions, perpetuating the set precedence of the colonial era. Establishment of restorative and regular preventive oral services for maintenance of oral health was never attempted. There were simply not enough oral health professionals to feasibly implement this and the medical-model of health was prevalent at that time, where health facilities were perceived as placed where you go only to "regain" your health.

Nonetheless, oral healthcare services are not uniformly available in the country. After independence, the government strived to avail dental services at regional hospitals. Gradually (starting in 1980s) the services were expanded to district hospitals although up to the year 2020; 30 out of 184 district councils had no oral healthcare services. Additionally, in large cities and towns, few health centers provide oral healthcare services. Along with the government's health sector reforms, permitting private healthcare services gave room to inauguration of private dental clinics which augment the government efforts in provision of oral healthcare. Illustrating the disproportionate distribution and the inability of the public health facilities to meet oral healthcare demand, the number of private oral health facilities outnumbers those of the public (Health Facility Registration System, 2021).

2.3 Cost-sharing

2.3.1 Moving away from "free" health in oral health

Cost-sharing is the term used to describe a co-payment scheme in which a user of a particular service contributes a certain amount towards its utilization. In the Tanzania health system context, users were expected to "top-up" on government-subsidized health services [5]. Cost-sharing was the first instance of introduction of user fees within the history of the United Republic of Tanzania. The rationale for its introduction was to increase the awareness of treatment costs and limit injudicious use of health services by the consumers. It also allows the healthcare users to function as contributors towards financing of their health system. Considering the slow economic growth and narrow taxable base for raising of required revenues, the idea appeared to have a lot of merit in context. Indeed, through cost-sharing and increasing government expenditure and investment in health generally, and oral health specifically- significant improvements have been made in recruitment and training of oral health personnel within the last fifteen years. Furthermore, many oral health facilities countrywide have been refurbished and equipped to modern standards.

However, as is usually the case, the actual reality of user-fees has now been shown to be more complicated than the fiction initially envisioned. Objective, multi-country assessments have shown that the introduction of user fees had increased health system revenues only modestly, but significantly reduced the access of low-income and underprivileged people to basic social and health services [6]. Furthermore, when assessing the impact of health expenditures of individuals, it was revealed that smaller proportions used dental services compared to medicines and outpatient care. A possible interpretation of this observation is that dental costs per visit may be too high that the households actively avoid them [7].

Removal or reduction of user fees has been found to increase the utilization of treatment and preventive services; however, it has also been shown to negatively impact service quality, especially in situations where the supplementing sources of health finances are to be derived from the government. On the other hand, introduction or removal of user fees was associated with rapid and immediate changes to the service utilization patterns [8]. Matee and Simon conducted a study in Tanzania to compare dental attendance and service utilization a year before and after introduction of user fees. There was a noted 33% reduction in dental attendance immediately after the introduction of user fees. The reasons for such a finding are potentially numerous, and it is difficult to ascertain the change in dental attendance solely due to the policy change regarding user-fees. Nevertheless, this study does highlight the rapidity with which utilization rates may change upon manipulation of financial barriers to healthcare use [9].

Poor countries and poor people that most need protection from financial difficulties are the least protected by cost-sharing policy and may prevent them from accessing needed care. To address this, provisions have been made and waivers placed for those identified as destitute or unable to pay for the services. However, difficulties remain on how to accurately and timely identify these individuals. At low incomes, out-of-pocket spending for healthcare is high on average and varies from 20 to 80% of the total cost of health service utilization [10]. Out-of-pocket payments place the burden of healthcare funding on an individual and translate into health service use, and hence benefits, being distributed according to ability-to-pay rather than need for healthcare [11].

One of the prominent effects of the cost-sharing policy can be vividly illustrated by the dental visit and service utilization patterns of the Tanzanian populations. A significant proportion of Tanzanians have oral symptoms but have never attended oral health facilities. More than 90% of all dental visits in Tanzania are due to symptoms, and frequently these symptoms have been present for a long duration prior to attendance. It is only when the symptoms become excessively severe or interfere with daily functions is attendance made. Upon attendance, most of the treatment utilized for dental caries is tooth extractions- even in situations where restorative care was amenable. In all these scenarios depicted, one factor can be drawn linking them together- a need of payment of health services prior to receiving health services. Therefore, although cost-sharing may have some positive consequences towards oral healthcare utilization, careful consideration needs to be made to tailor an optimum out-of-pocket payment structure [12]. What is undeniable too, is that in order to protect the most vulnerable and needy of the population, cost-sharing policy remains inadequate and inappropriate in the long term.

2.4 Health insurance

2.4.1 Moving towards "prepayment" model

Health insurance is defined as insurance against the risk of incurring medical expenses among individuals. Tanzania established the National Health Insurance

Fund (NHIF) through the Act of Parliament No. 8 of 1999 and officially began functioning in June 2001. The program was initially intended to cover public servants, although currently there are provisions and service packages which allow for self- enrolment of any individual/groups of individuals. The public formal employee pays a mandatory contribution as a percentage of their monthly salary with a government-matched percentage.

This program covers the principal member, spouse and up to four children below 21 years who are legal dependents. Unlike other health insurance models which may require a separate dental insurance; NHIF also provides oral healthcare services as part of the benefit coverage for its members. Initially, NHIF only offered very rudimentary oral health services, predominantly emergency care and some surgical procedures- however, it has steadily improved over time- and currently offers a wide range of services including complex restorative, prosthodontics and even orthodontic care. The usual caveats with accessibility remain, despite elimination of cost as a barrier. Utilization of oral services covered by NHIF will still largely depend on whether the oral health facility nearest the benefactor has the requisite skilled oral personnel and equipment to provide them.

Nevertheless, formally employed workers constitute about one-quarter of the total workforce in Tanzania. In recognition of this, in 2001, the Community Health Fund (CHF) Act mandated CHF implementation in all districts of mainland Tanzania. The aim of this fund was to provide health insurance to communities which were largely informally employed and thus not captured by the NHIF Act. The CHF is a district-based micro-health insurance scheme whereby members of the respective communities prepay for health services and the scheme receives a "matching grant" from the central government, which is equivalent to the premiums paid by the enrolled households [13]. Unlike NHIF which is mandatory, CHF is a form of voluntary community-based health insurance. CHF usually exist within localized communities, most often in rural areas: members make small payments to the scheme, often annually and after harvest time, and the scheme covers the fees charged by local health services [14]. CHF covers a slightly wider range of people and has been the predominant form of health insurance, although it is considered to have the least favorable benefit packages. The scheme generally only covers outpatient care at primary health-care level- although efforts are underway to improve the overall package offered to benefactors. Generally, this scheme continues to be plagued by low enrolment and dismal retention rates.

When people are enrolled into a health insurance scheme, they gain several rights regarding their healthcare. "The expectations of patients are that membership of the insurance scheme gives them rights and makes them customers of the healthcare providers" [14]. Therefore, it becomes exceedingly demoralizing when their health service expectations are not met. Generally, health insurance, particularly through NHIF, has significantly increased accessibility to oral healthcare services in Tanzania. The assurance of purchasing power has allowed a flourishing of private dental practices and increased motivation in training of oral health personnel within the country. However, careful consideration is needed to ensure that this democratization of access does not lead to greater oral healthcare inequities especially among the informally (majority) employed population.

2.5 Future perspectives

2.5.1 Universal healthcare

Universal health coverage (UHC) is the availability of quality, affordable health services for all when needed without financial impoverishment. Tanzania's aim of achieving universal health coverage is provided in the nation's 4th Health Sector

Strategic Plan (2015–2020). The plan provides for a new health financing strategy aimed at helping the country attain the goal by addressing the existing segregate health insurance market through providing health insurance to all citizens. The goal is underpinned in the nation's 5th Health Sector Strategic Plan (2020–2025). Expected outcome and impact of Universal Health Coverage is improved access, coverage, and quality of health services.

Developing effective mechanisms for identifying and protecting people with very low incomes is critical in Tanzania. Even if user fees were completely abolished, as is happening in a growing number of African countries, it would still be necessary to identify people with the lowest incomes to protect them in relation to other financing mechanisms (e.g. to partly or fully subsidize their health insurance contributions). In addition, if universal coverage is to be achieved, it is necessary to explore ways of achieving funding pools that are as large and integrated as possible, to maximize income and risk cross-subsidies and to allocate pooled resources in an equitable way [11].

2.5.2 Probable implications on oral health outcomes

According to the World Health Organization there are three main goals for a healthcare system: good health, responsiveness to the expectations of the population, and fairness of financial contribution [15]. While the first objective, overall improvement of health, is self-explanatory the other two require more clarification. Responsiveness addresses the question of how far the healthcare system responds to people's expectations of it. The concept of fairness can be defined as "the highest possible degree of separation between contribution and utilization". It demands financial responsibility to vary according to ability to pay, and access to the healthcare system to vary according to healthcare needs irrespective of ability to pay [16].

Health insurance for all Tanzanians is foreseen to facilitate access to healthcare services. Expectantly people will no longer have to endure health problems or to wait until the situation is beyond bearable before consulting a health facility. Generally, Tanzanian population's oral health is predicted to improve in diverse aspects.

Availing Health insurance for all Tanzanians is expected to ease accessibility of oral healthcare. Easy access will optimistically facilitate a shift of the reason for visiting a dental clinic from pain or potentially pain situation driven to regular dental visits for check-ups and observance to follow up schedules. In a long run plausible positive outcome will be early diagnosis of oral diseases, efficacious management and ultimately better prognosis and generally improved oral health of all citizens.

3. Conclusions

Tanzania has made significant strides in improving and expanding oral healthcare accessibility of her people. This progress has been achieved through implementation of various policies embedded within the evolution of the social-political context in the country. The current trajectory of oral healthcare delivery system clearly highlights the unsustainability of the status quo. Adoption of universal health coverage and health insurance for all in the near future seems promising in easing access to oral healthcare.

Acknowledgements

We are grateful to the support offered by Muhimbili University of Health and Allied Sciences. (MUHAS).

Conflict of interest

The authors declare no conflict of interest.

Author details

Kasusu Nyamuryekung'e and Febronia Kahabuka*
School of Dentistry, Muhimbili University of Health and Allied Sciences,
Dar es Salaam, Tanzania

*Address all correspondence to: febby.kahabuka@gmail.com

References

[1] M. Turshen, " The impact of colonialism on health and health services in Tanzania," *Int. J. Heal. Serv.*, vol. 7, no. 1, pp. 7-35, 1977.

[2] T. Y.-H. organization and undefined 1986, "Socialist development and primary health care: the case of Tanzania," *JSTOR*.

[3] H. Wang, M. A. Juma, N. Rosemberg, and M. M. Ulisubisya, "Progressive Pathway to Universal Health Coverage in Tanzania: A Call for Preferential Resource Allocation Targeting the Poor," *Heal. Syst. Reform*, vol. 4, no. 4, pp. 279-283, 2018.

[4] M. of H. and S. W. Tanzania, "Health Sector Strategic Plan: July 2015 – June 2020," 2015.

[5] L. Gilson, "The lessons of user fee experience in Africa.," *Health policy and planning*, vol. 12, no. 4. pp. 273-85, 1997.

[6] M. Whitehead, G. Dahlgren, and T. Evans, "Equity and heath sector reforms: can lo-income countries escape the medical poverty trap?," *Lancet*, vol. 358, pp. 833-836, 2001.

[7] E. Bernabé, M. Masood, and M. Vujicic, "The impact of out-of-pocket payments for dental care on household finances in low and middle income countries," *BMC Public Health*, vol. 17, no. 1, pp. 1-8, 2017.

[8] M. Lagarde and N. Palmer, "The impact of user fees on health service utilization in low- And middle-income countries: How strong is the evidence?," *Bull. World Health Organ.*, vol. 86, no. 11, pp. 839-848, 2008.

[9] M. Matee and E. Simon, "Utilisation of dental services in Tanzania before and after the introduction of cost-sharing.," *Int. Dent. J.*, vol. 50, no. 2, pp. 69-72, 2000.

[10] G. Carrin, "Basic patterns in national health expenditure," vol. 80, no. 01, 2001.

[11] D. McIntyre *et al.*, "Beyond fragmentation and towards universal coverage: Insights from Ghana, South Africa and the United Republic of Tanzania," *Bull. World Health Organ.*, vol. 86, no. 11, pp. 871-876, Nov. 2008.

[12] K. Kolasa and M. Kowalczyk, "Does cost sharing do more harm or more good ? - a systematic literature review," *BMC Public Health*, pp. 1-14, 2016.

[13] A. Kalolo *et al.*, "Implementation of the redesigned Community Health Fund in the Dodoma region of Tanzania: A qualitative study of views from rural communities," *Int J Heal. Plann Mgmt*, vol. 33, pp. 121-135, 2018.

[14] D. McIntyre, "Learning from experience – Health care financing in Low and mid-income countries," 2001.

[15] A. Wagstaff *et al.*, "Progress on catastrophic health spending in 133 countries: A retrospective observational study," *Lancet Glob. Heal.*, pp. 169-179, 2017.

[16] Word Health Organization. "Everybody's business--strengthening health systems to improve health outcomes: WHO's framework for action," 2007.

Chapter 15

Patients' (Clients) Satisfaction with Medical Laboratory Services Contributes to Health and Quality Improvement

Nkereuwem S. Etukudoh and Uchejeso M. Obeta

Abstract

Patients' (clients/customer) services and satisfaction in Medical Laboratory Services and general healthcare is one of the twelve (12) quality essentials of Total Quality Management System (TQMS) emphasized by quality standards as seen in ISO 17025, ISO 15189 and ISO 9001. The patients otherwise referred to as customers or clients to Medical Laboratory and healthcare in general, is the heart-beat and kings to the healthcare system. This chapter looks into the quality aspect of medical laboratory services from the patients' angle towards thorough satisfaction or dis-satisfaction index and otherwise creates room for improvement in the services and healthcare in general. The chapter therefore, identified medical laboratory clients to include patients and patients' relations, physicians and other healthcare workers, public health and government, communities and interested parties, and medical laboratory profession. There is a need to administer services satisfaction survey developed by Director of Medical Laboratory Services or human resources/quality officers in line with the ISO 15189, ISO 17075 and ISO 9001 to customers/clients from time to time so the outcome can be used to correct services errors and cause quality improvement. It is believed that patients' satisfaction causes improvement in healthcare, quick recovery of patients and willingness of the patient to return to the healthcare facility in future. Patients' and customers' in medical laboratory feedback contributes to quality management and improvement to Medical Laboratory services and healthcare as an ingredient of TQMS.

Keywords: patients satisfaction, Medical Laboratory clients, customers, quality improvement, healthcare

1. Introduction

The Medical Laboratory is a laboratory that is equipped with biomedical instrument/equipment, materials and reagent (chemicals) for performing different medical laboratory tests using biological specimen (whole blood, serum, plasma, urine, stool, swab, sputum, exudates etc.), for disease discovery management and healthy living assessment. In the medical laboratory, some services like arrangements for test requests, preparation of patients, patient identification, samples collection, transportation, storage, processing and examination, test validation, interpretation, reporting and advice, in addition to safety and ethics are carried out during medical laboratory services [1, 2].

Treatment by patients themselves or treatment as a result of prescription given by a physician or other healthcare givers without the medical laboratory test leads to self-medication and medical guess work respectively. Cost of diagnosis could probably have contributed to the poor attitude towards visiting medical laboratories for proper diagnosis [1].

Patients' satisfaction is imperative for success. Without the patient in the laboratory, there would not be medical laboratory testing and examination of specimens in the laboratory. Patient are the most essential values in the hospital environment, medical laboratory inclusive. Just as patients contribute to safety in healthcare [3], patients equally contribute to medical laboratory services and quality of healthcare in general.

Medical laboratories continuously strive to attain very high levels of customer's satisfaction thereby serving their clients, improving quality and maintaining accreditation. The concept of customer service has not yet been made popular and accepted in most medical laboratories [4].

Patients' satisfaction is a component of healthcare quality and is increasingly being used to assess medical care in many countries in the world. Until recently traditional assessments of medical care were done purely in terms of technical and physiological reports of outcomes [5–8]. This patient/client satisfaction in the medical laboratory services is equally needed especially in Nigeria and other African countries and no wonder this chapter.

2. Conceptual clarifications

Patients are referred to as the main value of the medical and clinical environment. They are the reason for all works and therefore work cannot be done without them. Patients' satisfaction has a positive effect on clinical improvement, patient's adherence and retention, job satisfaction and appropriate clinical care by physicians [5, 9].

Patients' satisfaction is an expression of the gap between the expected and perceived characteristics of a service. It is recommended that patients be asked to report on their experiences through specific questions. Technique of factor analysis has demonstrated that patients' satisfaction is chiefly determined by 6 dimensions which are; care and information, food and physical facilities, non-tangible environment, nursing care, quantity of food and visiting arrangements [8]. However, any quality and improvement in healthcare without consideration to medical laboratory services may be missing a lot. The quality improvement in healthcare is mainly proven by the high quality of medical laboratory results.

Medical laboratory services in Nigerian public health facilities, have been rated very poor by patients. This is because patients are faced with overcrowding, long waiting time, poor provider-patient communication, poor facilities and environment while the patients are expecting higher standard. There is no doubt that there is a shift from professional perception that patients are uneducated and with little healthcare choice, to the fact that they are educated consumers who have many service demands and healthcare choices to make. This sends a signal to respect the patients and their needs or wishes as patients' perception provides the standard of quality in medical laboratory services and healthcare in general. The patient's satisfaction with medical laboratory service involves satisfaction with laboratory staff-patient interaction, satisfaction with sample collection processes, satisfaction with waiting time, satisfaction with laboratory facilities and environment, and satisfaction with costs of service [10, 11].

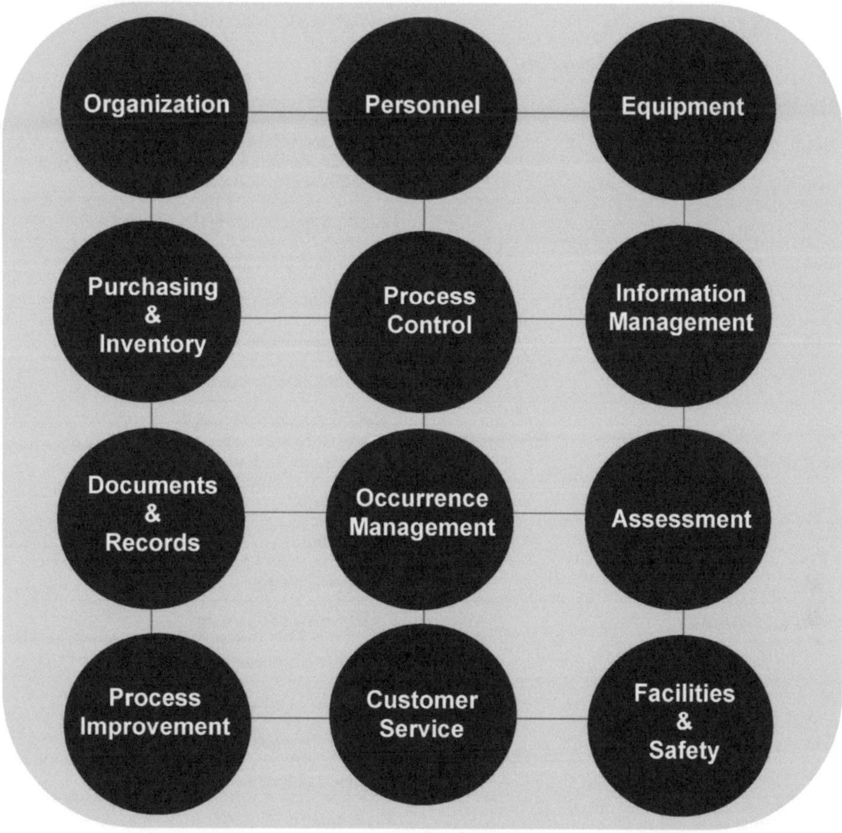

Figure 1.
Customer service is an essential inclusion in quality systems in the laboratory.

Patients satisfaction towards medical laboratory service is influenced by the quality of service and professionalism of the staff, provision of adequate information to collect sample and when and how to receive laboratory results, waiting time to receive laboratory results, availability of ordered laboratory tests, cleanness of the laboratory and accessibility of latrines [9].

Patients' satisfaction is core to quality of health and medical laboratory quality essential (**Figure 1**). It is always meaningless when it does not satisfy its users and clients. Measuring patients satisfaction plays an important role in the growing push towards healthcare, provide accountability and is critical in the implementation of continues improvement in medical settings. Patients satisfaction often reflect their perception of the healthcare offered as well as the process of giving that care compared to their expectations. In the laboratory, the connection between health service of quality and naturally experiencing quality leads to customer satisfaction. The customer satisfaction leads to the experiencing quality and experiencing quality also leads to customer satisfaction [12–14].

3. Discovering clients as the king in medical laboratory practice

The universal saying that the client (customer) is the king is also applicable in medical laboratory science. The clients in the medical laboratory practice are the pioneer of all work that are been carried out in the laboratory.

Medical laboratories found in	Possible customers (clients)
Hospital (Tertiary, Secondary/Specialist)	Physicians
	Other healthcare professionals
	Patients and relatives
	Hospital facility and management
	Community inhabiting the hospital
Primary Health Care (PHC)	Community healthcare workers
	Other healthcare professionals
	Patients and relatives
	PHCs and management
	Community and her people
Public health	Public health professionals
	General public
	Government
	Interested groups
Healthcare Industries	Healthcare professionals
	Industry and management
	Community and the people
Other Industries	Industry and staff
	Product customers
Private Medical Laboratories	Physicians
	Other healthcare professionals
	Patients and relatives
	Laboratory facility and management
	Community inhabiting the laboratory
	Medical laboratory regulating bodies
	Medical laboratory professional Associations

Table 1.
Categories of medical laboratories and possible customers (clients).

There is an increase attention to the clause "customer is the king" which relates the companies and their customer market. This new era of world economy globalization presents customers and the public as having the ears of the sellers based on the ability to choose, intervene and cause changes and improvement through buying power and definitions of necessities in the offers made by various companies and their marketers [15].

The emphasis on customer is the king is on satisfaction and a major reason of companies (health facility) existence. While the want of customers of interest to companies, marketing strategies should not be neglected even in the healthcare arena. Though customers may indicate what they want at any point, a time will come when there would be a need for new things and no wonder there is shape, design and size change by good marketing companies and this can be adopted in healthcare services especially in medical laboratories in other to satisfy their customers [16].

The increase in the buying experience is largely dependent on how the customers are being treated. That is why the failure to make transaction is majorly based on poor quality customer service. The existing customers are majorly the king as the patronage continues excellently than have new customers. The customer is the king when all the services needed are met and improved upon to suit every condition and time. No wonder some products are modified after a while in companies and marketing areas. This is not excluded from medical laboratory services, ranging from how services are being rendered to all the facility components that needs renovation and improvement from time to time [15].

The standard at which the healthcare provider and the customer ensure the laboratory function in a valuable way for their needs to be served. Clients in the medical laboratory practice expects that all works are done accurately and perfectly. The healthcare system does not function without the clients as the main trust or target for the work.

The customer is the king in medical laboratory services based on what the various categories of customers (**Table 1**) can get from such facility at any time of patronage.

4. Categories of medical laboratory clients and customers

The laboratory has several clients otherwise called customers that expects much from the medical laboratory [17].

For the sake of this chapter, the customers shall be classified into five (5) as their expectations are shown in **Table 2**.

i. Patients and patients' relatives: Patients are individuals that are registered to receive medical treatment in any healthcare facility or hospital. The patient accesses healthcare and makes payment where necessary. The patient relatives are equally family members, friends and well-wishers that accompany or stays with the patients during the time of accessing healthcare. The laboratory services rendered to the patients can be better explained by patients or their relatives thereby exploring the satisfaction levels.

ii. Physician and other healthcare providers/workers: Physicians or clinicians and other healthcare workers are customers because they request medical laboratory services for their patients for better clinical management. They may be satisfied or dissatisfied in such services based on the patients' response to treatment.

iii. The Communities and interested parties: The communities patronize facilities closer to them. They are the immediate subjects and patients depending on the degree of medical laboratory services required. The community and interested parties equally expects a low risk environment that may be used by the laboratory facilities. Satisfaction is necessary for them to continue to patronize and advertise the facility to others for such medical laboratory services.

iv. Public health and government: Then medical laboratory testing is mostly carried out to meet the public health need of a people thereby making government, public health officials or workers become customers/clients of the laboratory. There is no doubt that the medical laboratory service is a critical partner in disease surveillance, detection and prevention, and in other public health issues. Medical laboratory services must meet the needs of the public health workers in addressing any public health problems. The information gotten from the laboratory is germane to public health safety of which there must be satisfaction in all cases to ensue improvement.

Customers	Expectations
Physicians	Good request/result forms
	Short turnaround time to get result
	Quality result towards patient improvement
Other healthcare professionals (Medical laboratory Scientists, Nurses, Pharmacists, Community health workers, etc.)	As Above
Patients and patients relatives	Quality result
	Short turnaround time
	Health status discovery
	Good laboratory environment
	Humane and collaborative care from laboratory staff
	Less painful experience
Public health and government	Discovery of disease outbreaks and possible recommendations for eradication
	Provision of good result to the public and interested professionals
Community and interested parties	Quality results
	Good turnaround time
	Clean and hazard free environment
	Proximity and excellent practice
Medical laboratory profession	Quality results for confidence in professional services
	Respect from other customers due to service quality
	Community awareness and hazard free service delivery

Table 2.
Categories of customers and their expectations from medical laboratories.

v. The medical laboratory profession: The medical laboratory profession is also a client in the sense that the regulatory body like medical laboratory science council of Nigeria (MLSCN) or the professional body like association of medical laboratory scientists of Nigeria (AMLSN) gets satisfied with medical laboratory services based on quality results released by qualified professionals from various medical laboratory facilities. This is because, the quality results released to the clients provides satisfaction to the patients and to the profession. This generally promotes the profession among others.

5. Quality standards that dwell on patient satisfaction towards improvement

Philip Crosby defined quality practice as meeting the requirements of the customer. He applied this practice to business and manufacturing, but it is equally important for a medical laboratory. The medical laboratory needs to know who its clients are, and understands clients need and requirements [17].

The laboratory must produce the a product and a test result for its customers, if the customer is not given the ultimate care and is not well served as needed, then the laboratory is not achieving the primary goal.

Customers' satisfaction is a major component which dwell on quality management system [18–21], and a significant focus in the international organization for standardization (ISO).

Laboratory staff should understand the importance of customer satisfaction, and should interact with the customers in an appropriate way and giving information that is needed, and being courteous [22].

Implementing some of the standards [1, 23–25] as medical laboratory quality initiatives with regards to the laboratory customers [26–28] provides both laboratory and business benefits such as:

i. More customers' patronage for testing and/or calibration.

ii. Providing opportunity for accreditation which builds confidence to the public clients towards patronage

iii. There is improved community, state, national and global reputation and as well protects the image of medical laboratory

iv. Continuous data quality improvement and effectiveness of medical laboratory

v. Forming the basis for quality systems of medical laboratories like good medical laboratory practices.

6. The customer focused services in line with quality standards ISO 17025, ISO 15189 and ISO 9001 in medical laboratories

Some of the customer focused services as noted [1, 23, 24] are:

- The laboratory should communicate with customers to clarify requests and get customer input.
- The laboratory should have a formal program to collect feedback from customers on an ongoing basis.
- The laboratory should allow customers to audit the laboratory.
- There should be a policy and procedure for the resolution of complaints received from customers.
- Records of complaints and all steps taken when resolving the complaint should be maintained. This includes documentation of investigations and corrective actions.
- If necessary, customers should be notified nonconforming testing and corrective actions.
- Audit findings related to the quality of test and calibration results should be reported to customers.
- Customer complaints and suggestions should be part of management reviews.

7. Medical laboratory clients and patients survey instruments

The medical laboratory service clients/patients' survey should address pertinent satisfaction and quality issues [29, 30] as presented in the **Table 3** below.

SN	Dimension	Definition	Review codes
1	Medical laboratory service effectiveness and outcomes	The extent to which medical laboratory services are qualitative and services produce positive outcomes in patients including effectiveness and competence of providers.	• Evidence of quality diagnosis and revealing the status of the patient • Evidence of effective /ineffective practice • Evidence of competence/incompetence of staff • Access to all laboratory services
2	Access to medical laboratory services	The extent to which patients are able to access required laboratory services when needed including waiting times, patients' ability to find out about, get referred to and physically get to services, accessibility to all, and the range of services provided.	• Physical access; locations and parking spaces; • Responsiveness; waiting times and lists • Service without boundary • Range of services in the laboratory available
3	Medical laboratory organization of care	The extent to which users move smoothly between the necessary service departments or units throughout the medical laboratory services including pay points with adequate coordination, appropriate education and communication about quality service transition and continuity.	• Experience of humane and informed consent episode • Experience of sample collection and diagnosis care episode • Experience of turnaround time episode
4	Humanity of care	The extent to which clients are treated with dignity and respect including the provision of emotional support, alleviation of fear and anxiety, the provision of information and appropriate communication about the service.	• Privacy and confidentiality • Patient involvement to reduce pain • Promoting wellbeing • Delivery of diagnosis; respect and dignity; staff attitudes
5	Environment	The extent to which the physical setting within which laboratory services are rendered as safe, comfortable and appropriate to diagnostic needs and the clients.	Physical state of facilities such as rest rooms and waiting room

Table 3.
Client dimension of experience, definitions and director medical laboratory service review codes.

7.1 Preparation and examples

In preparation of medical laboratory service survey instrument, there is need to have a background of the client of interest. Patients and patients' relatives, Physicians and healthcare providers, public health and government, communities and interested parties and medical laboratory professionals as the client of interest give the picture of the adequate demographics and question content necessary at any time of survey. Equally, the survey may be prepared in three, four or five likert scale as may be structured by the auditor or the investigator. It shall be prepared to the standard and language the participant shall understand. Example of such survey is for the patient visiting a diagnostic centre in Jos (Template of Customer survey instrument) as seen below with three likert scale.

7.2 Administration of survey tools

The status of the medical laboratory service provider and her clients determines the way the survey tool can be administered. The survey tool can be administered in hard or soft copies to customers of a laboratory facility that is interested in the assessment. Hard copies can be given to customers after services delivery before departure from the facility while soft copies or online survey using survey monkey for instance or soft copies can be shared to clients via e-mails or social media such as Whatsapp, Twitter, facebook, etc. for convenience.

7.3 Data analysis

Data analysis of medical laboratory services survey of customers can be analyzed by the assessor or auditor or quality officer in charge. The analysis may be in percentages, means or use of SPSS or other statistical tools. This may involve the services of a statistician.

7.4 Implementation of findings from the patients

Having carried out the medical laboratory customers/patients' survey, implementation is very important by the quality officer or the human resources manager or Director, medical laboratory services. Any attempt to disregard patients' feedback may cause persistent disruption of testing because by the patient in the case of repeated visits. If not well handled, patients' medical laboratory experience can turn them off from allowing the physician to send them to the same laboratory and in turn makes the physician or other healthcare workers to stop or reduce referring of patients. The survey gives patients/customers a voice, about their needs and expectations and equally aids improvement.

The implementation of findings may be in the positive or negative depending on the variable involved. Oja et al. [30] puts it that "Customer satisfaction surveys cannot result in quality improvement, if proper corrective actions are not carried out".

8. Template of customer survey instrument

The template may be for patients alone, patients and patients' relatives, physicians and or other healthcare workers, public health experts or a combination of all medical laboratory customers. For this chapter, the template below (consent form and questionnaire) is for only the patients.

CONSENT FORM AND QUESTIONNAIRE

Etukudoh N.S. and Obeta M.U., of the Federal School of Medical Laboratory Technology (Science), Jos., would like to assess your satisfaction with the "**Federal School Diagnostic Centre**" so as to create a room for satisfaction and improvement in the services.

The survey will involve giving you a questionnaire to answer your choice in options provided or make comment where necessary. You are free to participate in this survey but if you decide not to, there is no penalty attached and this study will not in any way affect the outcome of your visit to the establishment or result for the test you requested.

All information filled in the questionnaire will be kept strictly confidential and your identity will not be disclosed.

If you accept to participate in the study, kindly sign in the space provided below;

Thank you.

Signature of participant/Date ....

Signature of investigator/Date ....

Instructions for the Questionnaire.

Filling the Questionnaire: The questionnaire takes within 5–15 minutes.

TICK your option box [√] or all that applies to you based on given options. Be frank and honest. Please answer every item. Give a true picture possibly with presentation of any available evidence.

Contact person: Please for any question, contact the assessor via 08039664892.

Thank you for participating.

Part 1. Demographics.

Age (Yrs): [≤20] [21–30] [31–40] [41–50] [51–60] [≥61].

Sex: [male] [female].

Marital status: [single] [married] [divorced] [widow/widower].

Education: [no form of school] [primary] [secondary] [polytechnic] [university].

Occupation: [farmer] [business] [private] [public] [others].

Residence: [rural] [urban].

Number of visits: [1st] [2nd] [3rd] [more than 3].

Distance to facility: [≤ 30 mins] [31–60 mins] [61–90 mins] [≥90 mins].

Part 2. Patients' Satisfaction Validated Constructs.

SN	Variables	Agree	Undecided	Disagree
Medical laboratory service effectiveness and outcomes				
1.	General satisfaction by the medical laboratory service			
2.	Improvement of laboratory service from time to time			
3.	Welcoming approach/friendliness/ competence of staff			
4.	Laboratory personnel's professional appearances (neatness, professional dressing)			
5.	Respect and courtesy of the staff			
6.	Availability of requested laboratory tests			

SN	Variables	Agree	Undecided	Disagree
Access to medical laboratory services				
7.	Location of cashier office and proximity to laboratory			
8.	Availability of laboratory staff on working hours			
9.	Waiting time for specimen collection			
10.	The cost of the laboratory service			
11.	Cleanliness of the facility			
12.	Location of rest rooms			
Medical laboratory organization of care				
13.	Test results received on time as told/not missing			
14.	Information given before specimen collection outside the laboratory room			
15.	Completeness of information on how and when to receive laboratory results			
16.	Ability of person drawing blood to put client at ease			
17.	Bruise development after phlebotomy procedures			
18.	Number of needle stick attempts			
Humanity of care				
19.	Maintaining privacy and confidentiality			
20.	Ability of the laboratory personnel to answer questions			
21.	Application of informed consent			
Environment				
22.	Availability of place in the blood drawing room to put personal things			
23.	Adequacy of sitting arrangement in waiting room			
24.	Problem of overcrowding			
25.	Cleanness and comfort of waiting room			
26.	Cleanliness of the blood drawing area			
27.	Latrine accessibility and availability			
28.	Latrine cleanness and comfort			

9. Proffering a way for patients/clients satisfaction in Nigerian medical laboratory administration

Patients and patients' relatives, Physicians and healthcare providers, public health and government, communities and interested parties and medical laboratory profession in general needs satisfaction from medical laboratory services. Such satisfied services needs team work among all healthcare workers [31, 32] including patients [33, 34]. In Nigeria for instance, the following could improve customers' satisfaction:

a. Ensuring high levels of satisfaction among the team members and customers on delivery of health services.

b. Improving communication in the provision of healthcare services while interacting with patients and caregivers.

c. Improving communication and partnership among all health providers and patients.

d. Improved response processes in addressing issues in determination of healthcare of client based on survey outcomes.

e. Ensuring clarity of the roles of all health providers working with the patients/clients.

f. Patients are less likely to receive the best possible care if medical laboratory services are not of high quality.

g. Minimizing guess work in healthcare management, rather address quality issues and use medical laboratory services in all health cases.

h. Address leadership challenges in health sector, especially towards using health administrators and human resource managers.

i. Address labour crisis and incessant strikes.

j. Equip, quality control and maintain medical laboratory installations.

k. Government should address cost implications of medical laboratory services and if possible create subsidy packages for public health laboratory services just as it is done for COVID-19 testing across the world, Nigeria inclusive.

10. Conclusion

Medical laboratory clients ranging from patients and patients' relations, physicians and other healthcare workers, public health and government, communities and interested parties, and medical laboratory profession deserves satisfaction and quality improvement. Such customer service and satisfaction should be in line with the ISO 15189, ISO 17075 and ISO 9001. There is a need to administer services satisfaction survey to customers/clients from time to time so the outcome can be used to correct services errors and cause quality improvement. In healthcare, satisfaction of patients (customers/clients) in medical laboratory services actually contributes to health and quality improvement and this should be sustained.

Acknowledgements

The authors wish to acknowledge MLT Ibrahim Asiya for initial assistance in the typing of the manuscript.

Conflict of interest

The authors declare no competing interests.

Notes/thanks/other declarations

Obeta M. Uchejeso conceptualized the Chapter, Both authors contributed equally in the chapter preparation, editing and approved the final manuscript for submission.

Author details

Nkereuwem S. Etukudoh and Uchejeso M. Obeta*
Federal School of Medical Laboratory Science, Jos, Nigeria

*Address all correspondence to: uchejesoobeta@gmail.com

References

[1] ISO (2003) Medical laboratories—Particular requirements for quality and competence. ISO 15189.

[2] Obeta MU, Maduka KM, Bassey IO, and Mary-Jane ON. (2019). Improving quality and cost diminution in modern health care delivery: The role of medical laboratory scientists in Nigeria. International journal of business and management invention. 8(8-19).

[3] WHO (2013). Exploring Patient Participation in Reducing Health-Care-Related Safety Risks. WHO Europe.

[4] Fondoh VN, Awasom CN, Enow-Tanjong R, Richard M. Fondoh RM, Njukeng P, Shang J, Ndasi J, Samje M, Muluh CN, Kinge TN. (2020). Evaluation of corrective actions of feedback from clinicians on clinical Laboratory Services at Bamenda Regional Hospital Laboratory, Cameroon. Afr J Lab Med. 2020;9(1), a843. DOI:10.4102/ajlm.v9i1.843

[5] Obeta MU, Udenze C, Goyin LP, and Ojo J. (2019). Assessment of job satisfaction indices among health professionals in Jos University teaching hospital: An analytical study. Journal of Business and management. 21(38-50).

[6] Almatrafi D, Altaweel N, Abdelfattah M, Alomari A, Yaseen W, Alsulami M, Abonaji F, Alqazlan M, Darrar H. (2018). Assessment of customer satisfaction with the clinical laboratory services provided in king Abdullah Medical City, Makkah. The Egyptian Journal of Hospital Medicine. 70 (11), 2029-2037. DOI:10.12816/0044864

[7] Bamidele AR, Hoque ME, and Van der Heever H. (2011). Patients satisfaction and factor of importance in primary health care services in Botswana. Afr. J. Biomed Res. 14(1-7).

[8] Lochoro P. (2004). Measuring patient satisfaction in Uganda Catholic medical bureau health institutions. Health Policy and Development; 2 (3) 243-248.

[9] Alelign A, Belay YA. (2019). Patient satisfaction with clinical laboratory services and associated factors among adult patients attending outpatient departments at Debre Markos referral hospital, Northwest Ethiopia. BMC Res Notes (2019) 12:517. DOI:10.1186/s13104-019-4558-8

[10] Olusina AK, Ohaeri JU, Olatawura MO. (2002). Patient and staff satisfaction with the quality of in-patient psychiatric care in a Nigerian general hospital. Soc Psychiatry Psychiatr Epidemiol 37: 283-288 DOI:10.1007/s00127-002-0548-5

[11] Briggs J and Tang C. (2011). Teaching for Quality Learning at University. Maidenhead, UK: Open University Press

[12] Teresa M, Bekele S. (2016). Assessment of patients' satisfaction towards general medical Laboratory Services at Shenen Gibe Public Hospital, Jimma town, south West Ethiopia. Journal of Health, Medicine and Nursing 31; www.iiste.org

[13] Georgieva E, Tsankova G, Kaludova V, Ermenlieva N. (2014). Patients' satisfaction with Laboratory Services at Selected Medical – Diagnostic Laboratories in Varna. Journal of IMAB – Annual Proceeding (Scientific Papers), 20(2) DOI:10.5272/jimab.2014202.500

[14] Harnet MJP, Correll DJ, Hurwitz S, Bader AM, Hepner DL. (2010). Improving efficiency and patient satisfaction in a tertiary teaching hospital preoperative clinic. Anesthesiology 2010; 112:66-72

[15] Craven R.(nd). Customer is the King; How to exceed expectations. Warwick, The High Street, Bath, BA1 8AR www.Robert-craven.com

[16] Vieira FGD (2004). The 'Customer as King' as a Myth in the Brazilian Market: Description and Analysis of Situations. Revista de Práticas Administrativas, 1(1), 69-76, 2004. ISSN 1807-1147

[17] WHO (2011): Laboratory quality management system.

[18] Emilia G, Gabriela T, Violina K, and Neli E. (2014). Patients satisfaction with laboratory services at selected medical diagnostic laboratories in Varna. Journal of IMAB. Vol. 20.

[19] Kinkus CA. (2012). Laboratory Management; Quality in Laboratory Diagnosis. Demos Medical Publishing, LLC New York.

[20] Abera RG, Abota BA, Legese MH, Negesso AE. (2017). Patient satisfaction with clinical laboratory services at Tikur Anbessa specialized hospital, Addis Ababa, Ethiopia. Patient Preference and Adherence 2017:11 1181-1188.

[21] Harnett M, Daren JC, Shelley H, Angela MB, and Hepner DL. (2009). Improving efficiency and patients satisfaction in a tertiary teaching hospital preoperative clinic. American society of anesthesiologists. 112:66-72′

[22] Rodas GA, Boaz AA, Melese HL, and Edao AN. (2017). Patients' Satisfaction with Clinical Services at Tikur Anbessa Specialized Hospital, Addis Ababa, Ethiopia. Dove press journal.

[23] Huber L. (n.d). Understanding and Implementing ISO/IEC 17025; A Primer

[24] Schneider F, Maurer C, Friedberg RC. (2017). International organization for standardization (ISO) 15189. Ann Lab Med; 37:365-370 DOI:10.3343/alm.2017.37.5.365

[25] Jocelyn CJ, Ward C, Thorndike A, Donelan K, Wexler DJ. (2020). Social factors and patient perceptions associated with preventable hospital readmissions. Journal of Patient Experience. 7(1) 19-26. DOI:10.1177/2374373518825143

[26] Paula K, Timo K, and Arto P. (2010). Health centers' view of the services provided by a university hospital laboratory: Use of satisfaction survey. Scandalinavian Journal of primary health care. 28(24-28)

[27] Koh YR, Kim SY, Kim IS, Chang CL, Lee EY, Son HC, Kim HH. (2014). Customer satisfaction survey with clinical laboratory and phlebotomy Services at a Tertiary Care Unit Level. Ann Lab Med; 34:380-385. DOI:10.3343/alm.2014.34.5.380

[28] Guo S, Duan Y, Liu X, Jiang Y. (2017). Three-year customer satisfaction survey in laboratory medicine in a Chinese university hospital. Clin Chem Lab Med. DOI:10.1515/cclm-2017-0787.

[29] Hailu HA, Desale A, Yalew A, Asrat H, Kebede S, Dejene D, Abebe H, Gashu A, Yenealem D, Moges B, Yemanebrhane Y, Melese D, Gurmessa A, Mohammed A, Getu Z, Ayana G, Kebede A, Abate E. (2020). Patients' satisfaction with clinical Laboratory Services in Public Hospitals in Ethiopia. BMC Health Services Research. 20:13. DOI:10.1186/s12913-019-4880-9

[30] Oja P, Kouri T, Pakarinen A. (2010). Health centres' view of the services provided by a university hospital laboratory: Use of satisfaction surveys. Scandinavian Journal of Primary Health Care, 2010; 28: 24-28. DOI:10.3109/02813431003672594

[31] Obeta MU, Etukudoh NS, Mantu EC. and Ime DM. (2020). Challenges of Inter Professional Teamwork in Nigerian Healthcare. DOI:10.5772/intechopen.95414

[32] Obeta MU, Etukudoh NS, Udenze C, and Eze ME. (2020). Inter professional teamwork in public organisations, a paradigm shift to crisis in Nigerian hospitals. London journal of medical and health research, vol. 20.

[33] Ashdown LC. (2020). Patient: A tool to assist in creating a patient-Centered team approach to health-care delivery: Lessons from a physician patient. Journal of Patient Experience. 7(1) 16-18. DOI:10.1177/2374373518812048

[34] Consumer protection council CPC, Federal Ministry of Health, Patients' bill of health.

Chapter 16

The Modern Universal Total Knee Arthroplasty: Maximized Value, Streamlined Efficiency

Bryant Bonner, Jesua I. Law, Erin Hofmann and Eric Dacus

Abstract

A universal total knee arthroplasty system able to accurately resurface either left or right knees of all shapes and sizes is compelling as there is an increased need for improved efficiency and value. With a modern universal total knee system, a single instrument tray can be utilized for more than 90% of cases and doesn't require any specific customization or disposable instruments. This streamlined workflow is accomplished with unique instrumentation that features a symmetrical femoral and tibial implant for all patients. Symmetrical tibial implants have been shown to have equivalent outcomes and low complications compared to asymmetric tibial trays. The universal symmetrical femoral implant, with its deepened trochlear groove, allows for optimal patellar tracking and recent studies have demonstrated this symmetrical femoral implant to have comparable femoral rollback and axial rotation to native knees. This efficient instrumentation reduces overall inventory, decreases turnover times, and exposes fewer instruments that may otherwise be susceptible to contamination. All without detriment to the patient outcome or surgeon workflow. Studies have shown clinical scores of the modern universal total knee arthroplasty system are a great value not only to the surgeon but also to the healthcare system as a whole—a necessity in modern healthcare.

Keywords: total knee arthroplasty, universal total knee, symmetrical component, efficient design, economics

1. Introduction

Total knee arthroplasty (TKA) is one of the most successful elective surgical procedures available [1], allowing for the treatment of end-stage osteoarthritis and functional limitation to restore patient mobility and functional activity. Recent reports project that elective joint replacement surgery will be the most common surgical procedure over the next 10 years [2, 3], and the number of TKAs performed in the United States (US) is estimated to increase exponentially—approximately 401% by 2040 compared to the 2014 US National Implant Services (NIS) database [4]. Meanwhile, according to the Centers for Medicare and Medicaid, healthcare expenditures are projected to grow at a rate of 5.8% per year [5] with a significant number of hospital costs being derived from operating room expenses [6]. Consequently, there is a push to maximize efficiency, including streamlining operating room flow (set up, surgical time, turnaround time) while reducing cost and risks of infection. This improved efficiency must come without sacrificing patient outcomes in an effort to rein in ballooning healthcare costs. In this chapter, we will highlight the significance of a modern universal total knee arthroplasty system in helping to simplify the OR and save on healthcare expenditures.

2. Design history

Total knee arthroplasty has evolved significantly since its first inception in the late 19th and 20th centuries; implant designs have improved and advances in surgical tools have born less invasive techniques. Originally, the first arthroplasty was conceived as a simple resection arthroplasty in the 1860s. Excess bone was removed to improve motion, but this was limited by the recurrence of bone formation, at times, knee fusion and this arthroplasty often lead to instability if too much bone was removed [7]. This technique evolved to interposition arthroplasty, by which the insertion of soft tissue was used to reconstruct the joint surface and help prevent bone formation; this method was abandoned due to continued pain and failure of the interposition [8]. The hinged prosthesis of the 1950s was the first to replace the femoral and tibial surfaces, and patients experienced significant pain relief. Unfortunately, these linked prostheses were unable to replace complex knee kinematics and had high failure rates due to early loosening from stress shielding [9]. The 1970s saw the evolution of the condylar TKA prosthesis from Ranawat, Coventry, and Townley, which set the foundation of the less constrained and more anatomic modern implants of today [10–12].

Initially designed with a symmetrical femoral component, these condylar implant systems offered pain relief but featured a shallow, straight trochlear groove, and struggled to replicate natural patellar tracking. The 1980s brought a shift to an asymmetric, side-specific design [13] to better match the normal bony anatomy

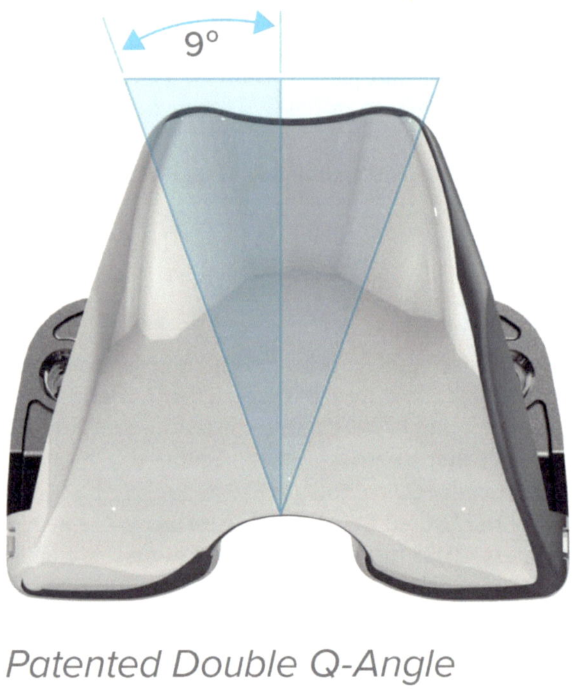

Figure 1.
Total Joint Orthopedics, Inc.'s (TJO) Klassic® Femur featuring a 9° double Q-angle to optimize patellofemoral tracking for both left and right-sided anatomy.

of the distal femur of a patient and thus improve knee kinematics [13]. Multiple studies have failed to show any significant difference in knee clinical or functional scores in patients with a modern universal femoral component when compared to those with asymmetrical femoral design [14–17].

While the symmetrical femoral component fell out of favor due to patello-femoral complications that were encountered during the design evolution, such as poor tracking and dislocation, these issues have since been corrected with modern universal designs [13]. For example, one implant company, Total Joint Orthopedics, Inc.'s (TJO) patented Klassic Femur has a unique deepened anatomical trochlear groove, allowing for optimal patellar tracking along a 9° double Q-angle for both left and right-sided knees while still retaining a neutral outside profile of the anterior flange and restoring native kinematics (**Figure 1**) [18, 19].

3. Design and rationale

There are a number of ways surgeons can address surgical techniques to help improve efficiency, including, but not limited to, patient-specific instrumentation, navigation assistance, and type of implant. A universal knee system is one way to help improve efficiency and reduce operating room costs. This system optimizes efficiency in a number of ways, one of which involves the implant design itself, which allows the surgeon to utilize the same system for the majority of primary TKA, but also allows the flexibility to progress from a cruciate-retaining primary TKA to a maximally stabilized revision TKA with the same family of instrumentation.

The femur is designed with a specific trochlear groove to accommodate patellar tracking for both left and right knee anatomy. This trochlear groove design is based on the quadriceps, or Q-angle, which describes the vector of the pull of the quadriceps on the patella and is fashioned so that its angle allows for optimal tracking for both left and right knees. Moreover, the universal knee system femur is designed to be compatible with a variety of polyethylene inserts, such as cruciate-retaining (CR); posterior cruciate ligament (PCL) sacrificing (PS) in both a posted posterior-stabilized, or ultra-congruent (UC), with a raised anterior lip for cruciate stabilization; and a varus/valgus constrained; polyethylene inserts, offering a full evolution of stability with one implant and instrumentation system. This alone significantly reduces the number of instruments and implants that must be shipped, sterilized, and stored at the hospital or surgical center. Because the system was designed holistically, cuts, peg locations, and trialing are standardized throughout the workflow, eliminating time-consuming steps when alternative sizing or additional stability is required. For example, a more constrained femoral trial can be utilized before making any further cuts to assess the need for a more constrained polyethylene insert.

The symmetrical tibial baseplate is optimized to fit both right and left proximal tibias using a potbellied design. Throughout development, design surgeons traced native tibial resections during routine TKA, and this gradual anterior bump optimizes fit in most patient anatomy. A plethora of studies have examined the universal tibial design, which suggests there is improved tibial coverage, improved external rotation, and decreased risk for overstuffing components [20, 21]. Additionally, consistent polyethylene thickness to the peripheral edges and matching conforming geometry of the baseplate and polyethylene insert optimize congruency, offering exceptional mid-flexion stability [19]. All baseplates, whether cemented or cementless, offer modularity so that they can accommodate a stem extension in either a primary or revision setting. Studies have shown that stemmed tibial components offer enhanced fixation and additional stability, and improve outcomes in heavier patients [22, 23].

In addition to the components, the instruments and number of trays utilized during the case can also significantly affect efficiency and cost. A majority of the instruments in the tray have multiple functions and are utilized at different times throughout the case. This universal knee system design allows up to 90% of cases, regardless of a workflow (e.g., gap balancing or measured resection technique), to be completed with a single tray of instruments; revision cases require one or two additional trays depending on the level of stability needed (**Figure 2**).

This significant optimization in the number of required instrumentation results in a reduced amount of inventory needed for a TKA which can help improve surgeon and hospital efficiency as well as reduce costs. A recent Harvard Business School study demonstrated that hospitals often underestimate the costs of idle space and equipment resulting in errors in utilization [24].

By reducing the number of trays, studies have also demonstrated that surgeons are able to reduce OR time and sterilization costs, the incidence of infection as well as optimize efficiency and ergonomics [25, 26]. Fewer instrument trays require less time to set up and break down and need less space and time to sterilize. Moreover, with respect to cleaning and sterilization, fewer instruments mean that there is less total exposed instrumentation surface area that is susceptible to contamination. Additional studies have also confirmed that the decreased inventory and instrumentation do not adversely affect patient outcomes but may actually improve them [26].

Studies in Europe have analyzed the cost of sterilizing and packaging reusable instruments somewhere between $0.59 and $11.52 (USD) per surgical instrument [27–29]. If a surgeon is able to reduce the number of instrument trays the savings could be huge, with one study looking at a reduction from 7.5 trays in a TKA to three trays. This reduction led to an estimated annual savings of $159,600 in sterilization costs and $99,000 in improved turnover times [30]. Each tray costs between $60 and $150 dollars to sterilize, and each tray averages 2 minutes to open onto the

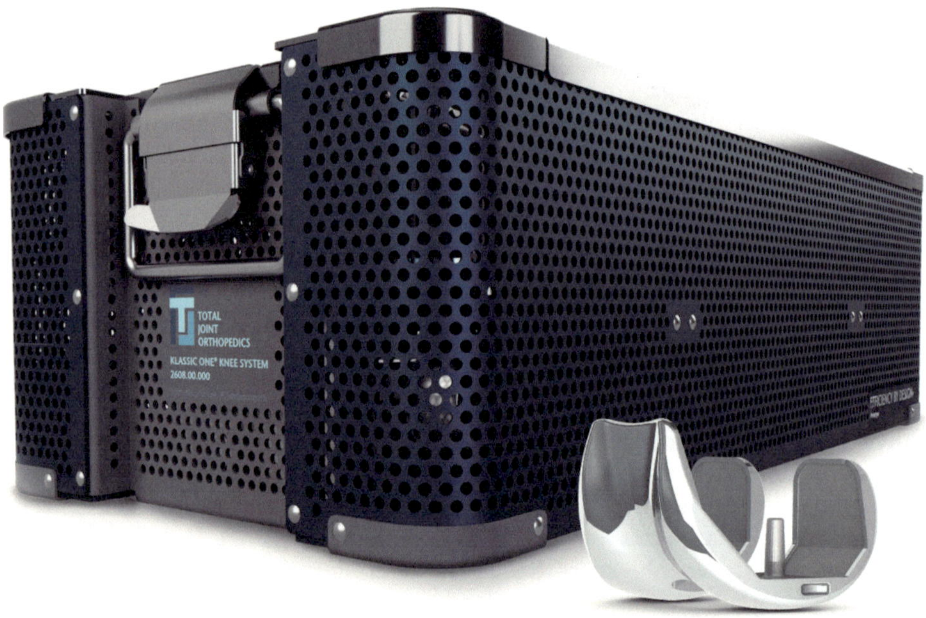

Figure 2.
With a modern universal total knee system, a single standard instrument tray may be used for up to 90% of primary total knee arthroplasty while following AORN guidelines to weigh less than 25 lbs. A second tray is offered for micro/macro trials, allowing a primary TKA to be performed with two trays or fewer 10% of the time. TJO's Klassic ONE® Knee System single instrumentation tray is featured as an example here.

sterile field; some systems have estimated a cost savings of up to $1350 per case compared to a typical eight tray implant system [1, 25, 26, 31, 32]. As a result, there is a significant opportunity to improve value through reducing and making hospital inventory more efficient.

4. Conclusion

Total knee arthroplasty remains one of the most successful elective operations and the number of cases is only expected to increase in the years ahead. Originally conceived as simple resection arthroplasty, total knee arthroplasty has seen many iterations through failures and redesigns to reach the condylar implant designs of today, however, the field remains hungry for further innovation in order to meet the anticipated demand of the future. One such method to maximize efficiency and reduce costs, while maintaining or improving patient outcomes, is the use of a modern universal total knee arthroplasty system.

Universal symmetrical tibial baseplates are already commonplace in many modern implant systems, with recent studies demonstrating the decreased inventory and instrumentation does not adversely affect patient outcomes, but it is the modern design of the universal femoral component that is especially intriguing. While there have been concerns in the past with patellofemoral tracking issues, the modern designs, such as those from Total Joint Orthopedics, Inc. (TJO), feature a patented trochlear groove allowing for optimal patellar tracking along a 9° double Q-angle for both left and right anatomy [18]. Furthermore, a modern universal total knee system features a reduced total number of instruments needed as the system is holistically designed using standardized connections and multi-use instruments. These innovations require less instrumentation for each TKA without sacrificing crucial steps or surgeon workflow, which provides significant cost savings, improvement in operating room efficiency, and a decreased infection risk. Fewer instrumentation trays require less inventory space, allow for faster sterilization, the decreased time needed for setup and breakdown, and less exposed instrumentation surface area that is susceptible to contamination. With these factors combined, some studies estimate a potential cost savings of around $250,000 annually, and some system manufacturers estimate potential savings of $1350 per TKA case. While some may see this as a relic of the past, the updated modern design of the components and revamped instrumentation of these systems provide cost savings and efficiency that is a premium in healthcare today. A modern universal total knee arthroplasty system is a crucial asset in any surgical setting, like hospitals and ambulatory surgery centers alike seek to reduce costs as healthcare expenditures balloon and sterile processing and storage space become more limited.

Author details

Bryant Bonner[1*], Jesua I. Law[2], Erin Hofmann[3] and Eric Dacus[4]

1 Hofmann Arthritis Institute, Salt Lake City, UT, United States

2 Valley Orthopedic Bone and Joint, Modesto, CA, United States

3 Total Joint Orthopedics, Inc., Salt Lake City, UT, United States

4 Independent Contractor (former TJO employee), Salt Lake City, UT, United States

*Address all correspondence to: bryant.bonner@gmail.com

References

[1] Guo EW, Sayeed Z, Padela MT, Qazi M, Zekaj M, Schaefer P, et al. Improving total joint replacement with continuous quality improvement methods and tools. The Orthopedic Clinics of North America. 2018;**49**(4):397-403

[2] Kurtz SM, Lau E, Ong K, Zhao K, Kelly M, Bozic KJ. Future young patient demand for primary and revision joint replacement: National projections from 2010 to 2030. Clinical Orthopaedics and Related Research. 2009;**467**(10): 2606-2612

[3] Cram P, Lu X, Kates SL, Singh JA, Li Y, Wolf BR. Total knee arthroplasty volume, utilization, and outcomes among Medicare beneficiaries, 1991-2010. JAMA. 2012;**308**(12):1227-1236

[4] Singh JA et al. Rates of total joint replacement in the United States: Future projections to 2020-2040 using the national inpatient sample. The Journal of Rheumatology. 2019;**46**(9):1134-1140. DOI: 10.3899/jrheum.170990

[5] CMS. National Health Expenditure Projections 2015-2025. 2015. Available from: https://www.cms.gov/Research-Statistics-Data-and-Systems/StatisticsTrends-and-Reports/National HealthExpendData/index.html [Accessed: 19 April 2017]

[6] Weiss A, Hollandsworth HM, Alseidi A, Scovel L, French C, Derrick EL, et al. Environmentalism in surgical practice. Current Problems in Surgery. 2016;**53**(4):165-205

[7] Ferguson W. Excision of the knee joint: Recovery with a false joint and a useful limb. Medical Times and Gazette. 1861;**1**:601

[8] Verneuil A. De la creation d'une fausse articulation par section ou re' section partielle de l'os maxillairde infer'rier, comme moyen de re' medier a l'ankylose vrai ou fausse de la machoire inger'ieure. Archives of General Medicine. 1860;**15**(5):174

[9] Walldius B. Arthroplasty of the knee joint using an endoprosthesis. Acta Orthopaedica Scandinavica. Supplementum. 1957;**24**:1-112

[10] Ranawat CS, Insall J, Shine J. Duo-condylar knee arthroplasty: Hospital for special surgery design. Clinical Orthopaedics and Related Research. 1976;**120**:76-82

[11] Townley CO. The anatomic total knee resurfacing arthroplasty. Clinical Orthopaedics and Related Research. 1985;**192**:82-96

[12] Coventry MB, Finerman GA, Riley LH, Turner RH, Upshaw JE. A new geometric knee for total knee arthroplasty. Clinical Orthopaedics and Related Research. 1972;**83**:157-162

[13] Robinson RP. The early innovators of today's resurfacing condylar knees. The Journal of Arthroplasty. 2005;**20**: 2-26. DOI: 10.1016/j.arth.2004.11.002

[14] Ashraf T, Beard DJ, Newman JH. Symmetrical vs asymmetrical total knee replacement—A medium term comparative analysis. The Knee. 2003;**10**:61-66

[15] Bindelglass DF, Dorr LD. Current concepts review: Symmetry versus asymmetry in the design of total knee femoral components—An unresolved controversy. The Journal of Arthroplasty. 1998;**13**:939-944

[16] Worland RL, Jessup DE, Vazquez-Vela JG, Alemparte JA, Tanaka S, Rex FS, et al. The effect of femoral component rotation and asymmetry in total knee replacements. Orthopedics. 2002;**25**:1045-1048

[17] Barink M, Meijerink H, Verdonschot N, van Kampen A,

de Waal Malefijt M. Asymmetrical total knee arthroplasty does not improve patella tracking: A study without patella resurfacing. Knee Surgery, Sports Traumatology, Arthroscopy. 2007;**2**: 184-191

[18] Mangiapani DS, Schaeffer JF, Myers AR, Hofmann AA. Less valgus alignment in total knee arthroplasty for the varus knee. Seminars in Arthroplasty. 2018;**29**(1):36-41

[19] Khasian M, LaCour MT, Coomer SC, Bolognesi MP, Komistek RD. In vivo knee kinematics for a cruciate sacrificing total knee arthroplasty having both a symmetrical femoral and tibial component. The Journal of Arthroplasty. 2020;**35**:1712-1719

[20] Mandalia V, Eyres K, Schranz P, Toms AD. Evaluation of patients with a painful total knee replacement. Journal of Bone and Joint Surgery. British Volume (London). 2008;**90**(3):265-271

[21] Bonnin MP, Saffarini M, Shepherd D, Bossard N, Dantony E. Oversizing the tibial component in TKAs: Incidence, consequences and risk factors. Knee Surgery, Sports Traumatology, Arthroscopy. 2016; **24**(8):2532-2540

[22] Morwood MP, Guss AD, Law JI, Pelt CE. Metaphyseal stem extension improves tibial stability in cementless total knee arthroplasty. The Journal of Arthroplasty. 2020;**35**(10):3031-3037

[23] Parratte S, Ollivier M, Lunebourg A, Verdier N, Argenson JN. Do stemmed tibial components in total knee arthroplasty improve outcomes in patients with obesity? Clinical Orthopaedics and Related Research. 2017;**475**(1):137-145

[24] Kaplan R, Porter M. How to Not Cut Health Care Costs. Harvard Business Review; 2014. pp. 117-122. Available from: https://hbr.org/2014/11/how-not-to-cut-health-care-costs and https://hbr.org/archive-toc/BR1411

[25] Watters TS et al. Analysis of procedure-related costs and proposed benefits of using patient-specific approach in total knee arthroplasty. Journal of Surgical Orthopaedic Advances. 2011;**20**(2):112-116

[26] Maathuis PGM et al. Perioperative contamination in primary total hip arthroplasty. Clinical Orthopaedics and Related Research. 2005;**433**:136-139

[27] Adler S, Scherrer M, Ruckauer KD, Daschner FD. Comparison of economic and environmental impacts between disposable and reusable instruments used for laparoscopic cholecystectomy. Surgical Endoscopy. 2005;**19**:268-272

[28] Demoulin L, Kesteloot K, Penninckx F. A cost comparison of disposable vs reusable instruments in laparoscopic cholecystectomy. Surgical Endoscopy. 1996;**10**:520-525

[29] Prat F, Spieler JF, Paci S, et al. Reliability, cost-effectiveness, and safety of reuse of ancillary devices for ERCP. Gastrointestinal Endoscopy. 2004;**60**:246-252

[30] Capra R, Bini SA, Bowden DE, et al. Implementing a perioperative efficiency initiative for orthopedic surgery instrumentation at an academic center: A comparative before-and-after study. Medicine (Baltimore). 2019;**98**(7):1-7

[31] Mont MA, Johnson AJ, Issa K, Pivec R, Blasser KE, McQueen D, et al. Single-use instrumentation, cutting blocks, and trials decrease contamination during total knee arthroplasty: A prospective comparison of navigated and nonnavigated cases. The Journal of Knee Surgery. 2013;**26**(4):285-290

[32] Siegel GW, Patel NM, Milshteyn MA, et al. Cost analysis and surgical site infection rates in total knee arthroplasty comparing traditional vs. single-use instrumentation. The Journal of Arthroplasty. 2015;**30**(12):2271-2274

Chapter 17

Teva Pharmaceutical: Generic Market Access to Global Healthcare Industry

Neta Kela-Madar

Abstract

The present paper represents a qualitative case study on the pharmaceutical company Teva, including an in-depth exploration of the company within the specific context of pharmaceutical industry. Being a qualitative case study in the business discipline, the company details regarding the shareholders, the stock price fluctuations in recent decades in comparison with other competitors will be presented. The objective of this article is to provide a thorough description of Teva, a global leader in the pharmaceutical industry, by assessing the evolution of the company considering the changes at the corporate level and in the market, like the appearances of new competitors. The results will contribute in providing an insight in how future pharma companies can avoid certain pitfalls and how they should reply to the market competition and different other changes on the market.

Keywords: Pharmaceutical, market access, healthcare, global industry

1. Introduction

Teva Pharmaceutical Industries Ltd. is Israel's first and largest multinational, reaching a dominant position on the global level, in generic pharmaceuticals. Teva has humble beginnings. Established in 1901, it was created out of a family endowment, immigrant loads, and a modest early investment. By 1990, it was one of the most prominent pharmaceutical companies in the world [1]. Teva's global meteoric rise was largely due to the development and patent of COPAXONE®, a novel treatment for multiple sclerosis.

Teva Pharmaceutical Industries Ltd. was one of the first companies to produce generic drugs and now it is one of the largest pharmaceutical companies in the world, with 16,000 products related to generics, novel drugs, and over-the-counter medications. Teva had been active in 60 countries internationally and supplied drugs to 200 million people worldwide. Manufacturing, research, and marketing sites were largely located in Israel, North America, and Europe.

The company had staff strength of 60,000 people, of which 6,500 were based in Israel. Since 1976, Teva has had eight chief executive officers (**Figure 1**). The year 1976 was a turning point for the company as Teva, Zori, and Assia united to create Teva Pharmaceutical Industries Ltd. It was a period of consolidation for the business [2].

The pharma industry suffered significant transformations over the last decades and a thorough analysis of how these changes impacted Teva company are worthy

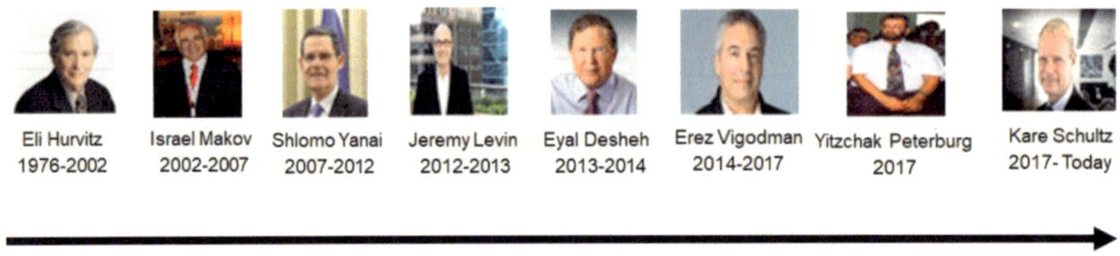
Eli Hurvitz
1976-2002
Israel Makov
2002-2007
Shlomo Yanai
2007-2012
Jeremy Levin
2012-2013
Eyal Desheh
2013-2014
Erez Vigodman
2014-2017
Yitzchak Peterburg
2017
Kare Schultz
2017- Today

Figure 1.
Teva C.E.O.s since 1976.

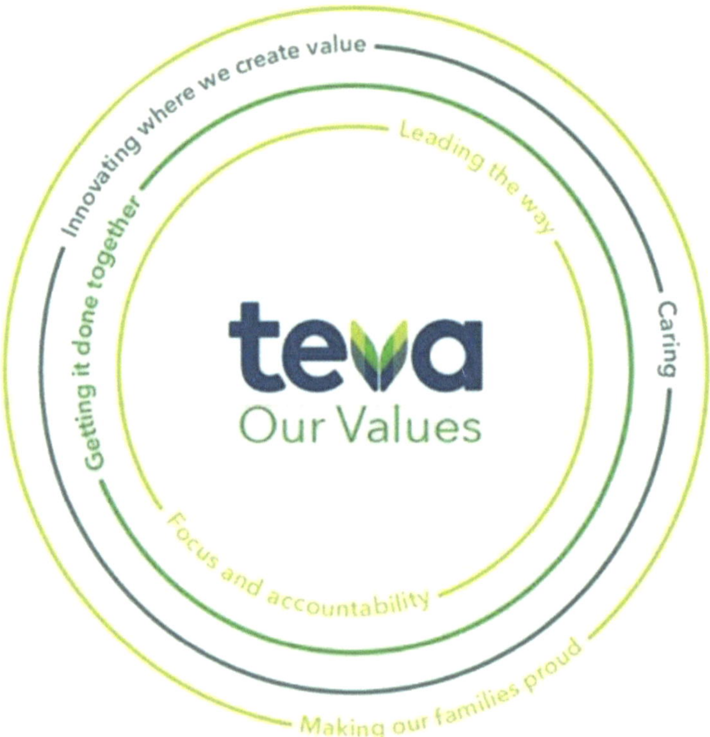
teva
Our Values
Innovating where we create value
Caring
Getting it done together
Leading the way
Focus and accountability
Making our families proud

Figure 2.
Teva's logo, describing Teva's values.

of study. Also, it is important to understand the new competitors from emerging markets, which are adopting aggressive tactics on the market. The present research describes an analysis of the case study on Teva company in the context of pharma industry, having as purpose to provide an insight in how future pharma companies can avoid certain pitfalls and how they should reply to the market competition and different other changes on the market (**Figure 2**).

2. Literature review

2.1 Company's values

With a mission to be a global leader in generics and biopharmaceutical, improving the lives of patients worldwide, Teva's core values were centred on corporate responsibility and transparency. During its initial successful decades, Teva consciously stressed a culture of employee satisfaction, and its message was that of a consumer brand to be trusted.

Teva emphasized the importance of drug safety, collaborations, health initiatives, and innovative research. The company had committed to various socio-economic initiatives, including donations, human rights, diversity, inclusion, occupational health, and safety, as well as the environment and pharmaceutical drugs [3].

2.2 History

The Teva production plant was established in Jerusalem on May 1, 1935, located in the neighborhood of Bayit Vegan. The factory was built with an investment of 4,900 pounds sterling, partially from the family endowment and partially from loans made by German immigrants. The immigrants wanted to support fellow German, Günther Friedlander, who was a pharmacist and botanist.

Banker Dr. Alfred Feuchtwanger became a partner in Teva when he funded a credit shortage in the company. He held a 33% share of Teva. In 1951, Dr. Feuchtwanger initiated Teva's initial public offering and entrance into the Tel Aviv Stock Exchange as a publicly listed and traded company.

During World War II, the factory supplied medicines to the Allied forces, in particular, to the British army in the Middle East. Sir Alan Gordon Cunningham, Colonial Minister and head of the British Mandate, visited the factory on behalf of the Secretary of State for the Colonies. His visit to the Teva factory significantly jumpstarted its reputation in the pharmaceutical industry.

In 1959, the pharmaceutical branch of the Israeli Manufacturer's Association conducted a survey among Israeli pharmaceutical companies, and the Teva plant in Jerusalem was ranked first. The results of the survey showed that the market approved of and supported Teva products, many of which were developed by Dr. Friedlander and the factory staff. The workers felt appreciated for their initiative and ideas. They took pride in their work and performed their tasks with strict execution.

In 1971, the Teva plant moved from Bayit Vegan to the industrial park in Har Hozvim. It was the first scientific factory that was established in Kiryat Atirot. Teva has expanded its operations over the years. For instance, in 1982, Teva received F.D.A. approval for its Kfar Saba plant in central Israel, which allowed it to market its generic drugs in the United States. The factories of Teva enabled the business to transform into a powerhouse drug maker. In 2019, the Kfar Saba plant of Teva received an F.D.A. approval stamp for the manufacturing of migraine drugs [4].

2.3 The company's main products

Regarding the commercialized products, the drugs produced by Teva can be used for migraines, pain management, cancer, and supportive care, and respiratory disorders. Some of the common generic drugs of the company are Alvimopan Capsules, Brinzolamide Ophthalmic Suspension, Colchicine Tablets, U.S.P., Dimethyl Fumarate Delayed-Release Capsules, Efavirenz, Emtricitabine, and Tenofovir Disoproxil Fumarate Tablets, etc. [5].

The company expanded into the treatment of a wide variety of disease types while simultaneously developing generic drugs. The goal was to provide faster and better solutions for patients battling various diseases. From a business perspective, Teva's strategy was to increase drug production to generate higher revenue.

In the mid-1990s, Teva introduced a novel drug called COPAXONE®, to treat multiple sclerosis. The drug was developed by a team of researchers at the Weizmann Institute of Science and was considered the world's best treatment against the condition. COPAXONE® received the United States Food and Drug Authority (F.D.A.) approval in 1996 and was regarded as one of the greatest achievements of Israel's scientific efforts.

This invention transformed Teva from a company that produced generic drugs to one that produced novel treatments. Since 2015, COPAXONE® was marketed to more than 50 countries worldwide. Teva's revenue from worldwide drug sales reached $4.2 billion, roughly 21% of the company's total revenue.

Another novel drug produced by Teva called Azilect was intended to treat Parkinson's disease. Teva launched the drug in Israel in 2005. A year later, the drug was launched and marketed in the United States. Teva discovered that Azilect was the only drug in the world that could treat the symptoms of Parkinson's disease and delay the physical deterioration due to the disease. Azilect has been sold in more than 45 countries around the world. In 2010, sales revenue for Azilect was $318 million.

At the end of 2016, Teva's novel drug portfolio was worth hundreds of millions of dollars. Considerable investments in R&D were critical to developing new novel drugs and maintaining Teva's current portfolio of novel drugs.

Patent protection has been an important tool for Teva to safeguard its innovation as well as to recoup the R&D invests in drug development. Various companies had tried to launch drugs in order to compete with COPAXONE®. In June 2015, the U.S. Federal Court of Appeals ruled that Teva's patent of its 20 mg dose of COPAXONE® was expired.

Teva's losses continued in 2017, as the U.S. Patent Commission in the Delaware District Court filed a motion to revoke the exclusivity of the patent from Teva that had accrued them $49 billion in revenue. This caused the company's stock to decline about 50 percent in 12 months' time. Additionally, the Federal Court of Appeals filed a request to cancel the validity of one of the company's patents for the lung cancer drug Alimta that earned the company $1.1 billion in 2016.

Teva had been looking at introducing a novel migraine drug to be a replacement of sorts for COPAXONE®. This new drug hoped to treat various iterations of migraines. Teva has introduced AJOVY, which is a pre-filled injection for the prophylaxis of migraines in adults. It received a nod from European Medicines Agency's Committee for Medicinal Products for Human Use in 2019 [6]. Despite patent challenges in the United States, in December 2015, the European Patent Office approved Teva's patent for the 40 mg dose of COPAXONE® until 2030.

3. Research method

To understand the evolution of a company in time, it is important to analyze the key factors which contribute to the success or to the fall of a company. The present paper is based on a qualitative research, aiming to provide an in-depth understanding on the correlation between the internal and external changes and the company's evolution.

According to Baskarada [7], the case study method is the most widely used method in academia for researchers interested in qualitative research, Baskarada [7] emphasizing the need to have a succinct guideline that can be practically followed.

This research presents a qualitative case study on Teva company in the context of pharma industry. Baxter and Jack [8] define a qualitative case study as a research methodology that helps in exploration of a phenomenon within some particular context through various data sources, and it undertakes the exploration through variety of lenses in order to reveal multiple facets of the phenomenon. In the case of Teva company, the used data sources are business reports, news media, as well as specialized articles on pharmaceutical industries. The company is analyzed from multiple facets like the evolution of the stock price, the corporate decisions, the appearance of new competitors on the market and how the company's revenues have been affected.

According to Yazan [9], in qualitative research, case study is one of the frequently used methodologies, in which a real-time phenomenon is explored within its naturally occurring context, with the consideration that context will create a difference [10]. In the present case, the real-time phenomenon is the historical evolution of the Teva company with the consideration that the context of the overall pharmaceutical industry plays an important part in this evolution.

The considered phases of the chosen methodology are the same as the one proposed by Rashid et al. [11] and they are the following: the foundation phase (analyze of what is relevant in assessing the success of Teva company in the context of pharma industry), prefield phase (deciding on the factors which will be measured, the case study protocol), field phase (in this case, gathering the relevant data from trustworthy resources), reporting phase (reporting the findings).

The factors which help in assessing the evolution of Teva company are the competitors, the company's business strategy, the stock performance and the company's overall performance. By analyzing these factors and reporting some of the quantitative data associated with them will help in painting a broad picture of the company's evolution.

4. Findings

4.1 Competitors

Teva has several competitors in the global market, like Momenta Pharmaceuticals, Mylan, Synthon, Unipharm and Rafa. Another name worth mentioning is Allergan, which, in 2015, became the largest shareholder of Teva after Teva acquired Allergan's generic pharmaceutical division.

One of the main products of Momenta Pharmaceuticals is Glatopa®, a generic form of COPAXONE®. In 2015 Glatopa® was approved by the US FDA and launched in the United States. Momenta Pharmaceuticals collaborated with Sandoz, a Novartis company, to produce Glatopa®. The intent was for Glatopa® to replace Teva's 40 mg dose of COPAXONE® [12].

The multinational drug development company, Mylan, was registered and based in the Netherlands, with branches in the U.K. and Pennsylvania. Until 2007, the American branch of Mylan only operated in the domestic market. However, after Mylan acquired German drug company Merck, and the Indian Laboratories of Matrix, Mylan became the second-largest generic drug company in the world, after Teva. Mylan started marketing their version of the 40 mg dose of COPAXONE® in October 2017 [13].

The Dutch company Synthon, is an international pharmaceutical company and one of the leaders in the field of generic medicines. In 2017, Synthon announced that it had successfully conducted clinical trials in order to prove that its glatiramer acetate (sold as Remurel by Alvogen) provided the same therapeutic benefit as Teva's 40 mg COPAXONE®. Synthon received the European Medical Agency's approval in a process in which all 29 E.U. Member states adopted the approval [14].

Regarding the key competitors in the domestic market, Unipharm and Rafa are worth mentioning. Unipharm, had been developing and marketing generic drugs since 1975. Founded by pharmacist Zvulun Tomer, the company was a pioneer in the generic drugs force. Unipharm's drugs targeted the treatment of a wide range of diseases and symptoms such as mental health, heart health, sleep, Alzheimer's, infectious diseases, urology, eyes, and more. In 2017, Unipharm launched a new plant in Mavo Carmel. At this manufacturing plant, Unipharm introduced new technologies and development processes to achieve production efficiencies and cost savings in generic drug manufacturing [15]. It uses innovative approaches to act as a one-stop solution for health manufacturing needs and thus poses challenges to Teva.

Rafa was founded in 1937 and is one of the leading pharmaceutical companies in the country. The company specialized in the marketing, manufacturing, and distributing of novel and generic drugs, prescription drugs, over-the-counter drugs, as well as therapeutic products. Rafa products were marketed to all Israeli health institutions, such as public and private hospitals, clinics, health clinics, and more, serving a wide range of ages in the population, from infants to the elderly [16]. The company focuses on research activities to introduce the latest drugs and therapies relating to different conditions and thus poses a challenge for Teva [17].

4.2 The business strategy

Since the 2000s, Teva had embarked on an acquisition strategy – buying over large generic drug companies to create value for the company. Some acquisitions seemed initially successful but proved otherwise later. Other acquisitions lacked clear plans. When Teva acquired U.S. drug company Cephalon in October 2011, Cephalon's R&D team took over the development of the anti-depression drug. Within a year, the R&D employees were laid off.

The acquisitions resulted in significant short-term financial gains because stock prices could be raised through acquisitions. Chief executives of that period had focused on creating shareholder value through mergers and acquisitions in the pharmaceutical market, rather than focusing their energy on their drug clientele and patients. They also channeled investments away from the research and development of drugs such as COPAXONE®.

4.3 Stock performance

Teva had a "dual stock," or a stock that traded in two trading areas: in the home country of the company, and in the stock exchange of another large country. Teva's dual stock was traded on the Tel Aviv Stock Exchange as well as the New York Stock Exchange.

At the beginning of the 2000s, Teva's share rose 20 times, which significantly impacted the Tel Aviv Stock Exchange. Investment in Teva had become extremely popular and was even referred to as the "people's share." However, Teva stock also experienced sharp declines during 1998, the middle of 2004, and after the publication of negative reports in 2006. A financial commentator at one point even said, the public suddenly understands that "Teva is also a share."

From the beginning of 2014 until the middle of 2015, Teva's share price almost doubled, but by the end of 2016, it returned to the level that it was in early 2014. In May 2017, Teva's share dropped to a level that it has not been since 2005.

4.4 Teva's overall performance

Since the end of 2015, Teva's shares are down by 64%, which has erased more than $40 billion in market capitalization [18]. The company's worsening performance led to a wave of layoffs. Teva cut 14,000 jobs worldwide, which was more than 25 percent of the company's international workforce. According to Teva, it plans to lay off 1,750 employees, and that's just the beginning [19]. The layoffs will occur as a result of the closure or sale of a significant number of R&D sites, headquarters, offices, and a number of the company's geographical divisions will also be reduced.

By the end of 2017, Teva closed or sold six plants. This was followed by the closure of another nine plants in 2018.

The company's two plants in Jerusalem, which employed 1,100 employees, have been closed, the factory in Kiryat Shmona sold, the R&D center in Netanya, which employed 350, people has also closed as of 2019 [20].

In addition, Teva ceased operations at the global logistics center S.L.A. from the Shoham Industrial Area, even though it employed 700 people [21].

While on the one hand, the reduction plan raised the value of the stock by creating the illusion of improvement, it damaged employee and customer trust and further contributed to the deterioration of the company's shares.

In 2019, Teva's total revenue fell by 8% to $16.9 million, which was a decrease of 8% as compared to 2018. This decline was mainly due to various reasons like the generic competition to COPAXONE®, a decline in revenues from U.S. generics business, BENDEKA®/TREANDA®, and Japan. However, this decline was partially offset by higher revenues from AUSTEDO, AJOVY, and QVAR® in the United States. COPAXONE® accounted for 11% of Teva's North America revenue from October to November 2019 [22].

5. Discussion

By combining the above-mentioned factors, a broad picture of the company's evolution can be painted.

Things took a downturn in the 2000s when Teva embarked on a strategy to create shareholder value through mergers and acquisitions. When Teva acquired U.S. drug company Cephalon in October 2011, Cephalon's R&D team took over the development of the anti-depression drug. Within a year, the R&D employees were laid off. The acquisitions resulted in significant short-term financial gains because stock prices could be raised through acquisitions. Chief executives of that period had focused on creating shareholder value through mergers and acquisitions in the pharmaceutical market, rather than focusing their energy on their drug clientele and patients. They also channeled investments away from the research and development of drugs such as COPAXONE®. Teva's reputation as an innovative and entrepreneurial Israeli company with a heart for its employees seemed to have lost its way (**Figure 3**).

In 2015, Teva's competitor, Allergan, became the largest shareholder of Teva after Teva acquired Allergan's generic pharmaceutical division. This resulted in much unhappiness among other shareholders, causing a corporate crisis. The other shareholders of the business were dissatisfied as the two leading generic businesses came together, and their fundamental needs and expectations overshadowed the needs of other shareholders [23].

After the U.S. Federal Court of Appeals ruled in 2015 that Teva's patent of its 20 mg dose of COPAXONE® was expired, the competitors launched their generic

Conditions	Description
Migraine[1]	A migraine is much more than just a headache. A migraine is an advanced neurological disease characterized by recurrent bouts of moderate to severe headaches. Teva's treatment for migraine is AJOVY which is a humanised monoclonal antibody[2].
Pain Therapy[3]	Pain is an unpleasant sensory and emotional experience, which is associated with actual or potential damage to bodily organs and tissue. Pain is sometimes a symptom, but it can also be an independent medical problem that requires treatment. Teva offers tools for dealing with pain in the form of literature, medical advice, and more. Pain therapy is intended to ease patients' suffering, improve their quality of life, and enable them to function better.
Central Nervous System (C.N.S.)[4]	Teva's C.N.S. drug collection included pain management treatments for adults with cancer, opiates, and products for muscle contraction for people with muscle and skeletal conditions. Investments were also made to develop non-opioid alternatives.
Cancer and Supportive Care[5]	The company has been working on new cancer treatments in the laboratory, which arebased on accurate diagnosis.
Breathing[6]	Teva provides respiratory products to increase the patients' quality of life and prognosis.

Figure 3.
Areas of care treated by Teva. (Sources: [1]Teva treatment for migraine, https://www.teva.co.il/Treatment-area/Migraine/, date accessed: 28 February 2020. [2]Teva launches AJOVY for the treatment of migraine with the YpsoMate autoinjector from Ypsomed, https://www.ypsomed.com/fr-CA/derniere-nouvelles/news-reader-detail-page/teva-launches-ajovy-for-the-treatment-of-migraine-with-the-ypsomate-autoinjector-from-ypsomed.html#:~:text=AJOVY®%20(fremanezumab%2Dvfrm),is%20affected%20by%20migraine%20worldwide, date accessed: 28 February 2020. [3]Teva treatment for pain, https://www.teva.co.il/Treatment-area/Pain/, date accessed: 28 February 2020. [4]Teva treatment for CNS, https://www.teva.co.il/Treatment-area/Central-Nervous-System/, date accessed: 28 February 2020. [5]Teva treatment for cancer, https://www.teva.co.il/Treatment-area/Oncology/, date accessed: 28 February 2020. [6]Teva treatment for breathing, www.teva.co.il/Treatment-area/BreathLobby/, date accessed: 28 February 2020. Teva Pharmaceutical Industries Limited, https://www.annualreports.com/HostedData/AnnualReports/PDF/NYSE_TEVA_2019.pdf, date accessed: 28 February 2020.)

DOI: http://dx.doi.org/10.5772/intechopen.97747

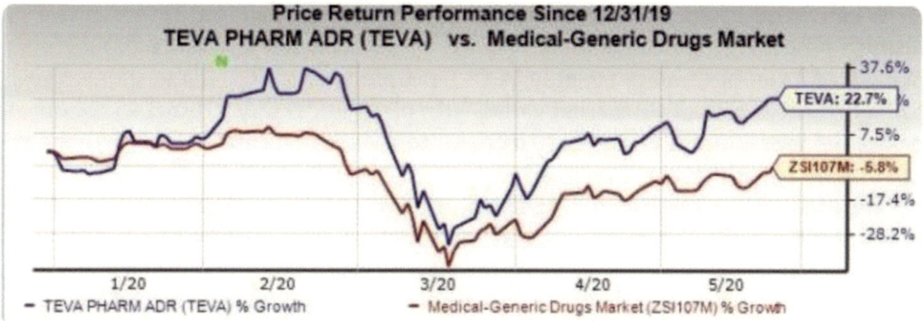

Figure 4.
Price return performance. (Source: Can Teva (TEVA) Return to Growth in This Year or Next?, https://finance.yahoo.com/news/teva-teva-return-growth-next-095909420.html?guccounter=1&guce_referrer=aHR0cHM6Ly93d3cuZ29vZ2xlLmNvbS8&guce_referrer_sig=AQAAAN5KQnTTIjE07PfncCLKNG0UwFpDU2vzUMoUxszodGcNCk5sv1NLAQ5MMRJ3ctF1Z9Rvi5QFhSDErtdGH6I66TL-5_HIFkVT_DpzonXFej10FdufNDxoUQdY2WbUJRUr89J9wa1vGEVR_pjI9sG7phD6PFgemJIZyfMUon5mZdno, date accessed: 28 February 2020.)

versions and the profitability of COPAXONE® eroded, and Teva's market share plunged. With the launch of Glatopa®, Teva had expected it to reduce Teva's revenue by 18% to 4.7 billion as well as further eroding prices [24]. This increased the competition of COPAXONE® significantly. Also, the competition generated by Mylan's generic version, sparked a competitive price war leading to Teva's US COPAXONE® revenue to fall by 20 percent (**Figure 4**). Regarding Synthon, one hit was when Synthon was accepted in European markets. Even though the European market was not the most important market for COPAXONE®, Teva had until then enjoyed patent protection and avoided competition. Synthon's announcement came just a few days after Mylan launched the 40 mg and 20 mg versions of glatiramer acetate in the United States [14].

Teva's troubles continued to mount. Its share value was reduced in the indices due to stock exchange reform. Teva was also denied a critical patent application which eroded the profitability of the flagship drug COPAXONE®. COPAXONE®faced growing competition after parallel pharmaceutical companies launched their generic versions in 2016, which triggered a precipitous decrease in Teva's market share (**Figure 5**).

One of the main reasons for Teva's losses is a result of being entirely dependent on the sales of one of the company's primary drugs, Copaxone, used as the treatment for M.S. This puts Teva in a weak position because any drop in drug sales can and will have a negative impact on the company.

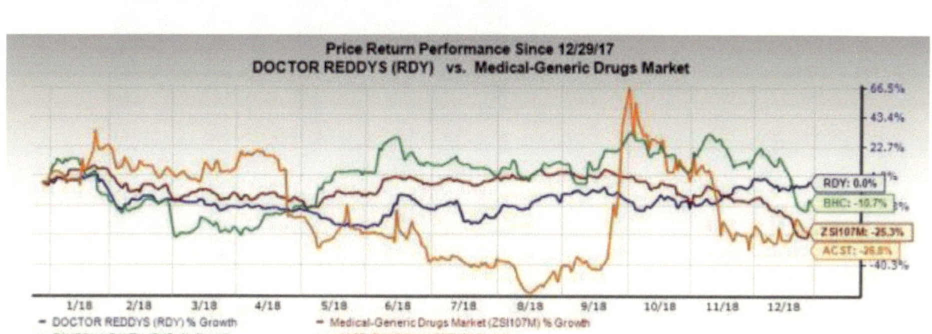

Figure 5.
Source: Zacks, Generic Industry on Path to Recovery: 3 Hot Picks for 2019, https://www.nasdaq.com/articles/generic-industry-on-path-to-recovery%3A-3-hot-picks-for-2019-2018-12-28, date accessed: 28 February 2020.

When Schultz joined the company, Teva's debt was $40 billion. Teva had also begun a process of significant streamlining, which included laying off about 25 percent of its employees, or roughly 14,000 people, and 1,750 in Israel alone. Teva had lost more than half its market value, with plans underway to leave 45 countries before the year is out. It is currently difficult to assess what can be done so that Teva can rebuild its reputation (**Figure 6**).

The acquisitions resulted in significant short-term financial gains because stock prices could be raised through acquisitions. Chief executives of that period had focused on creating shareholder value through mergers and acquisitions in the pharmaceutical market, rather than focusing their energy on their drug clientele

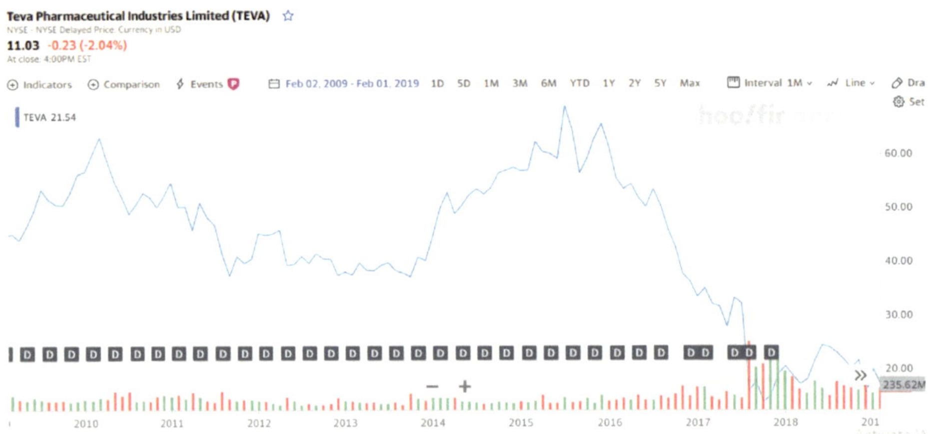

Figure 6.
Teva's stock performance. (Source: Teva Pharmaceutical Industries Limited, https://finance.yahoo.com/chart/TEVA, date accessed: 28 February 2020.)

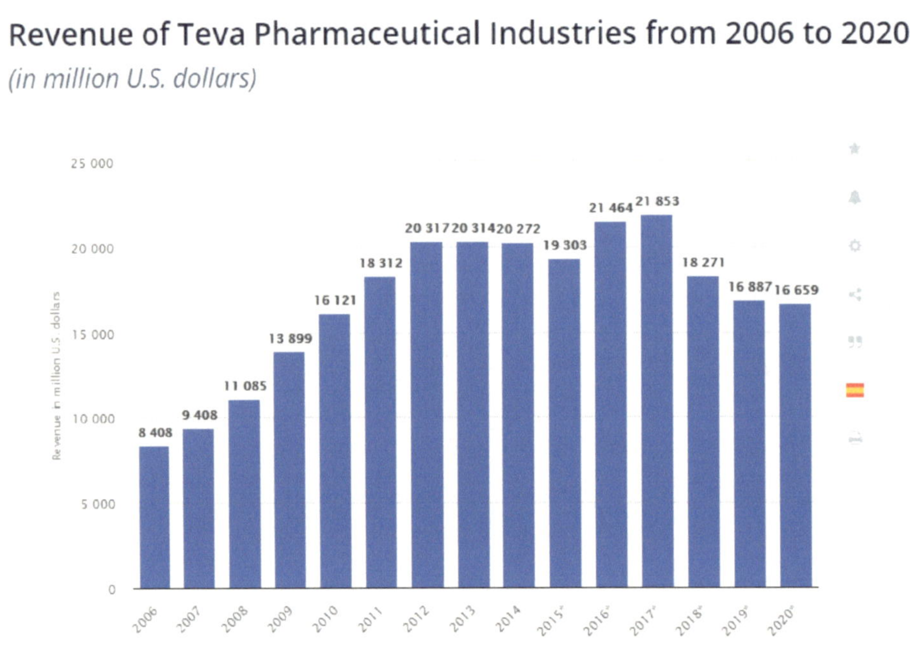

Figure 7.
Annual revenue of Teva Pharmaceuticals industries. (Source: Revenue of Teva Pharmaceutical Industries from 2006 to 2020, https://www.statista.com/statistics/272542/teva-pharmaceutical-industries-net-sales-since-2006/, date accessed: 28 February 2020.)

and patients. They also channeled investments away from the research and development of drugs such as COPAXONE®. Teva's reputation as an innovative and entrepreneurial Israeli company with a heart for its employees seemed to have lost its way (**Figure 7**).

In May 2017, Teva's share dropped to a level that it has not been since 2005; the decline was due to investors' concerns that in June 2017, Mylan would receive authorization to initiate the marketing of a generic version of Teva's profitable 40 mg COPAXONE® in the United States.

In the last decade, Teva has spent $70 billion on giant acquisitions, Cephalon and Actavis, and for that reason, it is expected that its value to be minimally $70 billion, but in reality, it is about half of that, and its share has plummeted more than the rest of the sector. The cutting of spending was not large enough to justify the acquisition.

In 2019, Teva's total revenue fell by 8% to $16.9 million, which was a decrease of 8% as compared to 2018. This decline was mainly due to various reasons like the generic competition to COPAXONE®, a decline in revenues from U.S. generics business, BENDEKA®/TREANDA®, and Japan. However, this decline was partially offset by higher revenues from AUSTEDO, AJOVY, and QVAR® in the United States. COPAXONE® accounted for 11% of Teva's North America revenue from October to November 2019 [22].

In spite of the many difficulties the company faced in the last decades, there is still the possibility that the company can rebalance again and learn from its mistakes. Teva is still a major pharmaceutical company that offers a broad range of drugs in the global market setting. It has been showcasing consistent performance and contributing to improve the health outcome of the general public. The firm's strategy plays a cardinal role in influencing its contribution to the dynamic industry.

Author details

Neta Kela-Madar
Industrial Engineering and Management, Sami Shamoon College of Engineering, Ashdod, Israel

*Address all correspondence to: neta.kela@gmail.com

References

[1] Reference for Business (2020). Teva Pharmaceutical Industries Ltd. - Company Profile, Information, Business Description, History, Background Information on Teva Pharmaceutical Industries Ltd. Reference for Business, URL:https://www.referenceforbusiness.com/history2/87/Teva-Pharmaceutical-Industries-Ltd.html#ixzz6p5SJOhuY (accessed on February 28, 2020).

[2] Teva Pharm 1 (2020). Improving health since 1901. Teva Pharm, URL:https://www.tevapharm.com/our-company/teva-history/#46361253 (accessed on February 28, 2020).

[3] Teva Pharm 2 (2020). Teva Core Values. Teva Pharm, URL: https://www.tevapharm.com/our-company/our-values/ (accessed on February 28, 2020).

[4] Zomer, N. (2019). Teva's Israeli Plant Receives FDA Stamp of Approval for Migraine Drug Manufacturing. Calcalistech, URL: https://www.calcalistech.com/ctech/articles/0,7340,L-3773870,00.html (accessed on February 28, 2020).

[5] Teva USA (2020). Generic medicines. Teva USA, URL: https://www.tevausa.com/our-products/article-pages/article-generic-medicine/ (accessed on February 28, 2020).

[6] Maggie Lynch, M. (2019). EU approval for Teva's quarterly dosed migraine drug. Biopharma Reporter, URL: https://www.biopharma-reporter.com/Article/2019/04/09/Teva-s-migraine-med-given-marketing-authorization#:~:text=Ajovy%20(fremanezumab)%2C%20developed%20by,its%20binding%20to%20the%20receptor. (accessed on February 28, 2020).

[7] Baskarada, S. (2014). *Qualitative case study guidelines*. The Qualitative Report, 19, 1-25.

[8] Baxter, P., Jack, S. (2008). *Qualitative case study methodology: Study design and implementation for novice researchers*. The Qualitative Report, 13, 544-559.

[9] Yazan, B. (2015). *Three approaches to case study methods in education: Yin, Merriam, and Stake*. The Qualitative Report, 20, 134-152.

[10] Kaarbo, J., Beasley, R. K. (1999). *A practical guide to the comparative case study method in political psychology*. Political Psychology, 20, 369-391.

[11] Rashid, Y., Rashid, A., Warraich, M.A., Sabir, S. and Waseem, A. (2019). *Case Study Method: A Step-by-Step Guide for Business Researchers.* Computer Science. International Journal of Qualitative Methods. DOI:10.1177/1609406919862424.

[12] National Multiple Sclerosis Society (2015). *An FDA Approved Generic Form of COPAXONE® (Glatiramer Acetate) For Relapsing MS Called Glatopa is Launched in the US*. National Multiple Sclerosis Society. URL: https://www.nationalmssociety.org/About-the-Society/News/An-FDA-Approved-Generic-Form-of-Copaxone-Glatira (accessed on February 28, 2020).

[13] Mylan, N.V. (2017). *Mylan Announces U.S. FDA Approval of First Generic for Copaxone® 40 mg/mL 3-Times-a-Week and May Be Eligible for 180-Day Exclusivity.* PRNEWSWIRE. URL: https://www.prnewswire.com/news-releases/mylan-announces-us-fda-approval-of-first-generic-for-copaxone-40-mgml-3-times-a-week-and-may-be-eligible-for-180-day-exclusivity-300530551.html (accessed on February 28, 2020).

[14] Macdonald, G. (2017). *Synton's generic version of Copaxone 40mg approved in Europe*. Outsourcing

Pharma. URL: https://www.in-pharmatechnologist.com/Article/2017/10/05/Synthon-s-generic-version-of-Copaxone-40mg-approved-in-Europe (accessed on February 28, 2020).

[15] Unipharm (2021). *News and Updates*. Unipharm. URL: http://unipharm.co.il/news-updates/?lang=en (accessed on February 28, 2020).

[16] Rafa (2021). A career in healing. Rafa. URL: https://www.rafa.co.il/ (accessed on February 28, 2020).

[17] Bloomberg (2021). Rafael Pharmaceuticals Inc. Bloomberg. URL: https://www.bloomberg.com/profile/company/1692961D:US (accessed on February 28, 2020).

[18] Roland, D. and Jones, R. (2017). *Teva Pharmaceutical's Stock Tumbles on Outlook.* Wall Street Journal. URL: https://www.wsj.com/articles/generic-competition-roils-teva-1501773117 (accessed on February 28, 2020).

[19] BBC (2017). *Teva Pharmaceuticals: Israeli drugmaker to cut 14,000 jobs*. BBC. URL: https://www.bbc.com/news/world-middle-east-42356115 (accessed on February 28, 2020).

[20] Greenberg, T. (2019). *Teva to Sell Northern Israeli Facility to Private Equity Fund FIMI*. Calcalistech. URL: https://www.calcalistech.com/ctech/articles/0,7340,L-3755808,00.html (accessed on February 28, 2020).

[21] Liu, A. (2019). *Teva sheds logistics center for $127M after 2 about-faces.* Fierce Pharma. URL: https://www.fiercepharma.com/pharma/teva-sheds-logistics-center-for-127m-after-2-years-2-about-faces (accessed on February 28, 2020).

[22] Teva (2019). Teva Reports Fourth Quarter and Full Year 2019 Financial Results. Teva Press Release. URL: https://s24.q4cdn.com/720828402/files/doc_financials/2019/q4/Q4.2019_PR.wtables_Final.pdf (accessed on February 28, 2020).

[23] Business Wire (2020). Teva Completes Acquisition of Actavis Generics. BusinessWire, URL: https://www.businesswire.com/news/home/20160802006666/en/Teva-Completes-Acquisition-of-Actavis-Generics (accessed on February 28, 2020).

[24] Cohen, T., Rabinovitch, A. (2018). *Teva Pharm shares sink as sales forecast disappoints market*. Reuters. URL: https://www.reuters.com/article/us-teva-pharm-ind-results-idUSKBN1KN1JO?edition-redirect=in (accessed on February 28, 2020).

Chapter 18

Impacts of Medical Tourism on Healthcare Access

Iskra Alexandra Nola and Zdeslav Radovčić

Abstract

Today, medical tourism is underrated and mostly perceived as a beauty tourism. However, except dermatological and dental services also organ transplantation, IVF and many other therapies are well present in medical tourism travel arrangements. Medical tourism without any doubt impacts access to healthcare. Healthcare system in many countries allows access to some of these services but all-around world approaches differ. We believe that healthcare access could greatly benefit by opening this kind of services to wider population while at the same time not endangering patient' safety. Harmonized propositions, accreditations and certificates for medical tourism industry access covered by both, private and public health insurances, would contribute to service transparency and patient' safety while taking care of moral aspects of such services. Therefore, if consciously incorporated, medical tourism, as a part of global healthcare could easily become an efficient and effective additional access to healthcare.

Keywords: accreditation, certificates, healthcare access, healthcare insurance, liability, medical tourism, patient's safety

1. Introduction

Medical tourism is an individual or organized journey outside of place of residence due to the use of medical service in another country. However, according to WHO, currently there is no internationally accepted official definition of medical tourism [1]. This could be seen as an obstacle while not having the uniform approach to the subject is often the reason why services differ all over the world. In addition, non-uniform approach to the given subject could slow or enable, depending on country, the process of establishing criteria for services that could or should be welcomed under the health and public health systems.

However, knowing that accessibility to healthcare in patients' places of residence can be limited for a number of reasons, including cost, distance to the closest health facility and waiting times, medical tourism represents a sector that could significantly improve healthcare access. Unmet care needs may result in poorer health for people forgoing care and may increase health inequalities especially if such unmet needs are concentrated among poor people. Traveling for health is a realistic option to overcome this issue.

The use of some kind of healthcare outside of place of residence is not a new phenomenon. Ancient Greeks, from the area around the Mediterranean, traveled to Epidaurus, to get the medical advice of Aesculapius. In the 18th century, patients from England visited various spas abroad, while they believed their immune system and overall health would be boosted by the different climate and water [2]. In the late 19th and at the beginning of 20th century Austro-Hungarian nobility discovered healing effects of water and air of the Croatian north coast, especially cities like Crikvenica and Opatija. However, finding balneal and climate therapy only, soon became insufficient. During the 20th century, wealthier people from less developed areas traveled to more developed regions to access better health facilities, highly trained medics, and new or more available procedures. Through the time, another group of medical travelers becomes more interested in finding good but less expensive institutions where they can get the same standard of specific medical care but for less money. This led to the new paradigm of medical tourism – patients that travel seeking for health service but also willing to combine they stay with the experiences that other country could give them. They became tourists with the plan [3].

Nevertheless, the shifts that are currently visible in the medical tourism show the main differences in services provided. Some countries develop specific "supply" of services based on specific "demands". In Europe Union (EU), there are countries that are much wealthier than the other European countries and thus some medical treatments are very expensive. For example, dental and dermatological services are often sought in eastern or southern European countries where the prices are much lower than in the northern and western countries [4]. The highest rate of hip replacement, which is most sought method when it comes to hip arthritis and related pain, are in Switzerland and Germany, among the countries members of Organization for Economic Co-operation and Development (OECD countries) [5]. This procedure has long waiting list if the healthcare access is organized through public clinics. Therefore, many patients opt to travel abroad to be operated sooner and at more affordable rate. In the past ten years, there is a visible in the number of outpatient hip replacements in United States of America (USA).

Not only the price is the cut-off value for the decision to go out of own country and seek the medical service. Sometimes the inability to get a specific medical help in one's own country is the main reason to travel for health (procedure or technology). In Europe, there are mutual agreements that cover such situations by existing national health insurances [6, 7], but the costs for rare diseases remain high. Sometimes, in certain countries, the procedures themselves or for certain group of people are not allowed due to cultural factors, as abortion, IVF or surrogacy, and thus some people reach for this kind of treatments available through medical tourism. Moreover, there is a controversy related to the transplantations of the organs and the completely new market developed for these procedures. Besides that, in poor countries, there is a risk of organ trafficking.

Different types of demands in medical tourism market and different laws applied in different countries create an environment of too many information, fear and uncertainty especially in relation to the aftermath, which is reasonable to expect to happen in some of the situations. Thus, the reasons why patients make the decision to use medical tourism is very important, especially for studying the possible implications related to [7].

Today, the market of medical tourism is valued at hundreds of billions of USD and is constantly rising, thus presenting multi-way matter of subject. In some countries the health systems are losing patients because of high prices which make the patients to go to other, nearby countries, and in some cases insurance system do not allow patients to use any non-conventional approach in their therapies and healing process [8]. In this case, patients often use all the procedures covered by their insurance and at the same time, they pay for different approach as well. Here we can say – the system (the government system) is losing again.

Medical tourism brings many advantages to patients, countries and governments, but also many negative consequences that affect the individual and public system. Obviously, the lack of internationally accepted official definition of medical tourism, of agreed definitions, of databases that record the total number of patients traveling abroad, of the procedures they undergo and of their outcome, is causing more problems as the time pass.

Without systematic monitoring and collecting data, it will be impossible to do the comparison of the quality of implemented services of medical tourism between countries and institutions. We believe that organized approach to this hot topic of medical tourism and implemented standards and measures through the health systems and services will not provide benefits only for the end-consumers, but also for the countries, governments and their economics as well.

2. Services

Medical services used by traveling patients are often elective interventions, complex surgery, procedures in the field of plastic surgery, dental medicine, as well as all other forms of medical care. Recently, there is a huge increase in search of second opinion outside of the country of residence and many internationally recognized clinics and hospitals see it as a lucrative side service.

However, the reasons that are behind the patients' engagement in medical tourism are complex. They include unmet care, the nature of services they are trying to find (including dental care), the manner by which the treatment is accessed (mainly dependable on resident's country healthcare system), available properly educated staff and waiting time related to the service to be done in the resident country.

2.1 Unmet care

Inadequate healthcare access and unmet care in their native countries has led to a significant increase in the number of people using medical services outside the borders of their country. For example, in all European countries, most of the population in 2018 reported that they had no unmet care needs for financial reasons, geographic reasons or waiting times (**Figure 1**).

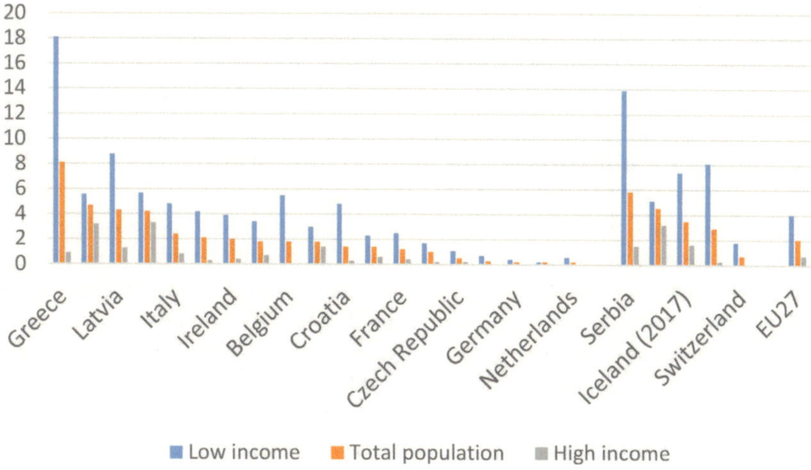

Figure 1.
Unmet need for medical examination due to financial, geographic or waiting time reasons, 2018. Source: This chart is made by authors by using data from Eurostat Database [9], (online data code: HLTH_SILC_08$DV_361; sdg_03_60; tsdph270) and OECD data.

However, in Estonia and Greece for example, at least 8% of the population reported some unmet needs for healthcare, with the burden falling mostly on people from low-income households, particularly in Greece. Nearly one in five Greek people in the lowest income quintile reported going without some medical care when they needed it and these unmet needs were mainly for financial reasons. In Estonia, long waiting times are the main reason for people to report unmet care needs, which are partly explained by the limited volume of some services (such as specialist consultations) fully reimbursed by public health insurance [9].

The gap in unmet medical and dental care needs between poor people and rich people remains large: on average across EU countries, people in the lowest income quintile are still four times more likely to report unmet medical care needs than those in the highest quintile, and six times more likely to report unmet dental care needs [9].

2.2 Staff shortage

The characteristics of national healthcare system will certainly define the overall demand for medical tourism in each country. In addition, the impact of medical tourism on national care system will depend on those characteristics as well. This double relation between medical tourism and healthcare system will finally affect the policy in this area.

Moreover, it is important to mention staff shortages especially in certain medical specializations or geographic areas [10]. In the coming decades, aged population is expected to be one of the major challenges for the health sector [11, 12]. The demand for healthcare will probably increase substantially in elderly population, particularly in the US and EU, and at the same time the proportion of the people in work will probably decline. In 2018, just over two fifths of all doctors in the EU were aged 55 years and over. According to the European Commission's Directorate-General for Health and Food Safety, more than 60 000 doctors (or 3.2% of the workforce) were expected to leave the profession each year during the period 2018–2020. There are countries more affected - in 2018, more than half of all physicians in Italy and Bulgaria were aged 55 years and over [13].

Proper healthcare access requires a sufficient number of doctors, with a proper mix of general practitioners and specialists and a proper geographic distribution to serve the population in the whole country. There were many concerns in the late 2000s about projected shortages of doctors arising from population aging and the aging of the medical workforce [9]. These concerns prompted many EU countries to take actions to anticipate the retirement of a large number of doctors, notably by increasing the number of medical students, to replace those retiring [9]. Several countries also took actions to postpone the retirement of current doctors and recruited more doctors from abroad [9].

In many countries, the main concern has been about growing shortages of general practitioners, particularly in rural and remote regions. Whereas the overall number of doctors per capita has increased in nearly all countries (**Figure 2**), the share of general practitioners (GPs) has come down in most countries.

In many countries, it remains a challenge to attract a sufficient number of medical students to fill the available training places for general practitioners. The uneven geographic distribution of doctors and difficulties in recruiting and retaining doctors in remote and sparsely populated areas is another persisting challenge in many European countries. In all countries, the density of physicians is generally greater in urban regions, reflecting the concentration of specialized services such as surgery in urban centers as well as physicians' preferences to live and practice in cities [9].

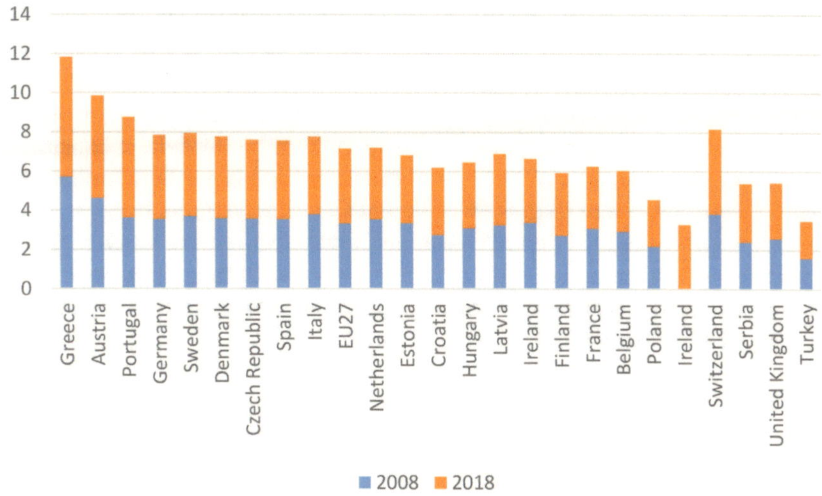

Figure 2.
Practising doctors per 1 000 population, 2008 and 2018 (or nearest year). Source: This chart is made by authors by using data from Eurostat Database [9], (online data code: hlth_rs_prs) and OECD data.

2.3 Waiting time

Some services in the international medical tourism are in more demand than others are. Services with long waiting lists are particularly influencing this demand. Moreover, long waiting lists for elective (non-urgent) surgery have been a longstanding issue in many European countries as they generate dissatisfaction in patients because the expected benefits of treatments are postponed. The COVID-19 pandemic will likely increase waiting lists for many elective surgeries, at least temporarily, as non-urgent interventions have often been postponed during the peak of the epidemic.

The median waiting time for people who received a cataract surgery in 2019 (or 2018) varied from about 30 days in Italy, Hungary and Denmark, to about 150 days in Estonia and 250 days in Poland. For hip replacement [5], the median waiting time ranged from 35 to 50 days in Denmark, Hungary and Italy, to 180 days in Poland and 250 days in Estonia. The pattern is generally the same for knee replacement, although in most countries the waiting time is slightly longer than for hip replacement [9].

2.4 Oral health

Oral health is an important, although often neglected public health issue. The global burden of dental diseases is mostly seen in caries and periodontal diseases being major public health problems in industrialized countries among children and adults [14].

The economic burden of oral diseases is substantial. With dental costs on the rise, a vast number of people across Europe and the USA are finding it difficult to afford proper dental care, especially when it comes to procedures that are more complex. This is the main reason people are deciding to spend their holidays in destinations that offer them the same quality of dental services at lower price rates. This cost-effectiveness principle is often the main principle in managing the choice of medical service and country of destination. There are different reasons why the prices in some countries are lower than in the other, but in most of the popular dental tourism destinations, it is due to lower labor and real estate costs. Dentists in these countries can afford themselves to have lower prices than their colleagues in big centers of

Europe and USA, while providing the same quality of dental work. Oral diseases account for more than 5% of total health spending on average across EU countries, and productivity losses due to oral diseases have been estimated at around EUR 57 billion a year [15]. The extent of public coverage for dental care costs can also partly explain some of the cross-country variations in the number of dentist consultations. In Romania for example, only 6% of dental care spending is publicly funded. By contrast, in Germany, more than 60% of dental spending is publicly covered [9].

The cost for non-medical dental treatment, esthetic ones, are much higher. This is specially related to the fact that there is no country with the public health coverage for esthetic dental treatments – those are covered mainly in children and for the visible teeth, if they are at all.

2.5 Healthcare access

Healthcare access mirroring the state organization and social sensitivity. Still, it is usually related to money and availability of services. Nevertheless, there are concerns that low- and middle-income countries will suffer the inequity and worse accessibility to healthcare if the medical tourism prevail [16]. The reasons, as elaborated in earlier paragraphs, are numerous: staff shortage or drain to the private sector [10], long waiting time, higher prices. However, healthcare access does not show only the shortcomings in countries where medical tourism applies [2]. There are benefits related to the growing medical tourism in such countries: money obtained from medical tourism services often spills to the secondary and tertiary sectors thus producing economic expansion. Even though, we need to be conscious on different aspects of medical tourism' impact on healthcare access [2].

The equity could be the main factor for reasonable approach to healthcare access and should be seen from two different angles. Firstly, equity in healthcare access for domestic population, which is not compromised by growing medical tourism while the systems are separate (national vs. private). Secondly, equity, which is compromised by staff or money drain into medical tourism' services which leaves healthcare access for residents inadequate.

The way of access to healthcare in relation to medical tourism is important parameter as well. Healthcare system in many countries allows access to some of these services but all-around world approaches differ. In addition, it differs widely according to healthcare diversity. The countries in which access to healthcare is guaranteed by the national policies will suffer less (or not at all, maybe even benefit) by growing presence of medical tourism. Those countries could experience more well-educated staff, new technologies and treatments present at their market, with no restrictions to use them. Competition could make this healthcare markets even better and more accessible. In countries where no national health insurance policies are present, the growing demand will allow medical tourism to expand, but the outcome could involve equation: more money – more services. Thus, the healthcare access will be as equal insofar as the differences between rich and poor are smaller. This does not necessarily mean that the presence of medical tourism will make more difference between rich and poorer. Maybe will be the reason for more output patients seeking the healthcare outside their country of residence.

Is the presence of medical tourism on healthcare market the reason to look the shortcomings or the benefits of it? Or we just should see the whole picture which shows the fact that medical tourism will not vanish, and the countries should only act in a sense of protecting patients, both incoming and domestic. We believe that healthcare access could greatly benefit by opening this kind of services to wider population while at the same time not endangering patient' safety. Good health insurance policies, certificates and well-defined services could best do this.

2.5.1 EU cross border healthcare directive 2011/24

Directive No. 2011/24/EU of March 9, 2011 [6] on patients' rights in cross-border healthcare aims to guarantee patient mobility and the free provision of healthcare services. The Directive contains provisions concerning the reimbursement of costs, the responsibilities of the Member States and their cooperation in healthcare. It has been applicable in the European member States since October 25, 2013, and in the European Economic Area* (Iceland, Liechtenstein, and Norway) since August 1st, 2015. However, it does not apply to Switzerland.

The main goal of this Directive is to facilitate access to "safe, high-quality cross-border healthcare and to promote healthcare-related cooperation between EU and EEA (Iceland, Liechtenstein, and Norway) member States, while maintaining each State's independent authority to organize and provide healthcare services".

According to the Directive, the patient is free to choose a healthcare provider or facility in either the public or the private sector, which correspond with the healthcare access, which does not make the difference between them. The patient will be reimbursed by the member State national health insurance, but the amount of money could differ – will be at least the price of the same service in resident county, or sometimes the full amount of the treatment received. If the patients receive the cross-border prescription for medication or medical device, the resident country must provide the follow-up care of same quality. State member is obliged to create National Contact Point responsible to inform patients of all of their rights. Directive also urged creation of updated "e-health" network in each country, which will enable continuity of care and access to high quality healthcare. Network among countries will also promote cooperation between competent centers and authorities, which was visible during COVID-19 pandemic, when EU states worked together and gave money for new treatment solutions (vaccines). Although we have witnessed intensive work on the vaccine in the last year, in previous years member States have also dealt with rare diseases, as one of the common concepts of access to health at European level. We can say Europe is already working on providing patients with "healthcare provider reference networks" and is promoting patient' mobility for expertise.

Directive 2011/24 EU covers all European Union citizens, nationals of the States of the European Economic Area (Iceland, Liechtenstein and Norway), refugees and stateless persons residing in a Member State of the European Union or the European Economic Area, who are or have been subject to the legislation of one or more Member States, as well as their family members and their survivors.

The Directive does not apply to long-term care (home care services), organ donations and public vaccination programs.

There are some good concepts in European' healthcare access policies that should be incorporate in medical tourism worldwide. However, we pointed out this Directive as a new medical tourism booster knowing that it will be difficult to copy-paste it in other continents lacking "Bismarck-like" health insurance model.

3. Health insurance

Medical tourism affects each country, but the challenges and advantages will differ based on specific health insurance. Likewise, state, non-state, individual, institutional levels of care and medical tourism market will engage healthcare system in different ways including profit, autonomy, and ethical aspects. All these relations will then ask for good funding and delivery models, incorporated in good insurance scheme.

Public healthcare systems are even more under the pressure to withstand the new era of globalized medicine [17]. Having in mind, that many countries do, and many do not have public healthcare coverage, the possible model for uniform approach to medical tourism insurances become questionable. In countries without public healthcare insurances, the use of external medical services could become more often but the system will not be burden – while the patients will pay for any consequence, visible after return, related to medical tourism treatment.

But those countries with public healthcare insurances will face another level of problems associated with medical tourism – the cost of all the consequences related to safety and efficacy that will emerge after the patient' return if he/she decided to use the treatment outside the country of residence. Notably, the patients from countries without national healthcare coverage will seek different treatments based on the price and availability [8]. This is something what Europe is prevented by its multilateral agreements on using national healthcare coverage across the border [6].

Health insurance is a data-driven business, and the more the data are organized and available, the more the insurance will be specific for the treatment. Traditional health insurance product design and pricing rely on gather and analyze the past data (e.g., past claims) of a healthcare access of certain population. The main question they answer is how many times? So, how many times a year the patient will use access to general practitioner, specialist, and hospital? The second question is how much? How much will each healthcare access cost? So, if there are not enough and/or reliable information on cross-border healthcare access than the health insurance policy could not be very precise. Then the next question is raised: How much such health insurance cost? Today' insurance companies offer coverage for expenses made due to medical tourism, making efforts to reduce costs, but mainly they do so by their own – no policies or laws almost nowhere are implemented in a way to protect nor the individual nor the system.

While there is difference between countries, the calculation is even more difficult. Today, the cross-border health insurance is typically a more rewarding product than a purely domestic product line. Thus, it is important to understand the local context of the country where the medical treatment is taking place, and to know how the healthcare access in this particular country is organized.

Most health insurance products cover treatment received solely in the customers' main country of residence. Some offer cross-border coverage, like those offered to the expatriate employees of multinational corporations, which give them healthcare access to the nearest centers of medical excellence in their region.

In time, the patients will increasingly be looking abroad for medical care, as they realize that the quality of treatment (physicians, drugs, devices, etc.) or the lower price, or the quicker access they are looking for is often not available locally (or the waiting list is too long). This also presents opportunities for hospitals, accreditation bodies and funders (e.g., insurance companies).

Safety and efficacy may not be the first parameter for choosing the treatment. Being used to get the appropriate care through the national healthcare system may make the patients to risk more. Therefore, the risks related to the medical tourism should be anticipated. For example, the entire documentation patient should carry with, the type of insurance, additional costs, post-operative care and complications. This is separate from medical malpractice insurance, which the doctors cover by own insurance - it only covers the consequences of "no fault" complications, not negligence. This will help the overall medical tourism industry to standardize all the elements related to the trip of their patients: travelers' choices, booking, treatments payment, insurance, language, etc.

A special section represents travel medical insurance. It pays for emergency medical expenses during a trip. If you are traveling and have an unexpected illness, injury or medical condition that is covered by your travel medical insurance, the plan will reimburse you, up to the plan limits. Travel medical insurance pays "reasonable and customary" charges for bills such as: ambulance service, doctor bills, hospital and operating room charges, X-rays, examinations, treatments, lab tests and anesthetics, drugs and medicines. However, this kind of travel insurance does not count as medical tourism as the main trigger for the trip taken was not a medical procedure of any kind.

4. Accreditations and certificates

Healthcare access enhanced and improved by assigned international accreditations and certificates could make a great impact on in- and specially out-patients service satisfaction.

Obviously, the global medical tourism will not affect all national healthcare systems and institutions in the same way, but a possibility of affecting the national healthcare access must be anticipated. Thus, the accreditations and certificates are needed.

There are world organizations referred as examples that publish accreditation. The oldest international accreditation organization is in Canada, accreditations Canada. They made the first accreditation in 1968 for a hospital in Bermuda. In USA operates accreditation body Joint Commission International (JCI), and this organization provides inspections and accreditation to institutions outside the USA since 1999. In United Kingdom (UK) operates Quality Healthcare Advice Trent Accreditation. The Australian Council on Healthcare Standards (ACHS) is a well-known authorized accreditation organization with the Australian Commission on Safety and Quality in Healthcare. The number of internationally accredited medical centres worldwide has witnessed substantial growth, for example, JCI accredits 100 new centres annually and covers 66 countries.

Unfortunately, there is no organization officially and universally recognized and responsible for such accreditation. Therefore, it is common to see health institutions that are interested in double/multiple accreditations, for US, UK and EU market, to reach patients from different parts of the world. Likewise, there are no necessary demands to obtain accreditation for service of medical tourism providers. This situation affects the consumers to choose the destination and the service without quantitative and/or qualitative information about clinical quality and related outcomes [3].

When a national healthcare system as a whole or an individual health institution is deciding on type of accreditation or certificate, they mostly ask for these main conditions and procedures to be covered by accreditation / certification process is standard of care and patients' safety including:

- ensure safe surgery
- reducing risk of healthcare-associated infections
- reducing the risk of patient harm resulting from falls
- improving the safety of high-alert medications
- improving effective communication.

However, what most present accreditation and certification organizations do not cover, as there is also no demand from healthcare systems or institutions at this time, is:

- hospital insurance coverage for all of its parts included in medical tourism services provided
- telemedicine, if incorporated in hospital work, should be seen as an advantage that reduce the cost of insurance, especially for post-treatment complications, while will allow doctors to follow-up their patients without additional cost of e.g., prolonged stay
- the number and severity of post-treatment complications tracked
- routine follow-up related to post-treatment care and complications arising from medical procedures performed abroad should be emphasized, identified and addressed
- secured funds that will assure medical tourist that any complication will be promptly covered, no matter insurance reimbursement protocol
- surveillance of contracts with agencies providing medical tourism services (buyers).

International accreditation also could be seen as a great marketing tool for incoming patients. However, problems related to accreditation process involve difference between countries (developed/non-developed), institutions in charge for accreditation (public/private or national/international), and the choice of criteria for accreditation. Good criteria for accreditation in medical tourism will incorporate the healthcare globalization processes preventing at the same time the unwanted consequences of medical tourism.

5. Conclusion

Today the term global health is mostly perceived as a part of public health where all the efforts are made to preserve overall health of the population due to socio-environmental impacts. However, the term reflects the efforts made by the national healthcare systems to protect the health of their citizens especially related to the global burden of disease (GBD). Thus, to understand the difference, it is important to see the medical tourism as a part of globalized medicine. It encompasses individual effort made by the single patient to improve his health. This makes medical tourism an important issue for national healthcare system in relation to in- and out-patients. In addition, it affects global health as well, while global health is easily imbalanced by supply/demand of medical services.

Numerous ethical questions on inequity of healthcare access for local residents could arise: drain of the professionals into private sector, fewer services in national sector, better technologies in private, etc. In vice versa situation, where patients are using medical treatments abroad, the system could easily be burden by costs arising from treating post complications due to medical tourism once they are back home.

However, these processes/challenges can help to facilitate creation of policies. Namely, knowing that different types of healthcare systems will be under the different types of demands for medical tourism could affect health insurance policies specifically.

Missing unified standards for, both, patients and organizations involved in medical tourism could bring enormous medical, legal and ethical risks in the future. Further on, having no unified terminology, or safety, legal and ethical standards is the reason why related problems remains unsolved. The accelerating growth in medical tourism industry, enhance urgent need for supporting measures that will ensure patient' safety at any level.

To create safe environment for this new, fast-growing industry, globally unified accreditation for all included services/facilities are needed. In order to preserve public safety, availability of healthcare and to give excellent service, global standardization and accreditation is expected to be most urgent processes that should be done in any country positioning itself as a medical tourism destination. Harmonized propositions for medical tourism industry access covered by both, private and public health insurances, would contribute to service transparency, physician' and management' liability, and patient safety while taking care of moral aspects of such services. Medical tourism without any doubt impacts access to healthcare. Therefore, if consciously incorporated, medical tourism as a part of global healthcare could easily become an efficient and effective additional access to healthcare.

Acknowledgements

Authors would like to thank Energy Clinic, luxury wellness spa chain in Croatia, for their donation for publishing this chapter.

Conflict of interest

The authors declare no conflict of interest.

Author details

Iskra Alexandra Nola[1] and Zdeslav Radovčić[2]*

1 School of Medicine, Andrija Stampar School of Public Health, University of Zagreb, Zagreb, Croatia

2 Energy Clinic Wellness Academy, Dubrovnik, Croatia

*Address all correspondence to: zdeslav@energyclinic.com

References

[1] Kelley E, WHO Patient Safety Programme Medical Tourism [Internet]. [cited May 19; 2019]. Available from: http://www.who.int/global_health_histories/seminars/kelley_presentation_medical_tourism.pdf

[2] Freire NA. The Emergent Medical Tourism: Advantages and Disadvantages of the Medical Treatments Abroad. Int Bus Res [Internet]. 2012 Jan 29; 5(2): p 41. Available from: http://www.ccsenet.org/journal/index.php/ibr/article/view/14582

[3] Radovcic Z, Nola IA. Medical tourism globe-trotting: Features, impacts, and risks. Vol. 13, International Journal of Healthcare Management. Taylor and Francis Ltd.; 2020. p. 94-100.

[4] Lunt N, Lunt N, Smith R, Exworthy M, T S, Horsfall D, et al. Medical Tourism: Treatments, Markets and Health System Implications: A Scoping Review, Paris: Organisation for Economic Co-operation and Development. 2011. Available from: http://citeseerx.ist.psu.edu/viewdoc/summary?doi=10.1.1.372.3673

[5] Hip replacement costs select countries 2019|Statista [Internet]. Available from: https://www.statista.com/statistics/450373/cost-of-a-hip-replacement-in-various-countries/

[6] EUR-Lex: Access to European Union law [Internet]. Directive 2011/24/EU of the European Parliament and of the Council of 9 March 2011 on the application of patients' rights in cross-border healthcare. Off J Eur Union. 2011. Available from: http://data.europa.eu/eli/dir/2011/24/oj

[7] Olkiewicz M. The impact of medical tourism on the quality of organizational and functional changes in the Polish healthcare system. UTMS J Econ/Univ Tour Manag Int Multidiscip J area south Southeast Eur. 2016; 7(1).

[8] Johnston R, Crooks VA, Snyder J, Kingsbury P. What is known about the effects of medical tourism in destination and departure countries? A scoping review. Int J Equity Health. 2010; 9.

[9] Health at a Glance: Europe 2020 [Internet]. OECD; 2020. (Health at a Glance: Europe). Available from: https://www.oecd-ilibrary.org/social-issues-migration-health/health-at-a-glance-europe-2020_82129230-en

[10] Snyder J, Crooks VA, Johnston R, Adams K, Whitmore R. Medical tourism's impacts on health worker migration in the Caribbean: Five examples and their implications for global justice. Vol. 8, Global Health Action. Co-Action Publishing; 2015.

[11] Ageing Europe - looking at the lives of older people in the EU - Eurostat 2019 report | AGE Platform [Internet]. Available from: https://www.age-platform.eu/publications/ageing-europe-looking-lives-older-people-eu-eurostat-2019-report

[12] Ageing Europe — 2019 edition - Products Statistical Books - Eurostat [Internet]. Available from: https://ec.europa.eu/eurostat/web/products-statistical-books/-/KS-02-19-681

[13] Eurostat. Your key to European statistics. Available from: https: //ec.europa.eu/eurostat

[14] Petersen PE, Bourgeois D, Ogawa H, Estupinan-Day S, Ndiaye C. The global burden of oral diseases and risks to oral health. Bulletin of the World Health Organization. 2005;(83):661-669.

[15] Platform for better oral health in europe [Internet]. Available from: http://www.oralhealthplatform.eu/

[16] Chen YYB, Flood CM. Medical Tourism's Impact on Health Care Equity

and Access in Low- and Middle-Income Countries: Making the Case for Regulation. J Law, Med Ethics [Internet]. 2013 Mar;41(1):286-300. Available from: https://pubmed.ncbi.nlm.nih.gov/23581671/

[17] Béland D, Zarzeczny A. Medical tourism and national health care systems: An institutionalist research agenda. Global Health. 2018 Jul 16;14(1).

Chapter 19

Ethical Deliberation in the Allocation of Respirators and Beds during the Covid-19 Pandemic in Brazil

Maristela Rodrigues Marinho, Sandra Pinto, Juliana Dias Reis Pessalacia, Priscila Kelly da Silva Neto, Marcela Tavares de Souza and Tatiana Carvalho Reis Martins

Abstract

This chapter proposes a theoretical reflection on the ethical deliberation process in the allocation of beds and respirators, in the light of the Theory of Health Justice, the Accountability for Reasonableness approach and the principle of health equity of the Brazilian Unified Health System (SUS, as per its Portuguese acronym), before the COVID-19 pandemic in Brazil. The pandemic has become a serious threat to health systems, as installed capacity has been exceeded whether in terms of material resources, equipment, technology and human resources. Thus, according to the theory of Accountability for Reasonableness, a fair and deliberative process aims to ensure resource allocation through limits and constraints (reasonableness), but government responsibility derived from human rights must be considered, allowing for health programming (accountability). Faced with this scenario, where the situation will often require us to make choices, this chapter intends to discuss the assumptions for ethical deliberation, taking into account the context of the act and its foreseeable consequences.

Keywords: Equity in Access to Health Services, Resource Allocation, Social Justice, Coronavirus Infections, Pandemic

1. Introduction

Throughout December 2019, in Wuhan city, Hubei province, Chinese health authorities identified pneumonia cases of unknown aetiology, which were subsequently attributed to the emergence of a new coronavirus (SARS-Cov-2) [1]. The World Health Organisation (WHO) has declared a state of public health emergency of international concern. Originally called 2019 - n - CoV, the infection caused by the new coronavirus was officially named COVID-19 on 11th March 2020, when it was declared a pandemic [2].

According to the Ministry of Health, in Brazil, until 28th April 2021, 14,521,289 confirmed cases of infection by COVID-19 had been notified, with 79,726 deaths [3]. This advance has led government agencies to adopt strategies to control the spread of the virus, such as closing schools and shops, banning meetings, instituting teleworking, isolating people in their homes, and also banning international and even national travels [2].

The Brazilian Unified Health System (SUS, as per its Portuguese acronym) has always been at the front line of public health emergencies in Brazil and it has not been different in the context of facing the COVID-19 pandemic. It is one of the largest health systems in the world and the fight against the pandemic has integrated all levels of healthcare, based on its guidelines and principles described in the organic laws of health n° 8080 and n° 8142, dated 1990 [4, 5]. SUS must respond in a planned, systematised and equitable way to this new challenge imposed.

In an analysis of SUS, in its 30 years of existence, the system's lack of priority and underfunding, associated with the country's economic crisis and especially, the Constitutional Amendment 95 (EC-95/2016), which freezes the public budget for twenty years, were highlighted as factors detrimental to the system [6]. Thus, the system is overloaded and, faced with the new pandemic context, needs investment in material resources and equipment, as well as physical and human resources [7].

In the context of the pandemic in China, substantial regional disparities in the availability and accessibility of health resources were observed that could partially explain the low mortality rates (despite the large number of cases) in the more developed provinces, such as Zhejiang (zero deaths among 1,171 confirmed cases) and Guangdong (four deaths among 1,322 cases). Following analysis of this data, the Chinese government moved to rapidly build new local medical facilities in the less developed provinces, a key measure that helped control the epidemic, protect front-line health professionals and mitigate the severity of the disease in patients [8].

A reflection was introduced by health professionals from the United States on the need for resources to care for a large number of patients with COVID-19 after the declaration of the pandemic in the country, questioning how prepared the US hospitals were in relation to material and human resources in the face of uncontrolled transmission of the virus and consequent challenges in clinical decision making. In moments of crisis, health resources must be allocated in an ethical, rational and structured way, so as to benefit a greater number of patients. It is pointed out that the main conflict in decision making is the definition of ethical criteria for the allocation of mechanical ventilation equipment and beds in Intensive Care Units (ICU) [1].

We need to think about what ethical duties should be observed in this scenario, when the health system is being demanded beyond its capacity. How to allocate resources equitably, ensuring resources to all levels of care and regions? [2].

In pandemic contexts, there is a direct concern with equity in the use of resources as a moral and legal imperative to respect, protect and fulfil human rights in relation to health service delivery, based on international norms and standards. Nevertheless, in relation to the human rights-based approach, "even if attention is paid to the philosophical foundations linked to relevant rights recognised in international law, this does not provide guidance on how these relevant rights help determine priorities among claimants" [9].

General theories of justice alone do not provide adequate guidance for the problem of priority setting. This is because these theories are too broad to provide precise answers to the key distributional questions necessary for priority setting. However, the Accountability for Reasonableness approach, suggested by Daniels, guides prioritisation and is consistent with human rights due to its concern with justice and the social determinants in its process, which enables it to be applied to health systems [9].

Accordingly, this chapter proposes a theoretical reflection on the process of ethical deliberation in the allocation of ICU beds and respirators, in the light of the Theory of Health Justice [10] and Accountability for Reasonableness approach [9], both proposed by the American philosopher and politician Norman Daniels; and the principle of SUS equity, before the COVID-19 pandemic in Brazil.

2. Ethical models of justice and allocation of scarce resources in pandemic situations

In this theoretical reflection, the relationship between the allocation of health resources in the context of the pandemic in an equitable way was constructed based on the work *Just health: meeting health needs fairly* [10], proposed by Norman Daniels, which discusses his theory of health justice, and on the work *Justice and Human Rights: Priority Setting and Fair Deliberative Process* [9], produced by the author in partnership with the academic lawyer Sofia Gruskin, which introduce the Accountability for Reasonableness approach.

Norman Daniels is a philosopher who works at Harvard University in the United States of America (USA) and is specialist in Bioethics. In his first work that addressed the topic of justice for health, Daniels described a deliberative process based on human rights and the principle of justice, through which health priorities would be set up to guide political decisions [11].

Daniels [10] resumes this work through other constructions in which the ideas are reformulated responding to several criticisms from various authors, at which point he explains that certain theories of justice do not contemplate the premise of equity. The author explains that a fair health process should ensure the legitimacy and fairness of decisions involving the definition of limits in the distribution of resources. In the field of health sciences, his books and articles have been widely cited in scientific publications that discuss the allocation of health resources from the principle of justice. In one of his articles, he emphasises the need to gather scientific evidence on the results of applying the "accountability for reasonableness" model to improve the legitimacy of decision-making health processes [12].

As a human rights-based approach, we suggest the following ones as key elements of Accountability for Reasonableness: 1. Direct concern for equity in the use of resources; 2. Examination of factors that may constrain or support planned interventions, including the legal, political, economic, social, and cultural context; 3. Participation and negotiation among all stakeholders, even if the primary responsibility lies with government officials to facilitate these processes and determine which interventions can have the greatest and best health impacts; and 4. Government responsibility and accountability for the way decisions are made, resources are allocated, and programmes implemented and evaluated, including the impact of these decisions on health and well-being [9].

A fair and deliberative process developed as a form of procedural justice to set limits under resource constraints must be complemented with measures to ensure appropriate stakeholder involvement and governmental responsibility derived from human rights. This description of fair process provides a coherent rationale for emphasising the key components of a human rights-based approach. At the same time, the emphasis on government responsibility operationalises the outcome of calling for a fair process. The combined approach makes the content and justification for the progressive improvement or realisation of a human right to health clearer. It is believed that "the result is generally politically feasible and can provide appropriate guidance to policy planners and implementers concerned with improving the health of the population in a fair way" [9].

The main idea behind Accountability for Reasonableness is that people are able to agree and justify, even when resources are limited, the reasons for the priorities they determine are necessary to meet health needs fairly. The following four conditions make the notion of Accountability for Reasonableness [9] more precise: 1. Publicity condition: decisions that set priorities for meeting health needs and their justifications must be accessible to the public; 2. Relevance condition: decisions on priorities should be supported by a reasonable explanation of why they were selected and determined; thus, a justification is reasonable if it appeals to accepted evidence, reasons and principles, including a wide range of stakeholders in decision making; 3. Review and appeal condition: there should be mechanisms for contestation and dispute and, more broadly, opportunities for review and improvement of policies in the light of new evidence or arguments; and 4. Regulatory condition: there should be public oversight of the process to ensure that conditions 1, 2 and 3 are met [9].

Thus, by forming a public record of decisions and the reasons behind them, the reasoning applied to priority setting can be improved over time. The involvement of various stakeholders in the process is not only useful to ensure that a range of relevant arguments and interests are considered, but also enables adherence and enhances legitimacy, even when the difficulties inherent in ensuring the presence and hearing of vulnerable groups are recognised. All these conditions fit well with the main elements of a human rights approach [9].

The philosopher also addresses global justice and its implications for health inequalities and human rights, emphasising that it can be applied in the reform of health systems and in the definition of health priorities. He also reflects that we cannot speak of a theory of justice for health without understanding the importance of global justice and social determinants, and that these can be protected when the appropriate health policy is adopted. When reflecting on professional obligations related to justice, he questions whether they should follow the population's point of view, which addresses the issue of social justice, or whether they should meet health needs depending on severity criteria, not taking into account other facts about the individual. It also points out that medical professionals are not in a position to judge and should not consider their judgements to indicate their recommendations [13].

2.1 Ethical and fair deliberation in the allocation of scarce resources in the COVID-19 pandemic

A scenario devastated by COVID-19 is in place and we are living a great dilemma: how to allocate scarce health resources in the face of this situation? Although SUS has its foundations based on principles, it has been facing significant annual losses in budgetary resources. It is known that pandemics caused by viruses are serious threats to health systems by imposing excessive demands that exceed the installed capacity both in terms of material resources and human resources [13].

According to a reflective study, several healthcare services in Brazil suffer from a lack of essential materials and equipment for care in this pandemic. This risky situation, without advance planning, can lead to waste of resources, damaging the confidence of health service users and professionals, in addition to causing loss of life. In light of the above, the system and service providers must be prepared to make the most of limited resources in order to reduce the damage to the system, people and society [13].

Those faced with pressing practical decisions about priorities in health resource allocation need an approach that provides guidance and enhances perceptions of legitimacy and justice; however, neither human rights nor general principles of distributive justice alone are sufficient to solve disagreements when setting priorities.

Any legitimate solution must make its prioritisation path sufficiently clear, so that everyone involved perceive it as fair and justified [9].

The Pan American Health Organisation (PAHO) [14] analysed a database of patients with COVID-19 and found that 19.4% of cases will present a mild condition; 40% a moderate condition; 15% a severe condition, requiring hospital admission; and 5% a critical condition, requiring mechanical ventilation. Thus, the need for expansion of care capacity can be divided into: patients with a mild or moderate condition, requiring home isolation and monitoring of symptoms; patients with a moderate or severe condition, requiring pharmacological treatment and clinical admission; and critically ill patients, requiring admission with mechanical ventilation and specialised intensive care capacity.

According to Cabral *et al.* [7], most health institutions do not have the capacity to meet an excessively high demand, as happens in pandemics, causing a lack of equipment and beds. What can we do before this dilemma of scarcity of resources?

Some strategies are being held, such as social distancing, which promotes the flattening of the epidemic curve and reduces demand on the health system. There are other important strategies to be used to solve resource allocation issues, such as, for example, the exercise of authority by the managers of the various spheres, in the mobilisation of industries for the rapid supply of resources; displacement of inputs and human resources from more affected areas to those of higher incidence; postponement of elective and non-emergency examinations and procedures [2].

In Brazil, Law n° 13979 was published on 6th February 2020, providing for measures to address the public health emergency of international importance resulting from the new coronavirus. The law sets out some strategies such as isolation, quarantine, medical examinations, laboratory tests, vaccination and cancellation of elective surgeries and examinations. It also waives bidding for the acquisition of goods and services to address the public health emergency. Furthermore, it determines exceptional and temporary authorisation for the importation and distribution of any materials, medicines, equipment and inputs in the area of health subject to sanitary surveillance, without registration with the Brazilian National Health Surveillance Agency (ANVISA, as per its Portuguese acronym), considered essential to assist in combating the COVID-19 pandemic, provided that justified by the competent authority. Another measure adopted is the exceptional and temporary restriction of highways, ports or airports, as long as recommended by ANVISA [15].

Protecting public health can mean protecting people of greater social vulnerability and those who are institutionalised, considering that the spread of the virus occurs rapidly in these places. In addition, resources need to be rapidly allocated to places where outbreaks occur, thus reducing the transmission of the infection and the hospitalisation rate. Priority groups also deserve attention, especially people with comorbidities, since they are more likely to fall ill and pass away. Finally, we must not forget the demands of social justice, ensuring the poorest and most marginalised a fair distribution of resources [2].

Thus, Gruskin and Daniels [9] warn that it is necessary to implement a fair deliberative process, developed as a form of procedural justice to set limits under resource constraints. In addition, they argue that this process should be complemented with human rights measures to ensure exclusion of discrimination, requiring the participation of affected populations in relevant decision making.

In the context of the pandemic in Italy, in the period of the greatest contagion of the virus, although the health system was highly efficient, it was impossible to meet the needs of the high number of critically ill patients simultaneously, during the peak of the pandemic, because they required more complex and expensive technologies [16]. Due to examples of nations that have already experienced this situation of overloaded health services, the rulers of many countries are concerned about their population, considering that, if there is a high number of severe cases, many people may die because there will not be sufficient mechanical ventilators and ICU beds. In this type of public health emergency, the ethical obligation of health professionals to prioritise the well-being of individual patients may be overridden by public health policies that prioritise the greatest good for the greatest number of patients. These circumstances raise a critical question: when demand for ventilators and other intensive care far exceed supply, what criteria should guide these rationing decisions? [17].

Faced with this scenario, where the situation will often require us to make choices, we ask: what are the assumptions for deliberation at this juncture, taking into account the context of the act and its foreseeable consequences?

A fair and deliberative process aims to ensure resource allocation through limits and restrictions (reasonableness), but it must consider governmental responsibility by allowing for health programming (accountability) [10]. This ensures a fair correlation for the operationalisation of health resources. For PAHO, the implementation of public policies should consider aspects such as universality, equality and non-discrimination, access to ensure mechanisms and social participation [18].

Thus, in the light of the theoretical frameworks of this reflection, we propose practical guidelines for health decision making, considering the context of scarcity of intensive care beds and equipment during the pandemic period of COVID-19 in Brazil, highlighting that some recommendations are suggested by authors and organisations from various countries. In order to demonstrate this information in a clearer way, we designed the following flowchart (**Figure 1**).

In order to hold the allocation and use of resources in a more just and ethical way during the pandemic, some factors must be considered, such as: assessing life expectancy in the short and long term, taking into account the current illness and comorbidities, using validated instruments; estimating life expectancy, prioritising patients with the probability of surviving longer after treatment; considering the right to live the complete life cycle; and identifying irreversible cases that should be referred for Palliative Care [13].

Thus, moral deliberation can be seen as a systematised and contextualised means for the critical and public analysis of life events, considering the values and duties involved in a concrete fact and seeking to understand them by listening and exchanging opinions and arguments between the parties, in order to guide a situation along a reasonable, prudent and feasible path, but without claiming to find the ideal or right decision. For a solution, ethical problems need constant and continuous assessment. The use of the deliberative procedure proposed by Diego Gracia for clinical bioethics in 1992 and 2020 proposes three distinct moments of human intelligence: the cognitive moment (facts), the valuation, estimation or preferences (values) and the realisation (duty, voluntary act) [19].

Even though resource constraints may not allow for a fully deliberate and equitable process in all cases, accountability for reasonableness helps reduce much of this imprecision by providing an explicit record of how alternatives are chosen. Over time, this record can reveal the true commitments to change that a government is able and willing to make [10].

One of the necessary conditions of the Accountability for Reasonableness approach proposed by Norman Daniels is that decisions on priority setting should provide a reasonable explanation of why the selected priorities were determined to be the best approach. It is also important to consider that, specifically, a justification is reasonable if it appeals to evidence, reasons and principles accepted as relevant by fair-minded people. The inclusion of a wide range of stakeholders in decision making is closely linked to this condition [9].

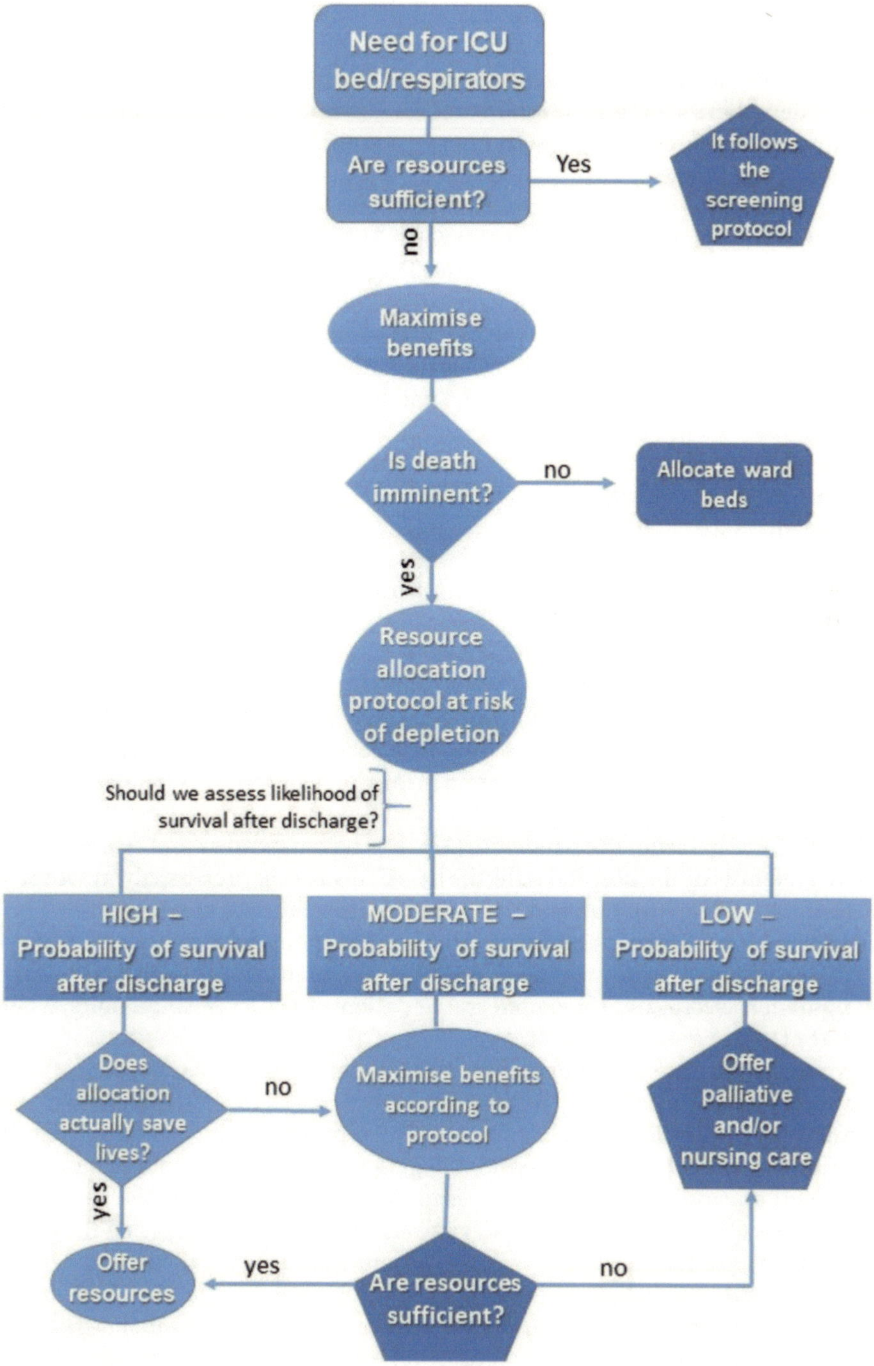

Figure 1.
Practical guidance for health decision making during the period of scarcity.

According to Gruskin and Daniels [9], a fair process, involving human rights, calls for negotiations among all stakeholders, even if the primary responsibility lies with government officials to facilitate these processes and determine which interventions may have the greatest health impacts. Thus, the involvement of various stakeholders in the process is not only useful to ensure that a range of relevant arguments and interests are considered, but also enables adherence and enhances legitimacy, even when the difficulties inherent in ensuring the presence and hearing of vulnerable groups are recognised. In addition, another condition pointed out by Norman Daniels in his approach is the condition of review and appeal where there should be mechanisms for contestation and dispute and, more broadly, opportunities for review and improvement of policies in the light of new evidence or arguments [12].

The allocation of scarce resources in the pandemic consists of four core values that have been applied in various ways such as: 1) benefit maximisation, offering priority to patients who are likely to survive longer after treatment; 2) treating people equally, implying random or first-come, first-served selection of people in similar conditions; 3) promoting instrumental value, prioritising those who can save others or rewarding those who have saved others in the past; and 4) prioritising those who are sickest or the youngest who will have a shorter life if they die without treatment [20].

Nevertheless, if resources are scarce, six recommendations are proposed that should be used to develop guidelines that can be applied fairly and consistently, these are: maximising benefits; prioritising health professionals; avoiding to allocate on a first-come, first-served basis; being responsive to evidence; recognising participation in research; and applying the same principles to all patients with or without COVID-19. It should also be noted that none of these recommendations alone will be sufficient to determine which patients will be prioritised [20].

In addition, the difficult decision on allocation of scarce resources should not fall on front-line professionals, since they are already overloaded with stress, which could cause failures. It is also necessary to prioritise health professionals in the allocation of treatments, aiming at their rapid recovery, due to the fact that they are the labour force in facing the pandemic [13]. It is recommended that two administrative references of the hospital hold the decision-making process, always informing the family of the situation and recording it in the patient's medical chart. The attributions of public health managers are also important in carrying out continuous monitoring of the resources used, enabling alignment of the protocol with the bed regulation system and timely referral of patients to other hospital units, when necessary [14].

We propose the use of protocols for decision making regarding the allocation of resources such as mechanical ventilators, considering situations where demand is greater than availability, and it is suggested that this policy be maintained while the pandemic lasts, always being decided together with the Superintendence/Board of Directors of each hospital. The process must be followed not only for cases of infection by COVID-19, but also for all critical cases [13]. Corroborating the previous statement, the fair allocation of resources must always be transparent, based on evidence and protocols and related to epidemiological data on morbidity and mortality. The population must always be included in the decision-making process [2]. The construction of an allocation protocol for depleting resources in situations of mass disasters and pandemics is not a merely technical task, but, on the contrary, must be grounded in ethical and legal principles commonly adopted at the international level [21].

Some values are fundamental in the development of protocols for resource allocation, the first value being that of justice in the distribution of resources, observing the duty to provide adequate care in any situation, managing resources, balancing equality and equity in their distribution. The second fundamental value is to ensure the maximisation of benefits, prioritising the good to the greatest number of people possible, recognising that resources should be directed to those who can really benefit, according to clinical evidence [13].

The US and UK advocate that resources should be allocated in a way that maximises the number of patients who survive treatment with reasonable life expectancy. Thus, experts state that removing a patient from a ventilator to provide it to other patients believed to be able to benefit rapidly, in order to maximise benefits, may be justifiable. Nevertheless, the potential for this decision disproportionately affects vulnerable populations, including older adults, people from minority communities or people with disabilities, and this decision is a major responsibility. Another concern is that pre-existing health disparities, fueled by inequitable social conditions, further harm certain vulnerable populations [22]. In April 2020, the first broad consensus of ethical recommendations for decision making in intensive care in pandemic situations was published by European scientific societies and institutes in the field of ethics. In general, the document proposes the application of the principle of distributive justice prioritising the best cost/opportunity and the principle of proportionality, eliminating conditions in which a minimal benefit is expected [23].

Managers and competent authorities are committed to increasing the supply of resources, making the need to use screening protocols as remote as possible, but we know that, with the progressive increase of severe cases, we must be prepared to use them [14]. The situation that several countries, including Brazil, have experienced due to the scarcity imposed by the COVID-19 pandemic highlights the need to develop a screening protocol based on ethical-legal principles. In addition, screening decisions must be made by independent teams that include medical specialists, legal counsel and health system administrators. These teams are responsible for repeatedly assessing the priority of patients. This practice is recommended in protocols widely adopted in the USA [22]. This team should be properly trained to perform its role, from protocol management to conflict resolution and communication with patients and families [21].

In order to protect vulnerable populations from injustice, health systems are encouraged to adopt transparent and evidence-based screening protocols that classify patients according to priority levels [22]. Nevertheless, such protocols use physiological variables to assess which patients will benefit most, allowing for a supposedly objective prognosis. In order make these protocols work effectively, health systems and physicians need to know which allocation decisions actually save the most lives. Furthermore, poorly designed screening protocols that treat the fact of having a disability as a contraindication to receiving scarce resources, or that prioritise categories of people for withdrawal, could leave health systems subject to ethical and legal claims of unfair discrimination [22]. In Italy, at the start of the pandemic, age, number of comorbidities, severity of respiratory failure and the likelihood of surviving prolonged intubation were being considered, with the purpose of offering limited resources to those who would benefit most and have the greatest chance of survival [16].

Health systems can mitigate discriminatory screening policies by ensuring that each patient is assessed individually and that the results are used to create a transparent, evidence-based prognosis. Pre-existing disabilities may be relevant to ventilator withdrawal and reallocation, but only if they arise from an individualised assessment [22]. It is recommended that the screening method should not use social factors but rather an initial screening based on survival criteria such as the Clinical Frailty Scale, which can be applied for all ages or disease type [13]. The scale is a physical, cognitive and functional assessment tool. In order to perform the allocation of resources, the scale score can be taken into account, generating a degree of priority. The Brazilian Intensive Care Medicine Association (AMIB, as per its Portuguese acronym) recommends the use of assessment instruments of severity scores such as Sequential Organ Failure Assessment (SOFA) and Acute Physiology and Chronic Health Evaluation (APACHE) by the screening teams. These instruments stratify the degree of severity of organ dysfunctions manifested by a patient. Screening protocols should include frequent and constant reassessment of ICU patients, avoiding dysthanasia [21].

The consensus of ethical recommendations related to intensive care, mentioned above, demonstrates the application of the principle of justice in a uniform way to all people suggesting to unlink the chronological age criterion as the only strategy, incorporating other variables such as the degree of frailty, biological age, as well as the patient's values and preferences, so that decision making occurs in a shared way among the team members and, whenever possible, with the patient and family through a respectful, transparent and trusting communication. For patients presenting acute respiratory failure, the consensus brings a screening model for ICU admission based on four prioritisation categories according to the patient's characteristics and current condition and for scarce allocation of respirators. Regarding mechanical ventilation of these patients, we propose an adaptation of the screening process based on the person's characteristics, encompassing the presence of several pathological processes different from the current ones and measurable by Charlson Severity Scale [23].

In its guiding document, AMIB considers that there are limitations to prepare screening protocols. First, preparing an ethically perfect protocol is impossible, considering that we live in a plural society. Another limitation is the absence of validated instruments to be used in screening. Nonetheless, in view of the pandemic situation of COVID-19 and the imminent depletion of equipment, especially mechanical ventilators, we must consider that there is not enough time for validation processes and, therefore, the use of instruments should always be monitored and followed-up through other assessment strategies. In light of the above, public debate and reviews of screening protocols are necessary to contribute to an ethical legitimacy of the process [21]. The Ethics Committees also work as deliberative advisors in moral conflicts of the clinic, in addition to helping health professionals and users in the learning of possibilities of alternatives of prudent solutions to be applied for each case [19].

3. Conclusion

This study has introduced theoretical reflections on the process of ethical deliberation in the allocation of beds and intensive care equipment, in the light of the Theory of Health Justice, the Accountability for Reasonableness approach and the principle of SUS equity, before the COVID-19 pandemic.

From the publications found, we observed that government, administrators and service providers have been mobilised to protect public health, making the most of limited resources and protecting the most vulnerable people and those who are institutionalised, in order to reduce damage to health systems, individuals and society. Even so, it is clear that it is impossible to meet the needs of the contingent of critically ill patients simultaneously.

As the crisis has evolved, generally speaking, nations have favoured public health policies that prioritise the greatest good for the greatest number of patients in allocating resources through reasonableness, adopting limits and constraints and government responsibility, thus enabling human rights-based health programming.

Regardless of the ethical support, if there is a scarcity of resources, there are many scenarios that will seem morally unsustainable, especially in the face of greater prognostic uncertainty. We should keep in mind the recognition that no screening protocol available will be perfect and that there may be a much better chance of approaching reasonable deliberations when adopting a proposal that seeks a good ethical and technical basis and that are open to public scrutiny and individualised reviews involving legal counsel and health system administrators and where decision making occurs in a shared way among the team and, whenever possible, with the patient. Responsibility, cooperation and preparedness are necessary attitudes at this critical time of COVID-19 pandemic.

Author details

Maristela Rodrigues Marinho[1], Sandra Pinto[1], Juliana Dias Reis Pessalacia[1], Priscila Kelly da Silva Neto[1*], Marcela Tavares de Souza[1] and Tatiana Carvalho Reis Martins[2]

1 Nursing, Federal University of Mato Grosso do Sul, Três Lagoas, Brazil

2 Health Sciences, Federal University of Mato Grosso do Sul, Três Lagoas, Brazil

*Address all correspondence to: priscila.baldonado@gmail.com

References

[1] Chopra V, Toner E, Waldhorn R, Washer L. How Should U.S. Hospitals Prepare for Coronavirus Disease 2019 (COVID-19)? Ann Intern Med 2020;172:621-622. DOI: 10.7326/M20-0907.

[2] Gostin LO, Friedman EA, Wetter SA. Responding to Covid-19: How to Navigate a Public Health Emergency Legally and Ethically. Hastings Cent Rep 2020;50:8-12. DOI: 10.1002/hast.1090.

[3] Brasil. Ministério da Saúde. Painel de casos de doenças pelo coronavírus 2019 (COVID-19) no Brasil [Internet]. 2020. Available from: https://COVID.saude.gov.br/. [Accessed: 2021-03-07].

[4] Brasil. Lei nº 8.080 de 19 de setembro de 1990. Dispõe sobre as condições para a promoção, proteção e recuperação da saúde, a organização e o funcionamento dos serviços correspondentes e dá outras providências. Diário Oficial da União. 20 set 1990.

[5] Brasil. Lei 8.142 de 28 de dezembro de 1990. Dispõe sobre a participação da comunidade na gestão do Sistema Único de Saúde (SUS) e sobre as transferências intergovernamentais de recursos financeiros na área da saúde e dá outras providências.

[6] Paim JS. Sistema Único de Saúde (SUS) aos 30 anos. Cienc e Saude Coletiva 2018;23:1723-1728. DOI: 10.1590/1413-81232018236.09172018.

[7] Cabral ERM, Bonfada D, Melo MC, Cesar ID, Oliveira REM, Bastos TF, Bonfada D, Machado LO, Rolim ACA, Zago ACW. 2020. Contributions and challenges of the Primary Health Care across the pandemic COVID-19. InterAm J Med Heal, 2020;3:1-6. DOI: 10.31005/iajmh.v3i0.87.

[8] Ji Y, Ma Z, Peppelenbosch MP, Pan Q. Potential association between COVID-19 mortality and health-care resource availability. Lancet Glob Heal 2020;8:e480. DOI: 10.1016/S2214-109X(20)30068-1.

[9] Gruskin S, Daniels N. Process is the point: justice and human rights: priority setting and fair deliberative process. Am J Public Health 2008;98:1573-1577. DOI: 10.2105/AJPH.2007.123182.

[10] Rid A. Just health: meeting health needs fairly. Bull World Health Organ 2008;86:653. DOI: 10.2471/BLT.08.054601.

[11] Daniels N. Just healthcare. Cambridge University Press. Nova York: 1985; 408p.

[12] Daniels N. Legitimacy and fairness in priority setting in Tanzania. Glob Health Action 2011;4. DOI: 10.3402/gha.v4i0.8472.

[13] Satomi E, Souza PMR, Thomé BC, Reingenheim C, Werebe E, Troster EJ, et al. Fair allocation of scarce medical resources during COVID-19 pandemic: ethical considerations. Einstein (Sao Paulo) 2020;18. DOI: 10.31744/einstein_journal/2020ae5775.

[14] Organização Pan-Americana da Saúde. COVID-19 Recomendações para atendimento em situação de pico de demanda por cuidados médicos e alocação de equipes médicas de emergência Documento preliminar - [Internet]. 2020. Versão 2. Available from: https://iris.paho.org/bitstream/handle/10665.2/52013/OPASEOCCOVID19200004_por.pdf?sequence=1&isAllowed=y. [Accessed: 2021-03-07].

[15] Brasil. Lei nº 13.979 de 06 de Fevereiro de 2020. Dispõe sobre as medidas para enfrentamento da emergência de saúde pública de importância internacional decorrente do coronavírus. Brasília: 2020. Available

from: http://www.planalto.gov.br/CCIVIL_03/_Ato n.d. [Accessed: 2021-04-18].

[16] Rosenbaum L. [Facing Covid-19 in Italy: ethics, logistics, and therapeutics on the epidemic's front line]. Recenti Prog Med 2020;111:192-197. DOI: 10.1701/3347.33179.

[17] White DB, Lo B. A Framework for Rationing Ventilators and Critical Care Beds During the COVID-19 Pandemic. JAMA 2020;323:1773-1774. DOI: 10.1001/jama.2020.5046.

[18] Organização Pan-Americana da Saúde. Guia para Implementação das Prioridades Transversais na OPAS/OMS do Brasil: direitos humanos, equidade, gênero e etnicidade e raça. Brasília: OPAS; 2018.

[19] Zoboli E. A aplicação da deliberação moral na pesquisa empírica em bioética. Rev Iberoam Bioética 2016:1-19. DOI: 10.14422/rib.i02.y2016.006.

[20] Emanuel EJ, Persad G, Upshur R, Thome B, Parker M, Glickman A, et al. Fair Allocation of Scarce Medical Resources in the Time of Covid-19. N Engl J Med 2020;382:2049-2055. DOI: 10.1056/NEJMsb2005114.

[21] AMIB (Associação de Medicina Intensiva Brasileira), ABRAMEDE (Associação Brasileira de Medicina de Emergência, SBGG (Sociedade Brasileira de Geriatria e Gerontologia) e ANCP (Academia Nacional de Cuidados Paliativos). Recomendações de alocação de recursos em esgotamento durante a pandemia por COVID-19 alocação de recursos [Internet]. 2020. Available from: https://www.amib.org.br/fileadmin/user_upload/amib/2020/abril/24/VJS01_maio_-_Versa__o_2_-_Protocolo_AMIB_de_alocac__a__o_de_recursos_em_esgotamento_durante_a_pandemia_por_COVID.pdf. [Accessed: 2021-03-10].

[22] Patterson R, Standing H, Lee M, Dalkin S, Lhussier M, Exley C, et al. Paramedic information needs in end-of-life care: a qualitative interview study exploring access to a shared electronic record as a potential solution. BMC Palliat Care 2019;18:108. DOI: 10.1186/s12904-019-0498-2.

[23] Rubio O, Estella A, Cabre L, Saralegui-Reta I, Martin MC, Zapata L, et al. Recomendaciones éticas para la toma de decisiones difíciles en las unidades de cuidados intensivos ante la situación excepcional de crisis por la pandemia por COVID-19: revisión rápida y consenso de expertos. Med Intensiva 2020;44:439-445. DOI:10.1016/j.medin.2020.04.006.

Chapter 20

Geospatial Clustering of Mobile Phone Use and Tuberculosis Health Outcomes among African Health Systems

Sunny Ibeneme, Nkiruka Ukor, Joseph Okeibunor and Felicitas Zawaira

Abstract

Background: While multiple studies have documented the impacts of mobile phone use on TB health outcomes for varied settings, it is not immediately clear what the spatial patterns of TB treatment completion rates among African countries are. This paper used Exploratory Spatial Data Analysis (ESDA) techniques to explore the clustering spatial patterns of TB treatment completion rates in 53 African countries as well as their relationships with mobile phone use. Using an ESDA approach to identify countries with low TB treatment completion rates and reduced mobile phone use is the first step towards addressing issues related to poor TB outcomes. **Methods**: TB notifications and treatment data from 2000 through 2015 obtained from the World Bank database were used to illustrate a descriptive epidemiology of TB treatment completion rates among African health systems. Spatial clustering patterns of TB treatment completion rates were assessed using differential local Moran's I techniques; and local spatial analytics was performed using local Moran's I tests. Relationships between TB treatment completion rates and mobile phone use were evaluated using ESDA approach. **Results**: Spatial autocorrelation patterns generated were consistent with Low-Low and High-Low cluster patterns and were significant at different p-values. Algeria and Senegal had significant clusters across the study periods, while Democratic Republic of Congo, Niger, South Africa, and Cameroon had significant clusters in at least two time-periods. ESDA identified statistically significant associations between TB treatment completion rates and mobile phone use. Countries with higher rates of mobile phone use, showed higher TB treatment completion rates overall, indicating enhanced program uptake ($P < 0.05$). **Conclusions:** Study findings provide systematic evidence to inform policy regarding investments in the use of mHealth to optimize TB health outcomes. African governments should identify turnaround strategies to strengthen mHealth technologies and improve outcomes.

Keywords: Africa, Health Systems, Tuberculosis, Mobile phone, Differential local Moran's I

1. Introduction

Mobile phones are becoming increasingly available and accessible globally. The global mobile phone subscription in 2009 was 68.0 per 100 inhabitants compared to 108 in 2019 corresponding to an overall 96% penetration rates[1]. In the African region, the estimated mobile phone penetration rate was 32.2% in 2008 compared to 85% in 2019 and is projected to rise to over 90% by 2025. The mobile broadband penetration rate also increased from 1.7% in 2008 to 30% in 2019 [1]. Many people who could not access fixed telephones for health informatics now use the mobile phone technology to access health services (mHealth). Compared to the wired information technology, the wireless technology is less expensive, more convenient, and readily accessible for individuals in many developing countries, including African countries [2, 3]. The mobile wireless technology has opportunities to facilitate communication among geographically isolated communities and could be harnessed to improve population health.

Mobile phones brought new opportunities for public health to Sub-Saharan Africa. With most of the African population in rural areas, mobile phone use has facilitated infectious disease management irrespective of geographical barriers [4–6]. Tuberculosis (TB) management is one area in which mobile phone use has shown great success because to effectively treat TB, patients must take four pills of anti-tuberculosis medications five times per week, for a period of 6 months [7]. This may create a high level of non-compliance to prescribed medications. Such protracted adherence could be facilitated by removing barriers to access and utilization through mHealth technologies [8]. In 2002, the South African government introduced the use of the mHealth technology, and computer databases to optimize TB treatment adherence. The database repeatedly lists patients who are due for their medications and an automatic Short-Message-Service (SMS) reminder sent to their mobile phones. This model enhanced treatment adherence and completion rates among sampled patients [7]. Thus, mobile phones provide platforms through which the SMS technology and other treatment-reminder protocols can be harnessed by TB patients to improve efficiency and optimize outcomes [6, 8]. Our study assumed that increased mobile phone use translates to broader access to TB services and represents the potential for impact on health with utilization of mobile phones to send/receive TB-related health information [9].

This study provides insight into the geospatial clustering of TB and mobile phone use among African health systems. Using an Exploratory Spatial Data Analytic (ESDA) approach, this study explored the spatial relationships between TB treatment completion rates and mobile phone use. Geospatial analytics of these concepts have opportunities to inform TB surveillance, intervention mapping and resource allocation. Moonan et al. conducted a geospatial epidemiological TB surveillance among newly diagnosed TB patients at the Tarrant County Health Department, Fort Worth, Dallas. Their model facilitated the identification of TB transmissions not identified during routine contact tracing. Thereby enabling the identification of at-risk populations, with an intervention mapping recommended for screening, treatment, and rehabilitation [10].

Conceptually, mobile phones facilitate information exchange and transfer without spatial barriers at high efficiency and low cost [4, 5]. Chadha et al. evaluated the effectiveness of the ComCare mobile application in coordinating TB referrals among patients in the Khunti District of India. It was discovered that the mobile

[1] Mobile phone penetration rate is the degree of diffusion of mobile phone use.

technology increased provider accountability and led to improved patient referral, retention, and treatment completion rates among network members [11]. Other researchers showed similar successes demonstrating the use of geospatial analytics in TB control, prevention, and management. Mwila and Phiri using geospatial analyses, cloud computing and web technologies modeled TB prevention strategies among developing countries. They explored ways to optimize TB monitoring and tracking protocols using technologies that display geographic distribution of TB cases on an mHealth application, while providing policy reports to inform intervention mapping activities [12]. While Yakam et al. spatially identified smear-positive pulmonary TB clusters among poor neighborhoods in Douala, Cameroon using mHealth technologies; Herrero et al. spatially explored cluster patterns of TB nonadherence and treatment dropouts in the metropolitan area of Buenos Aires, Argentina. Risk areas of nonadherence were characterized by poverty, ignorance, and reduced access to mHealth technologies [13, 14].

Multiple studies have documented the impact of mobile phone use on TB health outcomes for varied settings [11–14]. However, it is not immediately clear of the geospatial clustering patterns of TB treatment completion rates and mobile phone use among African countries. Previous studies have focused on evaluating TB medication access using geospatial disaggregated datasets of population characteristics [13, 15]. Hassarangsee et al. investigated the spatial detection and management of TB using information systems in the Si Sa Ket Province, Thailand [16]. However, the focus of this study is to evaluate the geospatial clustering patterns of TB treatment completion rates and mobile phone use among African health systems. It presents an exploratory spatial analysis of the relationships between TB treatment completion rates and mobile phone use for the countries in Africa. Using an ESDA approach to identify countries with low TB treatment completion rates and reduced mobile phone use could be the first step towards addressing issues related to poor TB outcomes. Thus, this presents an opportunity to identify African countries with limited resources and a high need for a wireless technology intervention.

2. Materials and methods

2.1 Data sources

Data for TB outcome and mobile phone use for African countries were obtained from the World Bank database [17] for the periods 2000 through 2015 (Supplementary Material—A). This study excluded one country due to incomplete data. In total, 53 countries representative of the African continent were included in this study. De-identified information was collated and aggregated per country and published at the end of each year by the World Bank, qualifying it as Institutional Review Board exempt [18].

2.2 Comparative statistical analyses

ArcGIS and GeoDa statistical software were used in all geospatial analyses which were performed in three stages and completed in November 2020. Univariate local Moran's I and global Moran's I were run on TB treatment completion rates separately. This was followed by a differential local Moran's I analysis to ascertain differential cluster patterns for different time-periods. Finally, spatial relationships between TB treatment completion rates and mobile phone use for year 2015 was evaluated using ESDA. To investigate treatment completion cluster patterns, spatial and tabular data were uploaded into ArcGIS 10.5.1. Geographically referenced data for TB treatment completion rates and mobile phone use for four time-periods (2000, 2005, 2010, 2015) were extracted for each country. These were added and joined to the African map by country shapefile and analyzed using an ESDA approach to visualize patterns and trends among geographically referenced data.

The Local Indicator of Spatial Association (LISA) represents the localized equivalent of the global Moran's I [19, 20]. For any location on a map, the LISA statistic measures and statistically tests the similarity of the geographically referenced data for that location (e.g., TB treatment completion rates at the source country) with the values of its corresponding local neighbors in space (surrounding countries). According to standard practice for reporting geospatial analytics, positive spatial autocorrelation is placed into High-High and Low-Low clusters; and negative spatial autocorrelation is placed into High-Low and Low-High outliers. High-High clusters denote above-average values of core countries versus surrounding countries. Low-Low clusters represent below average values of core countries versus surrounding countries. Low-High clusters means small changes among core countries versus high changes in the surrounding countries. Conversely, High-Low clusters means high changes among core countries versus small changes in the surrounding countries [20, 21]. For this study, a randomization of 999 permutations was used prior to result interpretations, and this study only analyzed observations with neighbors [20–22].

The Local Differential Moran's I (LDMI) statistic Eq. (1) measures if a variable change in space over time is related to its neighbors, and is calculated thus:

$$I_{D,i} = c\left(y_{i,t} - y_{i,t-1}\right)\sum_{j} w_{ij}\left(y_{j,t} - y_{j,t-1}\right) \tag{1}$$

Where y represents treatment completion rates for country i and neighbor j. The differential local Moran statistic I_D is generated based on change over time and is represented by the difference between yt and $yt\text{-}1$. The geospatial matrix (W_{ij}) is a binary spatial weights matrix. Under the queen first order principle, contiguous geospatial neighbors with common borders and vertex weights equals one. Therefore, observations that share common borders are considered neighbors for the calculation– all other locations are equals to zero [20, 21]. LDMI determines spatial autocorrelation on change over time ($y_t - y_{t-1}$). For this study, differential cluster patterns were evaluated between base time 0 (year 2000) and time 1 (year 2005), time 2 (year 2010) and time 3 (year 2015) respectively. Year 2000 was chosen as the base time because of data availability, which has been consistently captured for the 53 African countries included in this study [17]. Also, notable access to free anti-tuberculosis medications commenced in 2000 among most African health systems [23].

3. Results

Using geospatial data for 53 African countries for the periods 2000–2015, univariate global Moran's I values and associated pseudo p-values were computed and documented (Supplementary Material—B). In addition, LISA analytics identified different cluster patterns (Low-Low and High-Low) that were significant at different p-values (**Table 1**).

Figure 1 shows the clusters and significance levels of TB treatment completion rates in year 2000. Thirteen countries had significant clusters at different p-values including:

Figure 2 represents the clusters and significance levels of TB treatment completion rates in year 2005. Nine countries had significant cluster patterns at different p-values.

The clusters and significance levels of TB treatment completion rates for year 2010 are shown in **Figure 3**. Eight countries had significant clusters at different p-values.

The cluster patterns and significance levels of TB treatment completion rates for year 2015 are shown in **Figure 4**. Eight countries had significant clusters at different p-values.

	Variables	Moran's I value	Pseudo p-value
	TB_TreatmentCompletionRate_Yr2000	0.0190	0.021
Univariate Global Moran's I	TB_TreatmentCompletionRate_Yr2005	0.0177	0.032
	TB_TreatmentCompletionRate_Yr2010	0.0196	0.025
	TB_TreatmentCompletionRate_Yr2015	0.0179	0.031

Table 1.
Univariate global Moran's I result for the years 2000–2015.

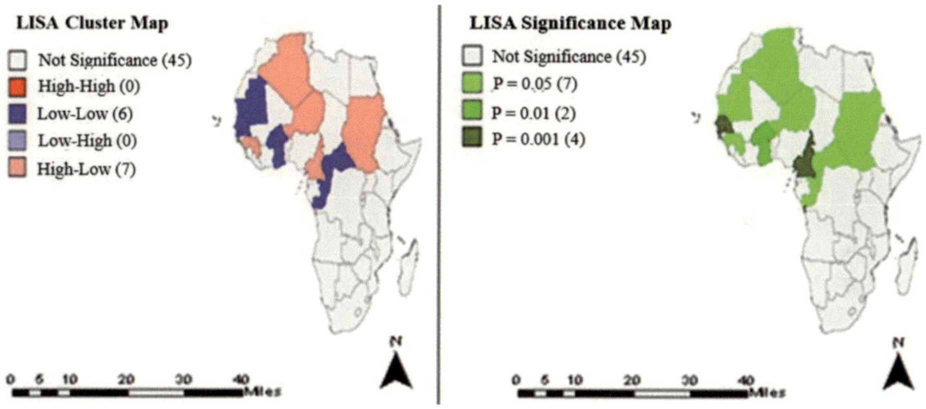

Figure 1.
Clusters and significance levels of TB treatment completion rates in year 2000.

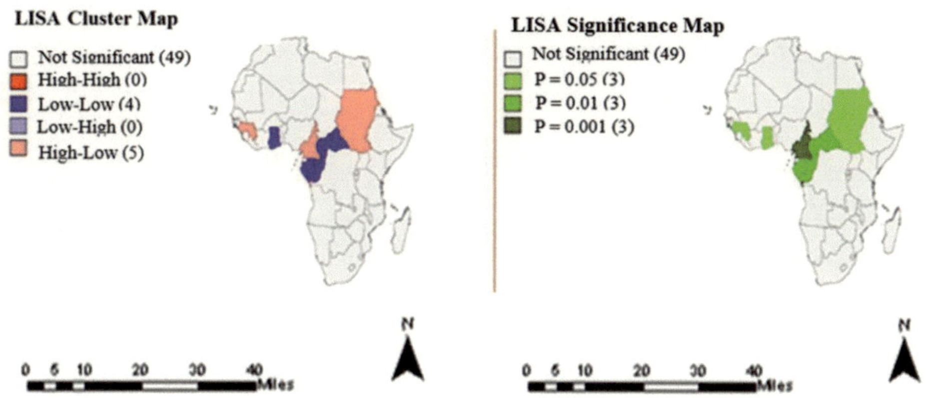

Figure 2.
Clusters and significance levels of TB treatment completion rates in year 2005.

3.1 Differential local Moran's I analyses

LDMI analytics identified different cluster patterns for the different time periods evaluated (**Tables 2–4**).

Table 2 represents LDMI results between time 0 (2000) and time 1 (2005). Algeria, Burkina Faso, and Senegal had significant clusters at different p-values (Supplementary Material—C).

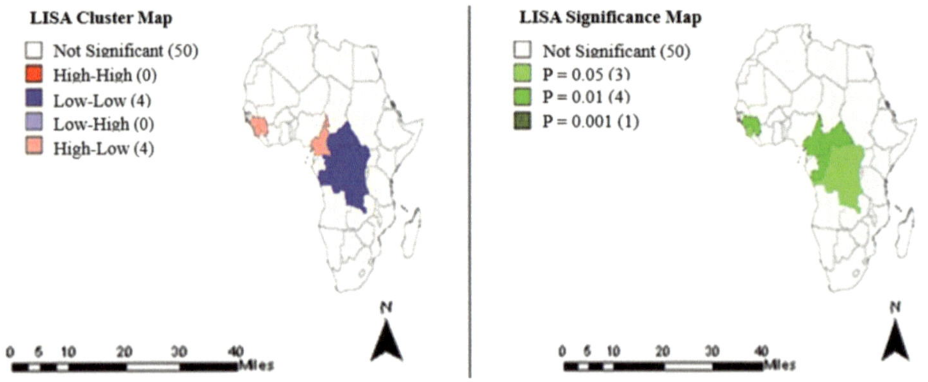

Figure 3.
Clusters and significance levels of TB treatment completion rates in year 2010.

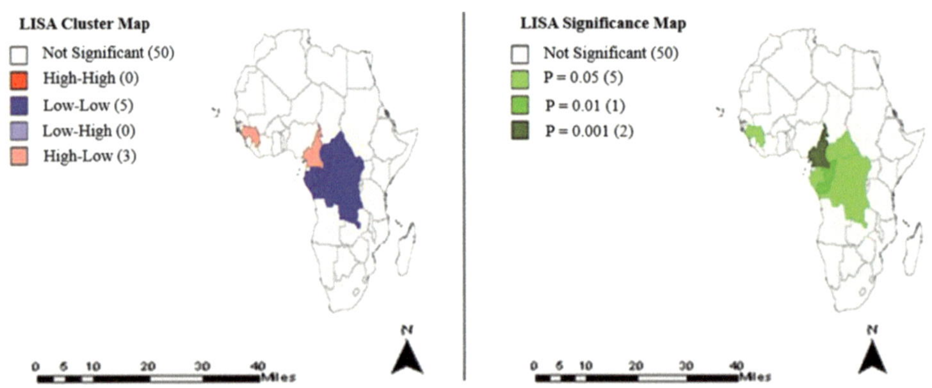

Figure 4.
Clusters and significance levels of TB treatment completion rates in year 2015.

	Countries	Cluster Type
Variable: TB_2000 & 2005	Algeria	High-Low*
	Burkina Faso	Low-Low*
	Senegal	Low-Low**
*Significance level: *p < 0.05; **p < 0.01.*		

Table 2.
Differential local Moran's I estimations of TB treatment completion rates between time 0 (2000) and time 1 (2005).

Variable: TB_2000 & 2010	Countries	Cluster Type
	Niger	Low-Low*
	Senegal	Low-Low**
	Gambia	Low-Low**
	Namibia	Low-High*
	Lesotho	Low-High*
	Djibouti	Low-High*
	Algeria	High-Low*
	Cameroon	High-Low*
	South Africa	High-Low*
	Dem Rep Congo	High-High*
	Kenya	High-High*
	Sierra Leone	High-High*

*Significance level: *$p < 0.05$; **$p < 0.01$.*

Table 3.
Differential local Moran's I estimations of TB treatment completion rates between time 0 (2000) and time 2 (2010).

Variable: TB_2000 & 2015	Countries	Cluster Type
	Niger	Low-Low*
	Burkina Faso	Low-Low*
	Senegal	Low-Low***
	South Africa	Low-Low**
	Algeria	High-Low**
	Cameroon	High-Low**
	Dem Rep Congo	High-High**

*Significance level: *$p < 0.1$; **$p < 0.05$; ***$p < 0.01$.*

Table 4.
Differential local Moran's I estimations of TB treatment completion rates between time 0 (2000) and time 3 (2015).

Table 3 shows the result between time 0 (2000) and time 2 (2010). Niger, Senegal, Gambia, Namibia, Lesotho, Djibouti, Algeria, Cameroon, South Africa, Democratic Republic of Congo (DRC), Kenya, and Sierra Leone had significant clusters at different p-values (Supplementary Material—C).

Table 4 represents estimation results between time 0 (2000) and time 3 (2015). Niger, Burkina Faso, Senegal, South Africa, Algeria, Cameroon, and DRC had significant clusters at different p-values (Supplementary Material—C).

Spatial Correlation Analyses.

Spatial relationship between TB treatment completion rates and mobile phone use identified High-High clusters, Low-Low clusters, and Low-High outliers (**Figure 5**).

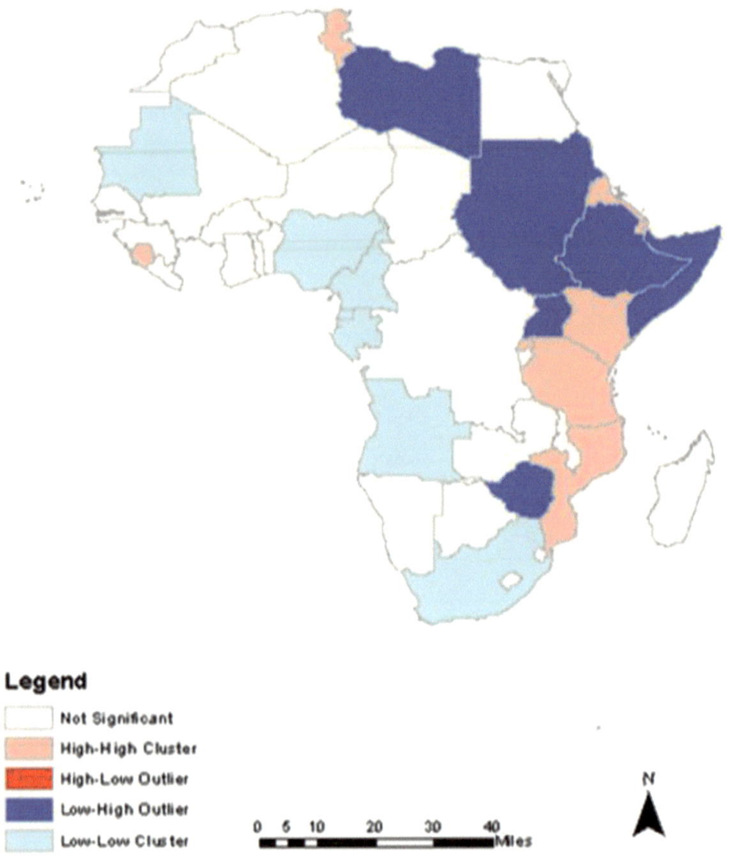

Figure 5.
Spatial correlation result between TB treatment completion rates and Mobile phone use.

4. Discussion

ESDA identified statistically significant clusters in TB treatment completion rates among some countries of Africa. Most African countries except those in the Southern region had significant clusters (**Figures 1–4**), predominantly Low-Low clusters (14 countries) and High-Low clusters (10 countries). Low-Low clusters suggest that TB treatment completion rates between 2000 and 2015 were low among identified countries and were surrounded by countries with similar low changes. High-Low clusters suggest high changes in the core countries versus low changes in their surrounding countries (18, 19). In year 2000, Algeria had a "High-Low" cluster tract (**Figure 1**). This suggests that the TB treatment completion rates for Algeria in 2000 was high, surrounded by countries with low rates. DRC had a "Low-Low" cluster tract in year 2010; suggesting that TB treatment completion rates was low for DRC, surrounded by countries with similar low changes (**Figure 3**). These findings could inform the formation of health policies for TB management strategies including resource allocation frameworks in countries. Study results also indicated that only a few countries had complete treatments for TB across Africa within the period of this study analyses. 13 countries out of 53 (**Figure 1**) had treatment completion rates in the year 2000, with all clusters being either outliers or cold spots. Nine countries in 2005 (**Figure 2**), eight countries in 2010 (**Figure 3**), and eight countries in 2015 (**Figure 4**). These suggest that poor compliance and nonadherence could impact treatment completion rates for which the mHealth technology could be harnessed to address issues related to access, utilization, and attrition [8, 14].

Differential Moran's I cluster maps identified hot spots, cold spots, and outliers among African countries. The base-case analysis identified three countries with significant clusters including Algeria, Burkina Faso, and Senegal. Cluster patterns for Burkina Faso and Senegal were Low-Low cluster tracts, which suggest low TB treatment completion rates surrounded by countries with similar low changes. Conversely, Algeria had High-Low clusters suggesting high changes in TB treatment completion rates versus low changes in surrounding countries (Supplementary Material—C, Figure 6). These findings could inform planning and suggest that the mHealth technology have opportunities to improve outcomes by facilitating fast, reliable, and updated health information.

While the time-period 2 analysis identified 12 countries with High-High clusters (Supplementary Material—C, Figure 7); the time-period 3 analysis identified eight countries with significant clusters (Supplementary Material—C, Figure 8). Altogether, two countries including Algeria and Senegal had significant clusters across the three time-periods of study evaluation (Supplementary Material—C). Nonetheless, of note is the fact that only three countries had significant clusters from LDMI analytics in year 2005 (Supplementary Material—C, Figure 6), compared to 2010 and 2015 where 12 countries (Supplementary Material—C, Figure 7) and seven countries (Supplementary Material—C, Figure 8) had significant clusters respectively. A possible explanation could be that 5-year period may not be enough time to appreciate significant changes in TB treatment rates (23). Conversely, the 15-year period may be too long to observe this trend. Thus, it appears the ideal time for this evaluation should be around 10-year time-periods. This gives credence to treatment guideline policy change introduced in 2009 by WHO that advocates following patients post treatment for longer periods irrespective of the form of TB [23]. In view of this, future studies should aim to do a sensitivity analysis to determine the precise time to explore TB treatment completion rates among African health systems.

It must be noted that identifying significant clusters in TB treatment completion rates in any country does not translate to TB-free nations. South Africa is one of the nations with good TB programs in Africa [22], corroborating this study findings (**Tables 2–4**). South Africa had significant clusters for TB treatment completion rates (Supplementary Material—C); which could possibly be attributed to the coordinated TB control measures introduced by the South African government [7]. However, despite government efforts to curb the incidence of TB in South Africa, recent study by the WHO identified South Africa as one of the seven countries that accounted for 64% of global new cases of TB [24]. Thus, notwithstanding significant TB treatment completion clusters identified by this study, the burden of TB in South Africa remains high.

Exploratory spatial data analyses identified significant association between TB treatment completion rates and mobile phone use rates. Countries with higher rates of mobile phone use, showed higher TB treatment completion rates suggesting enhanced program uptake. Dissecting this association with local level geographical data revealed differing cluster patterns suggesting that the diffusion was not consistent across the region.

High-High clusters indicate countries with high TB treatment completion rates surrounded by countries with similar high mobile phone use rates. Tunisia, Sierra Leone, Eritrea, Kenya, Rwanda, Tanzania, and Mozambique had High-High clustering of these two attributes (**Figure 5**). This suggests that the use of mobile phones may be facilitating TB treatment completion rates; and gives credence to findings by Chadha et al. which demonstrated how the mobile phone technology strengthened and optimized TB health outcomes [11].

Low-Low clusters indicate countries with low TB completion rates surrounded by countries with low mobile phone use rates. Mauritania, Nigeria, Cameroon, Equatorial Guinea, Gabon, Angola, and South Africa had significant Low-Low clustering of these two attributes (**Figure 5**). Such low uptakes may be contributory to the high burden of TB in Nigeria and South Africa and lends credence to reports by WHO that listed them among the six countries that contributed to the high burden of global new cases of TB in 2017 [24].

Spatial outliers indicate countries with either high or low TB completion rates surrounded by countries with either low or high mobile phone use rates. Identified Low-High outliers include Zimbabwe, Somalia, Ethiopia, Libya, Sudan, and Uganda (**Figure 5**). These are potential moderators and mediators for this study; and could possibly be related to factors that impede the use of mobile phones for health informatics including poverty, ignorance, and poor access to mHealth technologies [14].

This study had some limitations. It did not control for the presence or absence of factors that could influence access and utilization of services, which could impact the robustness of study findings. In addition, there were some limitations in the datasets used for this study. Geographical data for TB cases from the World Bank were at the country level only– granular spatial relationships could have been used and would have revealed cases at a finer resolution. More so, this study is exploratory in nature. It assesses correlation and not causation and becomes the first step in assessing the relationship between TB health outcomes and potential impacts of ICT tools such as mobile phone use on TB programs among African health systems.

4.1 Policy implications

Evidence-based decision making, monitoring of health status, tracking of expenditures and outputs for improving efficiency of investments are hallmarks of successful health programs. In recent times, public health intelligence platforms, such as the WHO's Epidemic Intelligence from open sources (EIOS), utilize strong data systems facilitated by digital technologies for health emergency preparedness and disease surveillance. Innovative digital technologies including mHealth have potential to offer new insights and tools to improve clinical decision making, data security and predictive analytics. Realizing the potential of mHealth to achieve development goals will require collaboratively addressing multiple challenges, including strengthening underlying digital infrastructure and digital health systems, working to improve data quality, responsible management and sharing of patient data, and eventually trust, security and utilization of data to inform strategic planning of health interventions. Thus, it is recommended that African health sector leaderships convene roundtable discussions to discuss critical policy dimensions of strengthening mHealth ecosystems, and lay the foundation for responsibly developing and adopting new innovations like mHealth-facilitated Artificial Intelligence (AI) applications in addressing privacy related issues. Such discussions should include but not limited to discussions on adopting latest advances in mHealth technologies including AI tools and telemedicine techniques in advancing population health. They should identify concrete actions for shaping policy and enabling environments to foster mHealth technologies for accelerated improvements in health and related development programs; showcase AI-driven innovative solutions for health, and share best practices from countries, including possibilities for customizations. Such approach could foster a deeper interest on the use of mHealth technologies to strengthen service delivery, improve the collection of quality data and promote data protection rights among African economies.

5. Conclusions

Exploratory spatial data analyses identified positive spatial autocorrelation for the periods evaluated, as well as varying cluster patterns of TB treatment completion rates across the periods of study evaluation. There was a direct spatial relationship between TB treatment completion rates and mobile phone use among related African countries. Spatial autocorrelation patterns generated were consistent with Low-Low and High-Low cluster patterns and were significant at different p-values. Algeria and Senegal had significant clusters across the study periods, while DRC, Niger, South Africa, and Cameroon had significant clusters in at least two time-periods. ESDA identified statistically significant associations between TB treatment completion rates and mobile phone use. Countries with higher rates of mobile phone use, showed higher TB treatment completion rates overall, indicating enhanced program uptake. Thus, there is need to strengthen national policies that promote TB medication adherence and completion using mHealth strategies among African health systems. African government should identify turnaround strategies to strengthen mHealth technologies and improve health outcomes.

Authors' contribution

SI, NU and JO conceived, coordinated, and wrote the first draft of the manuscript. JO and FZ participated in the study conception and overall study coordination. NK, JO and FZ contributed to writing the subsequent drafts of the manuscript. SI, NU and JO did the final review and edit of the draft manuscript. All authors read and approved the final draft manuscript before publication. All authors contributed to the article and approved the submitted version.

Competing interests

The authors declare that they have no competing interests.

Availability of data and materials

The dataset generated and/or analyzed during the current study are available in the World Bank database [http://data.worldbank.org/]; the International Telecommunication Union database [http://www.itu.int/en/ITU-D/Statistics/Pages/stat/default.aspx]; and the World Health Organization repository [http://www.who.int/countries/en/].

Abbreviations

SMS	Short Message Services
TB	Tuberculosis
WHO	World Health Organization
mHealth	Mobile Health
ICT	Information and Communication Technology

ESDA Exploratory Spatial Data Analytic
LISA Local Indicator of Spatial Association
LDMI Local Differential Moran's I.

A. Supplementary Material—A

African countries used in this analysis as listed by the World Health Organization. Available at: http://www.who.int/countries/en/ accessed April 2, 2020.

Algeria, Burundi, Burkina Faso, Benin, Angola, Cameroon, Botswana, Cape Verde, Central African Republic, Comoros, Chad, Congo, Democratic Republic of Congo, Côte d'Ivoire, Djibouti, Equatorial Guinea, Egypt, Eritrea, Ethiopia, Gabon, Ghana, Guinea-Bissau, Lesotho, Gambia, Guinea, Kenya, Liberia, Libya, Malawi, Mauritania, Mali, Madagascar, Mauritius, Mozambique, Morocco, Nigeria, Namibia, Niger, Sao Tome and Principe, Seychelles, Rwanda, Senegal, Sierra Leone, Somalia, South Africa, South Sudan, Sudan, Swaziland, Togo, Uganda, Tunisia, Tanzania, Zambia, Zimbabwe.

B. Supplementary Material—B

Univariate global Moran's I result for the years 2000–2015.

	Variables	**Moran's I value**	**Pseudo p-value**
	TB_TreatmentCompletionRate_Yr2000	0.0190	0.021
Univariate Global Moran's I	TB_TreatmentCompletionRate_Yr2005	0.0177	0.032
	TB_TreatmentCompletionRate_Yr2010	0.0196	0.025
	TB_TreatmentCompletionRate_Yr2015	0.0179	0.031

C. Supplementary Material—C

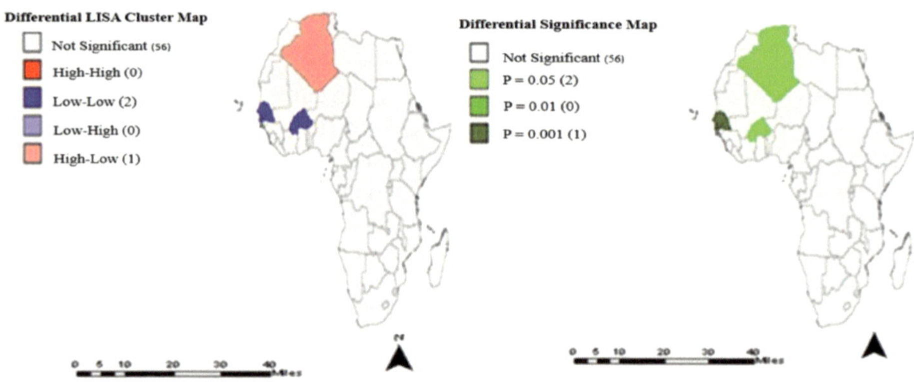

Figure 6.
Differential local Moran's I estimations of TB treatment completion rates between time 0 (2000) and time 1 (2005).

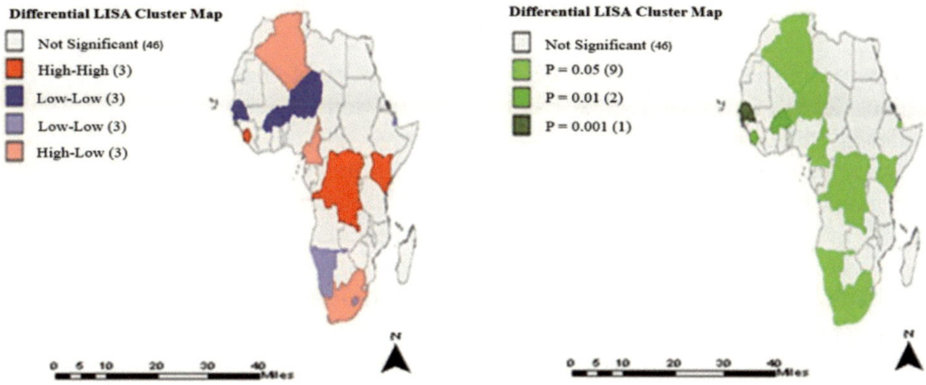

Figure 7.
Differential local Moran's I estimations of TB treatment completion rates between time 0 (2000) and time 2 (2010).

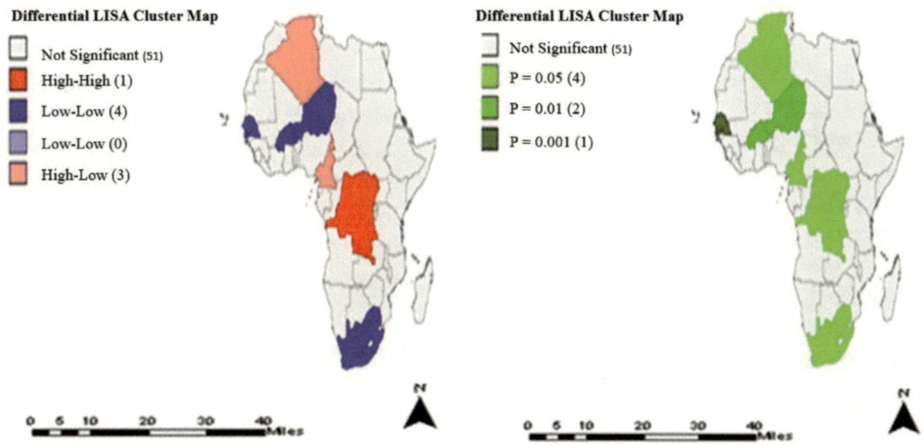

Figure 8.
Differential local Moran's I estimations of TB treatment completion rates between time 0 (2000) and time 3 (2015).

Author details

Sunny Ibeneme[1]*, Nkiruka Ukor[2], Joseph Okeibunor[1] and Felicitas Zawaira[1]

1 World Health Organization—African Regional Office, Brazzaville, Congo

2 World Health Organization—Country Office, Abuja, Nigeria

*Address all correspondence to: ibenemes@who.int

References

[1] International Telecommunication Union. (2020). Statistics. Available online at: https://www.itu.int/en/ITU-D/Statistics/Pages/stat/default.aspx (Accessed August 3, 2020.

[2] World Health Organization. (2016). Global diffusion of eHealth: Making universal health coverage achievable. Report of the third global survey on eHealth. Available online at: http://africahealthforum.afro.who.int/IMG/pdf/global_diffusion_of_ehealth_-_making_universal_health_coverage_achievable.pdf (Accessed May 29, 2020).

[3] Deloitte. (2012). Sub-Saharan Africa Mobile Observatory. Available online at: https://www.gsma.com/publicpolicy/wp-content/uploads/2012/03/SSA_FullReport_v6.1_clean.pdf (Accessed January 02, 2021).

[4] Clifford, G.D., Clifton, D. (2012). Wireless technology in disease management and medicine. Annual review of medicine. 63:479–492

[5] Shehata, A.M.H. (2016). Mobile phone and child mortality: The case of developing countries. The Business Management Review. 7:3

[6] Lee, M., Liu, P., Lio, M. (2016). The impact of the diffusion of information and communication technology on health: A cross-country study. Journal of Applied Research Quality Life. 11: 471–491.

[7] Kahn, J.G., Yang, J.S, Kahn, J.S. (2010). 'Mobile' Health Needs and Opportunities in Developing Countries. Health Affairs. 29: 252–258. doi: 10.1377/hlthaff.2009.0965.

[8] Micevska, M.B. (2005). Telecommunications, public health, and demand for health-related information and infrastructure. Journal of Information Technologies and International Development. 3: 57 – 72.

[9] Ibeneme, S., Revere, F.L., Hwang, Lu-Yu., Rajan, S., Okeibunor, J., Muneene, D., Langabeer, J. (2020). Impact of Information and Communication Technology Diffusion on HIV and Tuberculosis Health Outcomes among African Health Systems. Informatics 7:11.

[10] Moonan, P.K., Bayona, M., Quitugua, T.N., Oppong, J., Dunbar., D., Jost, K.C, Burgess, G., Singh, K.P., Weis, S.E. (2004). Using GIS technology to identify areas of tuberculosis transmission and incidence. International Journal of Health Geographics.

[11] Chadha, S., Trivedi, A., Nagaraja, S. B., Sagili, K. (2017). Using mHealth to enhance TB referrals in a tribal district of India. Journal of Public Health Action. 7(2):123 – 126.

[12] Mwila, I., Phiri, J. (2020): Tuberculosis prevention model in developing countries based on geospatial, cloud and web technologies. International Journal of Advanced Computer Science and Applications. 11:2.

[13] Yakam, N.A., Noeske, J., Dambach, P., Bowong, S., Fono, L.A., Ngatchou-Wandji, J. (2014). Spatial analysis of tuberculosis in Duoala, Cameroon: clustering and links with socio-economic status. *International Journal of Lung Disease*. 18:3. Available online at: https://doi.org/10.5588/ijtld.13.0573 (Accessed April 4, 2020).

[14] Herrero, M.B., Arrossi, S., Ramos, S., Braga, J.U. (2015). Spatial analysis of the tuberculosis treatment dropout, Buenos Aires, Argentina. *Rev. Saude Publica*. 49. Available online at: https://

doi.org/10.1590/S0034-8910.2015049005391 (Accessed June 4, 2020).

[15] Aker, J.C., Mbiti, I.M. (2010). Mobile phone and economic development in Africa. Journal of Economic Perspectives. 24(3):207 – 232.

[16] Hassarangsee, S., Tripathi, N.K., Souris, M. (2015). Spatial pattern detection of Tuberculosis: A case study of Si Sa Ket Province, Thailand. International Journal of Environmental Research and Public Health. 12:16005 – 16018.

[17] World Bank. (2017). Development indicators. Data Bank. Available online at: http://data.worldbank.org/indicator. (Accessed March 9, 2020).

[18] Gostin, L.O. (2008). Public Health Law; Power, Duty, Restraint. Second edition, University of California Press, Ltd. London, England.

[19] Moran, P. (1950). Notes on continuous stochastic phenomenon. Biometrika. 37:17–23.

[20] Anselin, L. (1995). Local Indicators of Spatial Associations – Lisa. Available online at: https://onlinelibrary.wiley.com/doi/epdf/10.1111/j.1538-4632.1995.tb00338.x (Accessed July 13, 2020).

[21] Anselin, L. (2002). Computing environments for spatial data analysis. Journal of Geographic Systems. 2:201 – 220.

[22] Highfield, L. (2013). Spatial patterns of breast cancer incidence and uninsured women of mammography screening age. The Breast Journal. 3:293 – 301.

[23] World Health Organization. Treatment of tuberculosis. (2010). Guidelines. Fourth edition, WHO press, Geneva Switzerland. Available online at: https://apps.who.int/iris/bitstream/handle/10665/44165/9789241547833_eng.pdf;jsessionid=2F6B414309443D2C741F2114F5CB7FB4?sequence=1 (Accessed May 27, 2020).

[24] World Health Organization. Global Tuberculosis Program. (2017). Available online at: www.who.int/tb/publications/GTBcorporate_factsheet.pdf. Accessed May 18, 2019.

Chapter 21

Improving Healthcare Access through Digital Health: The Use of Information and Communication Technologies

Najeeb Al-Shorbaji

Abstract

Healthcare has been going through major digital transformations due to the extensive use of information and communication technologies (ICT) in the sector. Many patients lack access to healthcare services due to lack of knowledge of the exitance of the service, physical or mental disability, distance, siege, lockdown and other possible reasons. Access to healthcare services has been impacted by a number of innovations including electronic health record, artificial intelligence, sensors, wearable devices, Internet of (medical) things, Blockchain, big data and other applications. COVID-19 has created new realities in accessing healthcare services through telehealth and telemedicine services as many countries have imposed lockdown and physical distancing. Digital health has been used to empower people, in general and patients in particular, to enable them to access healthcare services at the point of care or remotely. Healthcare professionals have been using digital health to enhance their knowledge, skills and more important to enable them to reach to patients to provide guidance and assistance. Using digital health solutions has a number of challenges which can be legal, ethical, infrastructural, human and material resources, training, education, attitude, cultural, organizational and behavioral. A number of national, regional and international agencies have adopted resolutions and developed strategies to support digital health implementation in countries. This chapter provides few examples to demonstrate how access to healthcare services is being enabled and facilitated by information and communication technology (ICT) through proper national planning of digital health.

Keywords: Healthcare services, information and communication technologies, eHealth, digital health, artificial intelligence, big data, telehealth, telemedicine, empowerment, patients, COVID-19, national planning

1. Introduction

Access to healthcare means having "the timely use of personal health services to achieve the best health outcomes. It consists of four components:

- Coverage: facilitates entry into the healthcare system. Uninsured people are less likely to receive medical care and more likely to have poor health status.

- Services: Having a usual source of care is associated with adults receiving recommended screening and prevention services.

- Timeliness: ability to provide healthcare when the need is recognized.

- Workforce: capable, qualified, culturally competent providers [1].

In 2001 Gulliford, et al. [2] provided a description of access to health services in which they said "Facilitating access is concerned with helping people to command appropriate healthcare resources in order to preserve or improve their health. There are at least four aspects, they said:

- If services are available, in terms of an adequate supply of services, then a population may 'have access' to healthcare.

- The extent to which a population 'gains access' to healthcare also depends on financial, organizational and social or cultural barriers that limit utilization. Thus, utilization is dependent on the affordability, physical accessibility and acceptability of services and not merely the adequacy of supply.

- The services available must be relevant and effective if the population is to "gain access to satisfactory health outcomes".

- The availability of services, and barriers to utilization, have to be evaluated in the context of the differing perspectives, health needs and the material and cultural settings of diverse groups in society

The Institute of Medicine (IOM) defined access to healthcare "as having timely use of personal health services to achieve the best possible health outcome [3]. According to The Agency for Healthcare Research and Quality's (AHRQ) [4] "access requires gaining entry into the health-care system, getting access to sites of care where patients can receive needed services, and finding providers who meet the needs of patients and with whom patients can develop a relationship based on mutual communication and trust". The National Academies of Sciences, Engineering, and Medicine [5] suggested that "People use healthcare services to diagnose, cure, or ameliorate disease or injury; to improve or maintain function; or to obtain information about their health status and prognosis". Anderson and Newman [6] presented a framework (4th phase) of health-care utilization that includes predisposing factors, enabling factors, and magnitude of illness. The framework suggests that an individual's access to and use of health services is considered to be a function of three characteristics:

1. Predisposing Factors: The socio-cultural characteristics of individuals that exist prior to their illness:

   a. Social Structure: Education, occupation, ethnicity, social networks, social interactions, and culture

   b. Health Beliefs: Attitudes, values, and knowledge that people have concerning and towards the healthcare system

   c. Demographic: Age and Gender

d. Enabling Factors: The logistical aspects of obtaining care:

e. Personal/Family: The means and know how to access health services, income, health insurance, a regular source of care, travel, extent and quality of social relationships

f. Community: Available health personnel and facilities, and waiting time

g. Possible additions: Genetic factors and psychological characteristics

2. Need Factors: The most immediate cause of health service use, from functional and health problems that generate the need for healthcare services.

   a. "Perceived" need will better help to understand care-seeking and adherence to a medical regimen,

   b. "Evaluated" need will be more closely related to the kind and amount of treatment that will be provided after a patient has presented to a medical care provider.

People go, or more important they do not go to healthcare services for different reasons. Three overarching categories of reasons emerged based on the necessity, availability, and desirability of care-seeking [7]:

1. low perceived need to seek medical care;

2. traditional barriers to medical care, in which people may want to seek care but are limited in their ability to do so; and

3. unfavorable evaluations of seeking medical care, in which people may perceive care-seeking as necessary and an available option, but not desirable.

Some of these reasons relate to the human nature of the people while others relate to the health facilities themselves. People go to these services to seek methods of prevention, protection, diagnosis, treatment, palliative care, education, research and a multiple of other reasons. Healthcare services may be provided in different ways and locations including hospitals in tertiary services, clinical and other professional services, dental services, home healthcare services which are at the increase as more patients move from hospital care to home care, nursing care services at the hospital or at home], pharmaceutical and medication dispensing services in addition to other over the counter medicines.

eHealth is one of the enablers of "access to healthcare services" along with a number of other factors. Social determinants of health represent a collection of factors that interplay in their influence of the health of people and therefore their ability to access health services using digital health technologies. It has become imperative to design and deploy such technologies in the communities to reduce inequity and improve ability to access health services. eHealth has been described as the "... use of information and communications technologies (ICT) in support of health and health-related fields, including healthcare services, health surveillance, health literature, and health education, knowledge and research" [8]. eHealth includes the ICT-enabled components of health informatics, healthcare informatics, medical informatics, biomedical informatics, mobile health (mHealth), and telehealth and telemedicine, as well as the human and non-electronic components which are essential for these systems to function. Digital health has been extensively used to mean all concepts included in eHealth plus the use of digital devices to capture, monitor and report health data images, and vital signs: body temperature, pulse rate, respiration rate and blood pressure) from individuals and the relevant signs from the environment. The World Health Assembly (WHA) adopted a resolution in 2017 [9] and then a global digital health strategy in 2020. The description provided by the two documents of digital health extensively referred to eHealth as the core component in national eHealth planning, integration of eHealth in health systems, application development, monitoring and evaluation. In a review of definitions of eHealth in 2005, [10] the reviewers found that technology was viewed both as a tool to enable a process/function/service and as the embodiment of eHealth itself. They expressed pleasure to note that technology was portrayed as a means to expand, to assist, or to enhance human activities, rather than as a substitute for them.

A diversified range of areas in which eHealth can be used as many studies indicate [11–13]. Some of these are directed to service providers while others are directly linked to patients. In all cases the ultimate benefit goes to the citizen.

This range of areas may include:

1. Improving access and exchange of information and data;

2. Improve the quality of care;

3. Reduce costs of healthcare;

4. Support research by academic and other researchers;

5. Building evidence for possible policy setting;

6. Safeguard patient empowerment and safety;

7. Health worker training and supervision: Pre-service and in-service and both remote and in-person mixed media training; mobile supervision checklists and observation data collection forms;

8. Data collection and reporting: At the household, community, facility, district, and national level; longitudinal patient tracking (electronic health records), patient registries, disease surveillance, contact tracing, vital events tracking, civil registration;

9. Supply chain management: Cold chain management, commodity tracking, counterfeit detection and prevention, equipment maintenance;

10. Financial transactions: Health savings accounts, insurance payments, provider reimbursements, salaries, per diems, conditional cash transfers, performance-based incentives, electronic vouchers;

11. Health workforce management: Tracking of training, certification, deployment and retention, provider work planning and scheduling;

12. Clinical care: Point-of-care intelligent diagnostics, remote clinical care, remote monitoring of patient compliance and status, clinical decision support (guidelines, algorithms, checklists);

13. Real-time communications: Between managers and providers (e.g., treatment guideline updates, routine health reporting), providers and providers (e.g., referrals, consultations), and clients and providers (e.g., symptom notifications, post-referral follow-up);

14. Public health information and behavior change: Public health education messages, appointment and treatment reminders, health provider point-of-care job aids, health information hotlines.

In a review of definitions of digital health [14], the findings showed that digital health, as has been used in the literature, is more concerned about the provision of healthcare rather than the use of technology. The reviewers added that "Wellbeing of people, both at population and individual levels, have been more emphasized than the care of patients suffering from diseases. Also, the use of data and information for the care of patients was highlighted. A dominant concept in digital health appeared to be mobile health (mHealth), which is related to other concepts such as telehealth, eHealth, and artificial intelligence in healthcare". Improving access to healthcare services: especially in rural and deprived areas with low (or no) availability of healthcare services, eHealth tools can enable remote consultations, therapies and rehabilitation [15].

eHealth and digital health will be used in this chapter interchangeably to mean the "use of information and communication technology in health". They are considered true interdisciplinary sectors that bring knowledge and practices from the fields of computer and information sciences, telecommunications, social sciences, health sciences (medicine, public health, pharmaceutical, dentistry, health management], health services research, communication, law and engineering. Success of eHealth depends on the extent and ability to integrate and function as an interdisciplinary system. Elements and applications of digital health have become an integral part of health services and information delivery. One cannot imagine a health service without the use of one or more of a digital health device or an eHealth application. eHealth is contributing to achieving Universal Health Coverage (UHC) and the Sustainable Development Goals [16]. eHealth has shown to enable national health system that use ICT to ensure that the people are aware of the availability of and accessibility to health services, that people are happy (satisfied) with the services they receive and that a monitoring and evaluation system is in place [17–20].

WHO (2013) [21] describes the goal of UHC as to ensure that all people obtain the health services they need- prevention, promotion, treatment, rehabilitation and palliation without risk of financial ruin or impoverishment, now and in the future. eHealth empowers patients and make services and providers more transparent and providers are become more efficient when they use eHealth technologies to manage or deliver healthcare services.

WHO (2016) [22] confirmed that "It has become increasingly clear that UHC cannot be achieved without the support of eHealth." The results of the Global eHealth Survey conducted by WHO in 2015 in which a total of 125 countries participated provided some key findings based on the themes that were covered in the Survey. These included:

1. More than half of WHO Member States now have an eHealth strategy, and 90% of eHealth strategies reference the objectives of UHC or its key elements. It is becoming mainstream for countries to have policies for managing information.

2. A large number of countries reported at least one mHealth initiative (83%). Despite the rapid growth, however, very few Member States reported

evaluations of government-sponsored mHealth programmes, thereby limiting knowledge of what works well and what mistakes to avoid.

3. By offering care at a distance, telehealth services enable greater equity in health coverage. The use of telehealth continues to grow, and teleradiology is the most widespread (77%). Other services, such as telepathology, remote patient monitoring, and tele-dermatology, are also in use in nearly half of countries.

4. eLearning, which encompasses a variety of interventions in terms of tools, content, learning objectives, pedagogical approaches, and setting of delivery, is used for medical students' and doctors' education in over 84% of countries. Implementation of eLearning is associated with a number of challenges. For example, there is a lack of robust and comprehensive health science eLearning evaluation standards, leading to haphazard evaluation and accreditation of eLearning programmes.

5. National electronic health record (HER) systems are now reported in 47% of countries.

6. In total, 78% of countries reported legislation protecting the privacy of personal information, and 54% reported legislation to protect the privacy of electronically held patient data.

7. Nearly 80% of countries reported that healthcare organizations use social media for the promotion of health messages.

8. 17% of countries already report having a national policy or strategy regulating "big data" use in the health sector.

As healthcare itself is data and information intensive sector it simply means that for this sector to achieve its objectives, it has to collect, exchange and utilize high quality data. Health data has a number of characteristics including:

1. Critical patient data and information remains scattered across different departments and systems;

2. Data is not accessible and handily available in times of need. Too much data, little information;

3. Multiple service providers (public, private, army, charities, etc.) in the system do not have a system in place for smooth process management;

4. Very little or no exchange (sharing) of information on patients, diagnosis, treatments, etc.;

5. Privacy, confidentiality and ownership of personal health data are compromised;

The above has led to potential misuse, no use or underuse of health data. Digital health strategies have become integral parts of the overall public health and healthcare delivery system in many parts of the world as health and digital technology seamlessly integrate. Planning, monitoring and evaluation of digital health have become essential to the health systems strengthening process. These have become part of the health system's resilience and learning. A country cannot afford to have a resilient health system that is responsive to current and future demands without using digital health technology to predict, protect, diagnose, educate and treat. Adopting digital health strategies carries the promise to improve the quality of health services, reduce costs, improve equity of access, and empower citizens in a person-centered healthcare system [23]. Evidence, to prove that all these are attainable at the same time, is still being built. Digital health technologies vary in form and utilization, but have a number of commonalties:

1. They are all made to help/assist healthcare professionals to better collect data, diagnose, educate and treat individuals;

2. They represent serious attempts to replace healthcare professionals in performing tasks that look tedious or dangerous, especially when a disease is difficult to diagnose or treat using traditional means;

3. They may work together to perform a task for the sake of both the healthcare provider and the patient. This simply means more than one technology functions with others to perform the same task of data collection, diagnosis or treatment.

Digital health has adopted a number of other "new" technologies that were not originally designed for the health sector. This has shown that this sector is in a real need for such technologies to enable safe, secure, affordable, timely and equitable access to health services.

2. Range of digital health solutions used to improve access to healthcare

The range of technological solutions that are used to enable access to healthcare services is endless. The attempt here is to provide details of the eHealth/digital health types of applications that are more used rather than the list of technologies themselves. These include:

2.1 Electronic health record

Electronic health record (EHR) is a repository of information regarding the health status of an individual in computer processable form which is collected primarily to support the provision of integrated holistic healthcare to that individual but may also be used, subject to legislation and consent, for secondary purposes that benefit the health of the wider community [24].

The EHR has been one of the most persistent and yet changing technology in healthcare. It's the cornerstone of any electronic health system which influences the rate of success of the digital health services in an institution or even a country. EHR systems come in different forms and sizes aiming at collecting, storing, sharing and utilization of health data by healthcare providers, the patient and other third-party players as the legal and ethical frameworks permit. The complexity of the record's structure, compliance with both semantic and syntactic standards, the interface, open vs. commercial suppliers, language version and many other issues pose challenges to implementation of EHR systems to enable access to health services.

Healthcare institutions may avoid implementing of such systems due to a number of issues they face, which automatically limit access to healthcare services by people (patients and non-patients):

1. Inaccurate patient identification in a record makes it extremely difficult and impractical to offer health services. Absence of a unique number for each patient may cause not only delay in provision of health services but could cause medical errors;

2. Lack of standard terminology and standard data exchange format hamper the efficiency of data exchange due to lack of semantic interoperability. This will cause both delay in service provision, inability to report, cost and more important medical errors;

3. Healthcare professionals, patients and the community have expressed concerns about privacy, confidentiality and the quality and accuracy of electronically generated information. The better secure technology, blockchain for example, legal and ethical awareness may reduce anxiety;

4. Patients may not trust the EHR due to both hardware and software reasons. Interrupted electrical (power) supply, wrong algorithms, lack of training on the system, etc. are all reasons limiting access to healthcare services.

Despite all these challenges, benefits of an EHR system to collectively enable fast and reliable access to healthcare services have been documented. These can be:

1. Health information and data. Immediate access to key information. This would improve caregivers' ability to make sound clinical decisions in a timely manner;

2. Result management. Ability of all providers participating in the care of the patient across multiple settings to quickly access new and past test results. This would increase patient safety and effectiveness of care;

3. Order management. Ability to enter and store orders for prescriptions, tests, and other services in a computer-based system. This should enhance legibility, reduce duplication, and improve the speed with which orders are executed;

4. Decision support. Using reminders, prompts, and alerts to improve compliance with best clinical practices, ensure regular screenings and other preventive practices, identify possible drug interactions, and facilitate diagnoses and treatments;

5. Electronic communication and connectivity. Efficient, secure, and readily accessible communication among providers and patients. This would improve continuity of care, increase timeliness of diagnoses and treatments, and reduce the frequency of adverse events.

6. Patient support. Tools that give patients access to their health records. This would provide interactive patient education and help them carry out home monitoring and self-testing, which can improve control of chronic conditions.

7. Administrative process. Computerized administrative tools such as scheduling systems. This would improve hospital and clinic efficiency and provide more timely service to patients;

8. Reporting. Electronic data storage that employs uniform data standards. This will enable healthcare organizations to respond more quickly to personal, federal, state, and private reporting requirements.

2.2 Telemedicine

Telemedicine is not a new concept but the technology has been extensively used in the last two years due to the corona virus (COVID-19) pandemic. This is not the place to enlist the history of telemedicine as a technology and as a method to enable access to healthcare services remotely. The World Health Organization [2009] defines telemedicine as "the delivery of healthcare services, where distance is a critical factor, by all healthcare professionals using information and communication technologies for the exchange of valid information for diagnosis, treatment and prevention of disease and injuries, research and evaluation, and for the continuing education of healthcare providers, all in the interests of advancing the health of individuals and their communities" [25]. Telemedicine and telehealth are two concepts that are exchangeable despite the fact they differ as telemedicine focuses on provision of health services to an individual while telehealth focusses on provision and assessment of healthcare services to a population. In their systematic review, Monaghesh and Hajizadeh (2020) they indicated that "telehealth can become a basic need for the general population, healthcare providers, and patients with COVID-19, especially when people are in quarantine, enabling patients in real time through contact with healthcare provider for advice on their health problems" [26]. The promise and potential of telemedicine have been to provide timely, safe, and less expensive care, where the patient/individual does not need to be in the same place/room with the healthcare provider. This simply means that access to healthcare services does not have to move from where the patient is to get into the point of care. During COVID-19 social/physical distancing, has resulted in radical increase in the use of telemedicine services in all countries. This mode of service was provided to avoid contact between patients and healthcare providers who might have been diagnosed as positive COVID-19 and to ensure continuity of primary or secondary healthcare services and in some case tertiary care. Telemedicine services have been provided to ensure timely access to high quality information and care, including prevention and protection services, provision of public health support, provides a form of patient engagement with other patients, family members and healthcare providers, the more advanced form of support includes screening for diagnosis and disease discovery and supports eLearning for both care providers and recipients [27–29].

2.3 Health on the Internet

A number of concepts are being used to mean information accessed and delivered through the use of the Internet. Among these is the web, which has been defined as "a techno-social system that allows individuals to interact on technological networks, thus improving individual's cognition, communication and cooperation" [30]. Other applications on the Internet include email services and social media platforms. Consumers of health information have found these applications in multilingual forms, easy to access and many of them have been found to be useful and relevant to their needs. The move from Web 1.0 to Web 4.0 has resulted in providing the end user with more power to control what is being posted and searched on the web using natural language processing. Consumer health, where web developers or owners directly reach out to people poses a challenge of quality of health information, timelessness and possible abuse by predators on the internet [31]. Eysenbach, and Diepgen, [32] provided a number of important issues emerging as a result of failure to control the quality of health information on the internet. They concluded:

1. The quality of information on the internet is extremely variable, limiting its use as a serious information source;

2. A possible solution may be self labelling of medical information by web authors in combination with a systematized critical appraisal of health-related information by users and third parties using a validated standard core vocabulary;

3. Labelling and filtering technologies such as PICS (platform for internet content selection) could supply professionals and consumers with labels to help them separate valuable health information from dubious information;

4. Doctors, medical societies, and associations could critically appraise internet information and act as decentralized "label services" to rate the value and trustworthiness of information by putting electronic evaluative and descriptive "tags" on it;

5. Indirect "cybermetric" indicators of quality determined by computer programs could complement human peer review.

The perceived value of information, the quality, usefulness, the level of trust and the language of the site are factors that influence the level of attraction to use a website to search for health information. The emerging quality management sites such as "Heath On the Net- HON" [33], that provides 8 principles (in 38 languages) to make a judgment of the web site is a good example of how health infuriation consumers may get guidance on quality of health information on the Internet. Meeting these principles will result in a certificate provided by HON to the website. It's important, however, to make sure that searching the web for health information, especially for self-diagnosis is no alternative to consulting ad as specialized healthcare professional as "the immediate and widespread sharing of medical and other scientific information outside of expert circles before it has been thoroughly vetted (eg, preprints) can be dangerous, especially in a pandemic [34].

As early as 1997 [35], the use of health information on the internet has been a major issue for consideration as a way to get information that may lead to further use of healthcare facilities and qualified health workforce personnel, while for others, it has been used as the sole source of information resulting to what has been described by WHO (2020) [36] as the "infodemic" being too much information including false or misleading information in digital and physical environments during a disease outbreak. It causes confusion and risk-taking behaviors that can harm health. It also leads to mistrust in health authorities and undermines the public health response. An infodemic can intensify or lengthen outbreaks when people are unsure about what they need to do to protect their health and the health of people around them. With growing digitization – an expansion of social media and internet use – information can spread more rapidly. This can help to more quickly fill information voids but can also amplify harmful messages." The use of social media has aggravated the situation due to availability and finding unvetted information.

There are different uses of health information on the web such as:

- Education and awareness for both healthcare providers and citizens;
- Self-diagnosis with all the disadvantages related to this;
- Access to diagnostic result reporting for clinical staff;
- Searching for healthcare sites location, profiles, personnel, services, etc.;
- Searching for health and medical products and services;
- Electronic ordering of laboratory services (pathology, radiology services);
- Patient event history via special forms or email services;
- Discharge letter production;
- Attending an appointment on the internet;
- Searching for health and medical information in books, journals and other information sources.

2.4 Mobile health (mHealth)

mHealth is a medical and public health practice supported by mobile devices, such as mobile phones, smart phones, the Internet, patient monitoring devices connected to mobile phones, personal digital assistants (PDAs), and other wireless devices. mHealth support includes patients, care-takers, pharmacists, or other healthcare providers making use of any digital technology in addition to the devices mentioned above specialized applications called APPs [37]. The top six areas of using mobile phones for health, according to the WHO global survey, include: toll-free emergency, health call centers, appointment reminders, community mobilization, information delivery, mobile telehealth and emergency management systems and mHealth applications [38]. Mobile APPs are software programs that run on smart phones and other mobile communication devices. They can also be accessories that are attached to a smartphone or other mobile communication devices, or a combination of accessories and software [39].

These APPs:

1. Help patients/users self-manage their disease or condition without providing specific treatment suggestions;
2. Provide patients with simple tools to organize and track their health information;
3. Provide easy access to information related to health conditions or treatments;
4. Help patients document, show or communicate potential medical conditions to healthcare providers;

5. Automate simple tasks for healthcare providers; or

6. Enable patients or providers to interact with Personal Health Records (PHR) or Electronic Health Record (EHR) systems.

A very wide range of mobile health APPs is available right now, which helps patients (and non-patients) to access healthcare services and information on their own convenience. There are infrastructural, cultural, legal and ethical challenges. In general, these APPs have been used in areas such as: sports and fitness activity tracking, diet and nutrition, weight loss coaching, pharmacy; sleep cycle analysis, stress reduction and relaxation, meditation, symptom checkers, access to personal health records, digital imaging, electronic chart review, laboratory results review, life scan for patients with diabetes, remote heart monitoring, ECG viewer, oxygen level remote check, telehealth services, prescription management, appointment reminders, International Classification of Diseases (ICD) reference guide, evaluation and management coding, specialized medical reference material, pregnancy and baby development, exercise and fitness, remote dictation, surgery scheduling and interoffice communication.

2.5 Big data

"Big data in health refers to large routinely or automatically collected datasets, which are electronically captured and stored. It is reusable in the sense of multipurpose data and comprises the fusion and connection of existing databases for the purpose of improving health and health system performance. It does not refer to data collected for a specific study" [40]. Leveraging big data to find patterns and predict diseases which helps both medical researchers and health leaders to better understand the disease distribution in a country or a community, which if properly used can contribute to building sustainable healthcare systems, collaborate to improve care and outcomes and eventually increase access to healthcare. It is to be noticed that the major bulk of medical data unstructured and is clinically relevant, that data resides in multiple places like individual electronic medical records (EMR), laboratory and imaging systems, physician notes, medical correspondence, claims, etc. [41]. Accompanied with big data concept is data analytics which is evolving into a promising field for providing insight from very large data sets and improving outcomes while reducing costs. The potential of big data to transform healthcare has been identified [42]. The study of data science and the emerging importance of data as a resource in health have influenced the way that healthcare is being studied and its cost-effectiveness, efficiency, disease prevalence and accessibility are predicted.

2.6 Geographic Information Systems (GIS) for health

Among the major challenges to accessing healthcare services is lack of knowledge of their existence, lack of knowledge of the distance between the place of residence and the healthcare centre and unaffordability to transport to the centre. Brown [43] enumerated five potential benefits of integrating GIS in healthcare IT: identifying health trends, tracking the spread of infectious disease, utilizing personal technologies, incorporating social media and improving (health) services. Brown concluded that "GIS is a powerful tool that has been successfully implemented to help address a number of significant health issues ranging from disease management to improved services". Geolocation technologies for health have made it easier to locate the nearest healthcare centre, provision of the full profile of the centre and the best method to reach it. Integration of geographic data elements (locations) and the thematic data in a database utilizes the best of the two worlds as it has become possible to locate the place where a specific type healthcare services exists. "GIS plays a critical role in determining where and when to intervene, improving the quality of care, increasing accessibility of service, finding more cost-effective delivery modes, and preserving patient confidentiality while satisfying the needs of the research community for data accessibility [44].

2.7 Blockchain in healthcare

Blockchain in healthcare which has been described as "a distributed system which records and stores transaction records. "... a shared, immutable record of peer-to-peer transactions built from linked transaction blocks and stored in a digital ledger" [45]. It allows to securely transfer the ownership of units of value using public key encryption and proof of work methods [46]. Security and data privacy have been among the major reasons for not trusting a system by the patients. Not trusting a system is one limiting factor to access to healthcare system. Increasing security and trust would encourage more people to come forward to use healthcare systems. For patients, in particular, block chain allows payments through crypto-currencies, which is becoming a trend in the money market. Patient safety is being monitored through drug traceability, especially tracing of counterfeit medicine. Patient data management as personal health data is growing at a very high rate and from multiple sources, many patients became more conscious that data about them needs to be more secure and less accessible by unauthorized parties.

2.8 The Internet of Things (ToT)

The IoT is described as a network of physical devices that uses connectivity to enable the exchange of data [47–49]. The Internet of Medical Things (IoMT) has allowed patients to stay at home or anywhere and yet provide health data about themselves to specialized centers for monitoring purposes. This amalgamation of medical devices and applications that can connect to healthcare information technology systems using networking technologies meant that patients can still access healthcare services enabled by technology without them leaving their places. Wearable devices for health monitoring are technologies that can be worn on the human body. This type of devices has become a more common part of the tech world as companies have started to evolve more types of devices that are small enough to wear and that include powerful sensor technologies that can collect and deliver information about their surroundings. A wearable device is often used for tracking a wearer's vital signs or health and fitness related data, location, etc. These may include continuous glucose monitoring devices, smart bandages, smart pills and remote patient monitoring, monitoring of patient's movement, dietary system, etc. Adherence to medication helps patients to take medications on time and even inform medical professionals if the patient fails to adhere to medications. In addition to the many advantages to patients, wearables aid healthcare providers in many ways, by simply improving access to healthcare services while having real time health data collection and time saving. Home care and monitoring are provided to many of the aging patients, patients with chronic diseases and those that are for economic or logistic reasons they are advised to stay at home while access to health services is enabled by digital health tools. Hospital to Home Healthcare (H2H) has become the solution of choice and is an integral part of health service delivery system. These technologies have been used to:

a. Reduce unnecessary hospital visits and the burden on healthcare systems by connecting patients to their physicians;

b. Allowing the transfer of medical data over a secure network;

c. Empowering individuals to better control their healthy lifestyle, well-being and fitness;

Landers, et al. [50] suggested four pillars as the key characteristics of the home health agency of the future: patient and person centered, seamlessly connected and coordinated, high quality of care and technology enabled that allows patients to more easily connect with healthcare professionals and receive more intensive services in new settings.

The mobile device (smart phone or an internet connection) connected to a medical device at home and linked to health centre provides the opportunity to send signals related to vital signs of the patient. The functionality of these devices depends on the type/reason for which this device is provided. These may include measuring body temperature, blood pressure, glucose level in the blood, heart beat rate, respiration and air flow in real-time mode, for patients that need kidney dialysis machines.

Medical wearables with artificial intelligence and big data are providing an added value to healthcare with a focus on diagnosis, treatment, patient monitoring and prevention. Access to healthcare is enabled by wearables as these provide a number of advantages. Wearable devices applied to healthcare offer multiple advantages to healthcare professionals as well as the patients [51]:

1. Premature diagnosis. Wearable devices allow the early detection of symptoms thanks to more precise medical parameters;

2. Personalization. The doctor, with the help of a software can quickly create a program based on the needs of the patient;

3. Early diagnosis. Precise medical parameters in the wearable devices allow early detection of symptoms;

4. Remote patient monitoring. Healthcare professionals can monitor patients remotely and in real-time through the use of wearable devices;

5. Control and monitoring of the patient: the medical professionals can monitor the patient's evolution in real time and, if necessary, make changes in the treatment remotely. In addition, patients can also control their health status by connecting the device whenever and wherever they want.

6. Adherence to medication. Wearable devices help patient to take medications on time and even inform medical professionals if the patient fails to adhere to medications;

7. Information registry. The data are stored in real-time, allowing a more exhaustive analysis of the information. This results in a more complete and precise report on the patient's medical history, which can be shared with other medical specialists;

8. Optimum decision by the doctor. The doctor is able to compare and analyze data to make a sharper clinical decision to enhance the patient's quality of life;

9. Saving healthcare cost. Remote healthcare via wearable devices mean saving time and mobility, as it removes the need for the patient to be continuously transferred to the medical center.

It is recognized that some patients require multiple technologies which resulted in the emerging of the technology that tends to streamline data collection, delivery and use. The Internet of Medical Things (IoMT) is an amalgamation of medical devices and applications that can connect to healthcare information technology systems using networking technologies.

2.9 Artificial Intelligence and Machine Learning in Health

According to a World Health Organization's survey (2017) [52], there are still 400 million people who do not even get essential healthcare support and services. Although artificial intelligence (AI) can reduce this number, the only hurdle is its implementation is the need for huge financial support. Among the reasons for this state of affairs is that patients cannot access healthcare services due to a number of social determinants of health. AI provides an opportunity for many of those who cannot access health services to be reached out "virtually" through image recognition and interpretation, diagnostic assistance, generating reminders and alerts and therapy planning. AI brings a number of benefits to the healthcare system, including to patients. It provides fast and accurate diagnostics, it reduces human errors, it contributes to cost reduction as the patient can get doctor's assistance without visiting hospitals/clinics which results in cost cutting. AI assistants provide online care and assist patients to add their data more frequently via online medical records, etc. and it supports the Virtual Presence of patients through telemedicine services which allow specialists to assist their patients who live in remote locations. Using a remote presence robot, doctors can engage with their staff and patients in hospitals or clinics and assist or clear their queries. More recently, WHO released its guidance on "Ethics and Governance of Artificial Intelligence in Health" [53]. The guidance provided the areas of application of AI in healthcare delivery as it has been used in:

1. Diagnosis and prediction-based diagnosis. AI is being considered to support diagnosis in several ways, including in radiology and medical imaging. Such applications, while more widely used than other AI applications, are still relatively novel, and AI is not yet used routinely in clinical decision-making.

2. Clinical care. Clinicians might use AI to integrate patient records during consultations, identify patients at risk and vulnerable groups, as an aid in difficult treatment decisions and to catch clinical errors.

3. Emerging trends in the use of AI in clinical care. The reports indicated that several important changes imposed by the use of AI in clinical care extend beyond the provider–patient relationship. Four trends described in the report are:

    a. the evolving role of the patient in clinical care;

    b. the shift from hospital to home-based care;

    c. the use of AI to provide "clinical" care outside the formal health system; and

    d. use of AI for resource allocation and prioritization.

The guidance also provided other areas in which AI has been contributing including health research and drug development, supporting health systems management and planning and in public health and public health surveillance that includes Health promotion, disease prevention and outbreak response.

2.10 Monitoring, evaluation and quality management of healthcare services

Monitoring is the periodic and ongoing operation to ensure that the healthcare services are on track while evaluation is designed to measure the relevance, efficiency and effectiveness of healthcare services and their impact on the health of people. In both cases quality data is essential and require setting the baseline by which progress or lack of it can be measured. A data system, usually computer-based health information system, that routinely collects and reports information about the delivery and cost of health services and patient demographics and health status. The major purpose of monitoring and evaluation (M&E) is to measure progress aiming at learning and improving the services. Reeve, Humphreys and Wakerman [54, 55] in the Australian context indicated that Integral to improving rural and remote health outcomes is the provision of appropriate, accessible and effective healthcare services relevant to the needs of communities, which requires a mechanism to monitor and evaluate the impact of health services on improving health outcomes for communities.

M&E requires data collection, its storage and analysis which transforms it into information, knowledge and evidence that can be used for making evidence-based policies, decisions and actions. M&E is based on a set of indicators and measurable targets, which makes it necessary to use ICT tools to fulfill these requirements of data collection, its storage, trends analysis, comparison of achievements with targets, evidence creation and application.

Quality of health services is generally understood to mean that, at all levels of a health system, there is an inherent and explicit recognition of the value of efforts to improve the quality of health services provided – and such efforts are systematically promoted within an enabling environment that encourages engagement, dialog, openness and accountability [55].

Fundamental success factors for provision of quality health services [56] were widely considered to be prerequisites for quality health services include: essential infrastructure, health workers and health management information systems and data systems (e.g. availability of quality measures and data collection templates to generate data, computer hardware/software to analyze data and synthesize the findings into actionable information for further improvement).

3. Challenges to digital health implementation

A number of country studies have listed challenges and opportunities of using digital health solutions from legal, ethical, infrastructural, human and material resources, training, education, attitude, organizational, cultural and behavioral points of view [57–66]. These challenges may include:

1. Infrastructure. Stable electric power supply, place to put computers, air conditioning, local area networks, and other logistics to host computers and their programmes;

2. Availability of ICT info-structure including computers, programmes, applications and internet that were designed with users in mind;

3. Connectivity (Internet, telephone lines, or else) represents a major constraint not only at the national level but could be at the local and even community and household level. The Internet penetration rate at global level is 59.5%. Major parts of Africa, for example, the major part of the continent needs access to the internet which creates a considerable obstacle in developing digital infrastructures. The very limited bandwidth in many communities makes it very difficult to download or even to properly access the Internet (web, email, social medial platforms, etc.);

4. Lack of financial incentives and priorities in countries where priority setting in the health field focusses on building hospitals, delivering drugs, caring of people during the pandemic and focusing of health workforce rather than investing in eHealth to serve the sector in a more cost-effective manner. It is believed in many countries that ICT in health is costly and investing in this area might not be the priority and a cost saving measures. The organizational financial, logistic and legislative support coupled with changes in the workflow of patient care may have a real impact of acceptance of technology as more investment in time and resources is being provided;

5. Difficulty in using the ICT for health to provide the necessary support of patients. System operators and patients alike have a sense that technology has potential to improve and is not really doing what it is supposed to do. If that technology is a little bit more user-friendly it could have a better chance of penetration and utilization in the healthcare setting;

6. Lack of well-trained workforce to manage eHealth programmes and projects. Human resources include not only the technicians who should be trained to operate ICT services but also policy-makers, managers and the public at large. Literacy rate that limit acceptance of digital tools to help in managing health resources hampers the progress in this area;

7. ICT professionals are, to a great degree, are disconnected from healthcare professionals. They both work in silos which limits the understanding and disagreement in the common objectives of helping people to get access to and having better healthcare services. Cultural barriers that exists between the ICT professionals, ICT investors, developers, and practicing physicians do exist and limit the potential to make full use of ICT resources for health. The lack of time from the healthcare staff point of view limits the ability to give feedback and utilize the technology;

8. The culture of monitoring, evaluation, creation and use of evidence are missing. The absence of these put a lot doubt in the minds of policy-makers, funders and even the community to accept ICT in health applications. In fact, a number of studies were developed which some of them call for development of M&E frameworks while others call for building and using evidence for eHealth;

9. Seamless integration of technology is health systems at the higher level and the implementation level where, for example the electronic health record or the mobile health application is not an integral part of health services provision. The absence of integration creates silos and a sense this technology is being for the "elite", for "testing" purposes, to comply with a donor wish or even "to enable data collection about patients for use in research and other purposes;

10. Sustainability of eHealth solutions where people get used to a service and then it is stopped as a result of shortage of funding, lack of enthusiasm by managers and lack of leadership and shortage of human resources to manage the investment. Lack of interest by people due to distrust and not meeting their expectations;

11. Data integration supported by interoperability standards is constraints that has been recognized not only by operators but also by patients. The question is why do operators have to fill in the same data more than once in the same healthcare facility? Why do patients have to provide even demographic information in multiple settings? More vicious than this the inability to share data about the same symptom with different codes being assigned to the same disease?

12. Ethical and legal constraints that hamper access to health information including privacy, confidentiality, data ownership and digital divide. The context in which eHealth is being implemented by individuals, communities and countries provides a better understanding of these constraints. Ethics and legal frameworks differ from one culture to the other making the accepted practices in one society not accepted in another which makes it more difficult to generalize among cultures. In their scoping study, James et al. [67] found that "Of greatest challenge to eHealth systems are ethico-legal factors, particularly privacy and research ethics concerns, such as informed and broad consent, secondary uses of data and return of results". The WHO guidance on ethics and governance of AI [68] addressed three parties: Healthcare providers (Ministry of Health and others, the manufactures of AI solutions and the Universal Declaration of Human Rights [69] provides an excellent framework for countries to use as ethical principles are laid down, which strongly promote the concept of "All human beings are born free and equal in dignity and rights." Privacy, confidentiality and personal information are all protected. Digital divide is persisting not only at global level as countries do have access to ICT resources, while others do not enjoy the same privileges. The same divide exists at the community level and at the gender level. All these issues have a serious impact of access to healthcare. One would not expect an individual or a community to have access to health resources if this person or community is deprived from basic human rights and suffers from a digital divide.

4. National planning of digital health

Over 85 countries have developed their national eHealth plans, strategies or policies [70]. It is noted that some of the these are for ICT in general and health is part of that. The toolkit provides a road map for eHealth applications development and services to enable secure, relevant and cost-effective utilization of ICT in health. The national eHealth strategies aim to help the healthcare sector to improve the health outcomes using the ICT resources at the national level while considering fundamental elements in terms of regulatory, governance, standards, human capacity, financing and policy contexts and more important it aims at ensuring coordinated effort by the two sectors: Health and ICT in the country to produce seamless integration of ICT in health sector. This integration results from defining the common threads and links between national health strategies and national ICT strategies, where coordination, compatibility and interoperability of national, sub-national and local plans are considered and the provision of a platform for integration and joint work to develop shared solutions and systems. The national eHealth strategy seeks high level of transparency, accountability and return on investment to allow for meager resources in a country to be fully used as it supports the rationale and basis for investment in eHealth by the different stakeholders. In most cases the Ministries of Health have a lead role in the development with ministries of ICT and other stakeholders taking part. Other stakeholders may include:

1. The community (patients and no-patients)

2. Healthcare providers in the private sector, non-government organizations and other healthcare providers;

3. Ministry of Information and Communication;

4. Departments of civil registration and national statistics;

5. Legislative bodies and legal authorities;

6. Ministry of Planning/Finance;

7. Academic institutions and research centers;

8. The relevant civil society organizations.

While countries should focus on a range of structured activities that lead to the progressive development of a national eHealth strategy, WHO and the International Telecommunication Union developed the National eHealth strategy toolkit [71] as a tool to be used y countries that already have strategies in place or those that have embarked on development of new strategies. The way forward as provided by the Toolkit suggests:

1. identifying the key health and non-health sector stakeholders who will need to be involved in the development of a national eHealth vision and plan and its subsequent implementation, and engaging with them;

2. establishing governance mechanisms to provide improved visibility, coordination and

3. control of eHealth activities;

4. establishing the strategic context for eHealth. This provides the foundation for the eHealth vision and plan, and enables the government to assess and make informed decisions on whether to pursue opportunities that present themselves from the ICT industry and other stakeholders;

5. assessing the current eHealth environment in terms of the eHealth components that already exist as well as existing programmes or projects that will deliver eHealth capabilities.

5. Conclusion

eHealth and digital health have been in use for many years. COVID-19 pandemic has accelerated the use of information and communication technology. Enabling access to healthcare during the pandemic has provided an opportunity not only to test the capabilities of health information systems and their delivery mechanisms but also to test their cost-effectiveness, efficiency, acceptance by healthcare providers and patients, compliance with international standards, interoperability and the ethical and legal principles that they use.

New innovations will continue to emerge and the healthcare sector will continue to make full use of these and has its own innovative approaches. All these innovations aim to support the health system to be more resilient and more capable of meeting the demands of people for more cost-effective and secure solutions. The dependence on data for policy development, decision-making and actions in the health sector will be strengthened as more data is being translated into information and knowledge for action.

Author details

Najeeb Al-Shorbaji
President, eHealth Development Association, Jordan

*Address all correspondence to: shorbajin@gmail.com

References

[1] Agency for Health Care Research and Quality. Access to care. https://www.ahrq.gov/topics/access-care.html (Accessed 10 April 2021)

[2] Gulliford M, et al. What does 'access to health care' mean? J Health Serv Res Policy 2002;7(3):186-8. doi: 10.1258/135581902760082517 (Accessed 07 April 2021)

[3] IOM (Institute of Medicine). Access to Health Care in America. Washington, DC: National Academy Press; 1993

[4] AHRQ (Agency for Healthcare Research and Quality). 2009 National Healthcare Quality and Disparities Reports. Rockville, MD: AHRQ; 2010. (June 13, 2017]. https://archive.ahrq.gov/research/findings/nhqrdr/nhqrdr09/qrdr09.html. (Accessed 4 April 2021)

[5] National Academies of Sciences, Engineering, and Medicine; Health and Medicine Division. Health-Care Utilization as a proxy in disability determination. Washington (DC): National Academy Press; 2018. https://www.ncbi.nlm.nih.gov/books/NBK500097/ (Accessed 30 March 2021)

[6] Andersen and Newman Framework of Health Services Utilization https://umanitoba.ca/faculties/health_sciences/medicine/units/chs/departmental_units/mchp/protocol/media/Andersen_and_Newman_Framework.pdf (Accessed 30 March 2021)

[7] Taber J M, Leyva B and Persoskie A. Why do people avoid medical care? A qualitative study using national data. Journal of general internal medicine 2015; 30(3), 290-297. https://doi.org/10.1007/s11606-014-3089-1 (Accessed 15 May 2021)

[8] WHA Resolution on eHealth 58.28 http://extranet.who.int/iris/bitstream/10665/20378/1/WHA58_28-en.pdf (Accessed 10 February 2021)

[9] WHA resolution on digital health https://cdn.who.int/media/docs/default-source/documents/gs4dhdaa2a9f352b0445bafbc79ca799dce4d.pdf?sfvrsn=f112ede5_75 (Accessed 20 May 2021)

[10] WHO. Global strategy on digital health 2020-2025. Geneva: WHO, 2021. 60 p. https://www.who.int/docs/default-source/documents/gs4dhdaa2a9f352b0445bafbc79ca799dce4d.pdf (Accessed 20 May 2021)

[11] Oh H, et al. What is eHealth?: a systematic review of published definitions. Journal of Medical Internet Research 2005; Vol 7, No 1 https://pubmed.ncbi.nlm.nih.gov/33227742/ (Accessed 5 May 2021)

[12] Bashshur R, Shannon G, Krupinski, E and Grigsby G. Taxonomy of Telemedicine, Telemedicine and e-Health 2011 http://deepblue.lib.umich.edu/bitstream/handle/2027.42/90498/tmj-2E2011-2E0103.pdf?sequence=1 (Accessed 20 May 2021)

[13] Labrique A, Vasudevan L, Kochi E, Fabricant R and Mehld G., mHealth innovations as health system strengthening tools: 12 common applications and a visual framework, http://www.ghspjournal.org/content/1/2/160.full.pdf (Accessed 20 May 2021)

[14] James S, et al. Benefits, Challenges and Contributors to Success for National eHealth Systems Implementation: A Scoping Review 2021 https://www.researchgate.net/publication/352477969_Benefits_Challenges_and_Contributors_to_Success_for_National_eHealth_Systems_

Implementation_A_Scoping_Review (Accessed 28 June 2021)

[15] Fatehi F, Samadbeik M and Kazem, A. What is Digital Health? Review of Definitions. Stud Health Technol Inform 2020; 275:67-71. doi: 10.3233/SHTI200696 (Accessed 20 May 2021)

[16] Barbabella F, et al. How can eHealth improve care for people with multimorbidity in Europe?.- Utrecht, NL, Nivel, 2016. https://www.euro.who.int/__data/assets/pdf_file/0007/337588/PB_25.pdf (Accessed 10 June 2021)

[17] The Millennium Declaration http://www.un.org/millennium/declaration/ares552e.htm (Accessed 15 May 2021)

[18] Novillo-Ortiz D, de Fatima Marin H., and Saigí-Rubió F. The role of digital health in supporting the achievement of the Sustainable Development Goals (SDGs). International Journal of Medical Informatics 2018; 114, pp. 106-107 (https://doi.org/10.1016/j.ijmedinf.2018.03.011) (Accessed 15 May 2021)

[19] Cisco. Reaching 650 Million: How Digital Technology is Key to Achieving Universal Health Coverage in ASEAN. Cisco and Access Health International, 2019. Cisco White Paper https://www.cisco.com/c/dam/global/en_sg/assets/pdfs/healthcare.pdf (Accessed 20 June 2021)

[20] Olushayo O, et al. How Can Digital Health Technologies Contribute to Sustainable Attainment of Universal Health Coverage in Africa? A Perspective. Frontiers in Public Health 2019; https://doi.org/10.3389/fpubh.2019.00341 https://www.frontiersin.org/articles/10.3389/fpubh.2019.00341/full (Accessed 20 June 2021)

[21] Universal Health Coverage 2030 Creating a Global Digital Health Dynamic Shaping the 21st Century Economy and Society https://static1.squarespace.com/static/56980b3805f8e20acb3cc322/t/5cdb90fbf4e1fcd31e494bf7/1557893372773/UHC+2030+May+21+WHA+72+Ministerial+Side+Event+-+Concept+Note+.pdf (Accessed 20 June 2021)

[22] World Health Organization. Research for universal health coverage: World health report 2013. Geneva: WHO, 2013, 169 p.

[23] World Health Organization. Global diffusion of eHealth: making universal health coverage achievable: report of the third global survey on eHealth. Geneva: WHO, 2016.- 156 p.

[24] Chaudhry B, Wang J, Wu S, Maglione M, Mojica W, Roth E, Morton SC, Shekelle PG. Systematic review: impact of health information technology on quality, efficiency, and costs of medical care. Ann Intern Med. 2006 May 16;144(10):742-52. http://www.ncbi.nlm.nih.gov/pubmed/16702590 (Accessed 10 June 2021)

[25] Standard Australia. http://www.e-health.standards.org.au/IT014SubjectAreas/EHRInteroperability.aspx (Accessed 12 May 2021)

[26] World Health Organization. Opportunities and developments: report on the second global survey on eHealth. Global Observatory for eHealth series - Volume 2: telemedicine in member states. Geneva: WHO, 2009. 96 p.

[27] Monaghesh E. and Alireza H. The role of telehealth during COVID-19 outbreak: a systematic review based on current evidence. BMC Public Health 2020; 20:1193. (Accessed 10 May 2021)

[28] Portnoy J, Waller M, Elliott T. Telemedicine in the Era of COVID-19. J Allergy Clin Immunol Pract. 2020;

8(5):1489-1491. doi: 10.1016/j.jaip.2020.03.008. (Accessed 10 May 2021)

[29] Marin A. Telemedicine takes center stage in the era of COVID-19. Life Science Technologies: Telemedicine 2020 https://www.sciencemag.org/sites/default/files/6NovTelemedicineFeature_0.pdf (Accessed 10 May 2021)

[30] Vidal-Alaball J, et al. Telemedicine in the face of the COVID-19 pandemic. Aten Primaria. 2020; 52(6):418-422. doi: 10.1016/j.aprim.2020.04.003. (Accessed 10 May 2021)

[31] Nimbalkar S B and Badodekar A R Survey of Future Technologies for Web Development. International Journal of Engineering Research & Technology (IJERT) Vol. 9 Issue 06,. https://www.ijert.org/research/a-survey-on-current-technologies-for-web-development-IJERTV9IS060267.pdf (Accessed 10 May 2021)

[32] Keselman A, et al. Evaluating the quality of health information in a changing digital ecosystem. J Med Internet Res 2019;21(2):e11129. doi: 10.2196/11129. (Accessed 5 May 2021)

[33] Eysenbach G, and Diepgen T L. Towards quality management of medical information on the internet: evaluation, labelling, and filtering of information. BMJ (Clinical research ed.) 1998;, 317(7171), 1496-1500. https://doi.org/10.1136/bmj.317.7171.1496 (Accessed 5 May 2021)

[34] Health on the Net. www.HON.ch (Accessed 5 May 2021)

[35] The COVID-19 infodemic: editorial. The Lancet Infectious Diseases, 2020; 20:8, p.875, https://doi.org/10.1016/S1473-3099(20)30565-X https://www.thelancet.com/action/showPdf?pii=S1473-3099%2820%2930565-X (Accessed 12 May 2021)

[36] Weisbord S D, Soule J B and Kimmel P L. Brief report: poison on line—acute renal failure caused by oil of wormwood purchased through the internet. N Engl J Med. 1997;337:825. https://www.nejm.org/doi/full/10.1056/NEJM199709183371205 (Accessed 15 May 2021)

[37] World Health Organization. Infodemic. https://www.who.int/health-topics/infodemic#tab=tab_1 (Accessed 19 May 2021)

[38] Free C, et al. The Effectiveness of Mobile-Health Technologies to Improve Health Care Service Delivery Processes: A Systematic Review and Meta-Analysis. PLoS Med 2013; 10(1): e1001363. doi:10.1371/journal.pmed.1001363 http://www.plosmedicine.org/article/fetchObject.action?uri=info%3Adoi%2F10.1371%2Fjournal.pmed.1001363&representation=PDF (Accessed 10 May 2021)

[39] World Health Organization. Opportunities and developments. Op Cit.

[40] US Food and Drug Administration. Device Software Functions Including Mobile Medical Applications, 2019. https://www.fda.gov/medical-devices/digital-health/mobile-medical-applications#a (Accessed 10 May 2021)

[41] European Commission. Study on big data in public health, telemedicine and healthcare: Executive summary. https://op.europa.eu/en/publication-detail/-/publication/5db46b33-c67f-11e6-a6db-01aa75ed71a1/language-en (Accessed 10 June 2021)

[42] Raghupathi W and Raghupathi V. Big data analytics in healthcare: promise and potential. *Health* Information Science and Systems 2014; 2:3 DOI: 10.1186/2047-2501-2-3 http://hissjournal.biomedcentral.com/articles/10.1186/2047-2501-2-3 (Accessed 15 June 2021)

[43] Institute for Health Technology Transformation, Transforming Health Care Through Big Data: Strategies for leveraging big data in the health care industry, New York, New York, 2013. http://c4fd63cb482ce6861463-bc6183f1c18e748a49b87a25911a0555.r93.cf2.rackcdn.com/iHT2_BigData_2013.pdf (Accessed 12 June 2021)

[44] Brown B. 5 benefits of geographic information systems in healthcare. HIT consultant https://hitconsultant.net/2015/10/29/5-benefits-of-geographic-information-systems-in-healthcare/#.ym4_lmgzaul. (Accessed 15 April 2021)

[45] ESRI. GIS for healthcare: today and tomorrow. https://www.esri.com/news/arcuser/0499/umbrella.html) (Accessed 15 April 2021)

[46] Blockchain. What is a blockchain? https://innovatemedtec.com/digital-health/blockchain (Accessed 10 June 2021)

[47] What is blockchain technology? https://support.blockchain.com/hc/en-us/articles/211160223-What-is-blockchain-technology (Accessed 10 June 2021)

[48] Yin Y. The internet of things in healthcare: An overview. Journal of Industrial Information Integration 2016; http://dx.doi.org/10.1016/j.jii.2016.03.004 (Accessed 15 May 2021)

[49] Medical Devices Network. The internet of things in healthcare: an overview. https://www.medicaldevice-network.com/ (Accessed 15 June 2021)

[50] Techopedia. Wearable Device https://www.techopedia.com/definition/31206/wearable-device (Accessed 15 June 2021)

[51] Landers S, et al. The future of home health care: a strategic framework for optimizing value. Home health care management & practice 2016; 28(4), 262-278. https://doi.org/10.1177/1084822316666368 (Accessed 10 May 2021)

[52] DyCare. Use of wearables devices in the health sector: What are wearables devices and what advantages do they offer? https://www.dycare.com/divulgation/use-of-wearables-devices-in-the-health-sector/ (Accessed 30 May 2021)

[53] World Health organization. Tracking universal health coverage: 2017 Global Monitoring Report: Joint WHO/World Bank Group report, December 2017. https://apps.who.int/iris/bitstream/handle/10665/259817/9789241513555-eng.pdf;jsessionid=605F944D46D031471A01732E1E53C7CB?sequence=1 (Accessed 10 June 2021)

[54] World Health organization. Ethics and governance of artificial intelligence for health: WHO guidance. https://www.who.int/publications/i/item/9789240029200. (Accessed 3 July 2021)

[55] Reeve C, Humphreys J. and Wakerman J A. comprehensive health service evaluation and monitoring framework. Evaluation and Program Planning 2015; Vol. 53, pp. 91-98 https://www.sciencedirect.com/science/article/pii/S0149718915000932#! (Accessed 30 June 2021)

[56] World Health organization. Quality health services: a planning guide. 64 p. https://www.who.int/publications/i/item/9789240011632. P. 6 (Accessed 15 June 2021)

[57] Ibid, p. 38

[58] Kostkova P. Grand Challenges in Digital Health. Frontiers in Public Health 2015; 3(134). DOI:10.3389/fpubh.2015.00134 (Accessed 20 June 2021)

[59] Statista (https://www.statista.com/statistics/269329/penetration-rate-of-the-internet-by-region/) (Accessed 25 June 2021)